The Renal Drug Handbook

Second Edition

Edited by

Caroline Ashley and Aileen Currie

UK Renal Pharmacy Group

Foreword by

Dr Aine Burns

Radcliffe Medical Press
Oxford • San Francisco

Radcliffe Medical Press Ltd
18 Marcham Road
Abingdon
Oxon OX14 1AA
United Kingdom

www.radcliffe-oxford.com
The Radcliffe Medical Press electronic catalogue and online ordering facility. Direct sales to
anywhere in the world.

British Library Cataloguing in Publication Data

A catalogue record for this book is available from the British Library.

ISBN 1 85775 873 0

Typeset by Advance Typesetting Ltd, Oxfordshire
Printed and bound by TJ International Ltd, Padstow, Cornwall

Contents

viii CONTENTS

Foreword

This second edition of *The Renal Drug Handbook* is a fantastic publication. Nephrology is a complex speciality and, increasingly, specialist nurses and paramedics are involved in the care of patients. Each of us needs to be wary of prescribing for renal patients and this handbook provides a highly practical, user-friendly method of ensuring that appropriate prescriptions are given to patients, whether they have normal renal function, renal impairment, transplants or are receiving renal replacement therapy. In addition, the authors give very helpful information on pharmacokinetics and common indications for the use of each drug described. This information is not available in any other single textbook. It is an invaluable resource for all healthcare professionals but particularly for those involved in the care of renal patients. A copy of the first edition can be found chained to note trolleys in all of the wards where renal patients are cared for in my hospital. This second edition is even more comprehensive.

Aine Burns FRCP
Consultant Nephrologist
Centre for Nephrology
Royal Free Hampstead NHS Trust
January 2004

Preface

Welcome to the second edition of *The Renal Drug Handbook*. The information contained in this book has been compiled from a wide range of sources and from the clinical experience of the editorial board of the UK Renal Pharmacy Group, all of whom are involved in the pharmaceutical care of renally impaired patients. As such, some of the information contained in the monographs may not be in accordance with the licensed indications or use of the drug.

The Handbook aims to:

- provide healthcare professionals with a single reference of easily retrievable, practical information relating to drug use, sourced from the practical experience of renal units throughout the UK. By referring to the monographs, the user is guided in how to prescribe, prepare and administer the drug with due regard to potentially serious drug interactions and any renal replacement therapy the patient may be undergoing
- provide a practice-based review of drug utilisation in renal units across the UK indicating, where appropriate, any local methods of use, licensed or otherwise.

The Handbook is not intended to offer definitive advice or guidance on how drugs should be used in patients with renal impairment, nor is it a comprehensive and complete list of all drugs licensed in the UK. The range of drugs covered will continue to grow with subsequent editions. The Handbook is not a guide to diagnosis or an indication of a drug's side-effect profile, except where adverse drug events are more pronounced in the presence of renal impairment. For a full account of the drug, users are advised to refer to the Summary of Product Characteristics, *British National Formulary*, package inserts or other product data for more in-depth information.

The use of drugs in patients with impaired renal function can give rise to problems for several reasons.

- Altered pharmacokinetics of some drugs, i.e. changes in absorption, tissue distribution, extent of plasma protein binding, metabolism and excretion. In renal impairment these parameters are often variable and interrelated in a complex manner. This may be further complicated if the patient is undergoing renal replacement therapy.

- For many drugs, some or even all of the altered pharmacokinetic parameters and modified interrelationships are unknown. In such circumstances, the informed professional judgement of clinicians and pharmacists must be used to predict drug disposition. This must be based on knowledge of the drug, its class, chemistry and pharmacokinetics in patients with normal renal function.
- Sensitivity to some drugs is increased, even if elimination is unimpaired.
- Many side-effects are particularly poorly tolerated by renally impaired patients.
- Some drugs are ineffective when renal function is reduced.
- Renal function generally declines with age, and many elderly patients have a GFR less than 50 mL/min which, because of reduced muscle mass, may not be reflected by an elevated creatinine. Consequently, one can justifiably assume mild renal impairment when prescribing for the elderly.

Many of these problems can be avoided by careful choice and use of drugs. This Handbook seeks to assist healthcare professionals in this process.

Using the monographs

- **Drug name**: the approved (generic) name is usually stated.
- **Clinical use**: a brief account of the more common indications in renally impaired patients is given. Where an indication is unlicensed, this is usually stated.
- **Dose in normal renal function**: the doses quoted for patients with normal renal function are generally the licensed dosage recommendations stated in the Summary of Product Characteristics for each drug. Where a product is not licensed in the UK, dosage guidelines are provided by the relevant drug company.
- **Pharmacokinetics**: basic pharmacokinetic data such as molecular weight, half-life, percentage protein-binding, volume of distribution and percentage excreted unchanged in the urine are quoted, to assist in predicting drug handling in both renal impairment and renal replacement therapy. '–' denotes 'not known' or 'no data available'.
- **Dose in renal impairment**: the level of renal function below which the dose of a drug must be reduced depends largely on the extent of renal metabolism and elimination, and on the drug's toxicity. Most drugs are relatively well tolerated,

have a broad therapeutic index or are metabolised and excreted hepatically, so precise dose modification is unnecessary. In such cases, the user is instructed to 'dose as in normal renal function'.

For drugs which are renally excreted, with a narrow therapeutic index, the total daily maintenance dose may be reduced either by reducing the dose or by increasing the dosing interval, or sometimes by a combination of both. Dosing guidelines for varying degrees of renal impairment are stated accordingly.

• **Dose in renal replacement therapy**: details are given for dosing in continuous ambulatory peritoneal dialysis (CAPD), intermittent haemodialysis (HD), and continuous arterio-venous/veno-venous haemodiafiltration (CAV/VVHD), where known. Drugs are categorised into dialysable/not dialysable/dialysability unknown, to aid the practitioner in making an informed decision for dosing within a particular form of renal replacement therapy. No specific guidelines are given for dosing in continuous arterio-venous/veno-venous haemofiltration (CAV/VVH). In general, dosing schedules are the same as for those quoted for CAV/VVHD, although it should be borne in mind that CAV/VVH may have a lower drug clearance capacity. Thus the clinician or pharmacist should use informed professional judgement, based on knowledge of the drug and its pharmacokinetics, whether to further modify dosing regimens.

The Intensive Care Group based at St Thomas' Hospital, London has an extensive database on drug removal by haemofiltration and haemodiafiltration, so any extra information can be obtained from them (Tel: 020 7928 9292, bleep 1863 or 1830).

• **Important drug interactions**: the interactions listed are those identified by a black spot in Appendix 1 of the *British National Formulary*. They are defined as those interactions which are potentially serious, and where combined administration of the drugs involved should be avoided, or only undertaken with caution and appropriate monitoring. Users of the monographs are referred to Appendix 1 of the *British National Formulary* for a more comprehensive list of interactions deemed to be not so clinically significant.

• **Administration**: information on reconstitution, route and rate of administration, and any additional comments are given. Much of the information relates to local practice, since the avoidance of the administration of large volumes of fluids is paramount. Only the most commonly used and compatible reconstitution and dilution solutions are stated.

• **Other information**: details given here are only relevant to the use of that particular drug in patients with impaired renal function or on renal replacement therapy. For further, more general information, please refer to the Summary of Product Characteristics for that drug.

Your contribution to future editions is vital. Any ideas, comments, corrections, requests, additions, local practices, etc. on the drugs in the Handbook should be put in writing to the Editors-in-Chief: Caroline Ashley, Pharmacy Department, Royal Free Hospital, Hampstead, London NW3 2QG *or* Aileen Currie, Pharmacy Department, Queen Margaret Hospital, Dunfermline KY12 0SU.

Caroline Ashley
Aileen Currie
January 2004

The following texts have been used as reference sources for the compilation of the monographs in this book:

• *Electronic Medicines Compendium.*
• *British National Formulary No. 44* (2002) Pharmaceutical Press.
• *Martindale: The Extra Pharmacopoeia* (33e) (2002) Pharmaceutical Press.
• Bennett WM et al. (1999) *Drug Prescribing in Renal Failure: Dosing Guidelines for Adults* (4e). American College of Physicians.
• *American Hospital Formulary Service* (2000).
• Knoben JE and Anderson PO (1993) *Clinical Drug Handbook* (7e). Drug Intelligence Publications Inc.
• Schrier RW and Gambertoglio JG (1991) *Handbook of Drug Therapy in Liver and Kidney Disease.* Little, Brown and Co.
• Dollery C (1999) *Therapeutic Drugs* (2e). Churchill Livingstone.
• Seyffart G (1991) *Drug Dosage in Renal Insufficiency.* Kluwer Academic Publishers.
• *Cyclosporin Interaction File* (Novartis Pharmaceuticals UK).
• *Drugdex Database.* Micromedex Inc., USA.
• Drug company information.

UK Renal Pharmacy Group

Editors-in-Chief

Caroline Ashley BPharm, MSc, MRPharmS
Principal Pharmacist, Renal Services
Royal Free Hospital, London

Aileen Currie BSc, MRPharmS
Senior Pharmacist, Renal Services
Queen Margaret Hospital, Dunfermline

Editorial Board

Robert Bradley BPharm, MSc, MRPharmS
Senior Pharmacist, Renal Services
University of Wales Hospital
Cardiff

James Dunleavy BSc, MSc, MRPharmS
Senior Pharmacist, Renal Services
Monklands Hospital, Airdrie

Clare Morlidge BPharm, Dip Clin Pharm, MRPharmS
Senior Pharmacist, Renal Services
University Hospital, Coventry and Warwickshire

List of abbreviations

ABC	advanced breast cancer	CYP	cytochrome pigment
ACE	angiotensin-converting enzyme	DIC	disseminated intravascular
ADH	antidiuretic hormone		coagulation
AIDS	aquired immunodeficiency syndrome	DVT	deep-vein thrombosis
ALG	antilymphocyte immunoglobulin	E/C	enteric coated
ALT	alanine transaminase	ECG	electrocardiogram
APTT	activated partial thromboplastin time	ECT	electroconvulsive therapy
ARF	acute renal failure	ED	erectile dysfunction
5-ASA	5-aminosalicylic acid	EDTA	edetic acid
AST	aspartate transaminase	ESRD	end-stage renal disease
ATG	antithymocyte immunoglobulin	ESRF	end-stage renal failure
AT-II	angiotensin-II	G-6-PD	glucose 6-phosphate dehydrogenase
ATN	acute tubular necrosis	GFR	glomerular filtration rate
AV	atrioventricular	GI	gastro-intestinal
BD	twice daily	GTN	glyceryl trinitrate
BMS	Bristol-Myers Squibb	HCL	hairy-cell leukaemia
BP	blood pressure	HD	intermittent haemodialysis
	British Pharmacopoeia	HIT	heparin-induced thrombocytopenia
BSA	body surface area	HMG CoA	3-hydroxy-3-methylglutaryl
BUN	blood urea nitrogen		coenzyme A
BWt	body-weight	HUS	haemolytic uraemic syndrome
CAPD	continuous ambulatory peritoneal	ICU	intensive care unit
	dialysis	IM	intramuscular
CAVH	continuous arterio-venous	INR	international normalised ratio
	haemofiltration	IP	intraperitoneal
CAVHD	continuous arterio-venous	IV	intravenous
	haemodiafiltration	LFT	liver function test
CIVAS	centralised intravenous additive	LHRH	luteinising hormone-releasing
	service		hormone
CL$_{CR}$	creatinine clearance rate	LMWH	low molecular weight heparin
CLL	chronic lymphocytic leukaemia	LVF	left ventricular failure
CMV	cytomegalovirus	MAO	monoamine oxidase
CNS	central nervous system	MAOI	monoamine oxidase inhibitor
COX-2	cyclo-oxygenase-2	MI	myocardial infarction
CRF	chronic renal failure	MMF	mycophenolate mofetil
CRIP	constant-rate infusion pump	MPA	mycophenolic acid
CSF	cerebrospinal fluid	M/R	modified release
CSM	Committee on Safety of Medicines	mw	molecular weight
CVVH	continuous veno-venous	NNRTI	non-nucleoside reverse transcriptase
	haemofiltration		inhibitor
CVVHD	continuous veno-venous	NSAID	non-steroidal anti-inflammatory drug
	haemodiafiltration	NSLC	non-small-cell lung cancer
CyA	ciclosporin		

OA	osteoarthritis	RhG-CSF	recombinant human granulocyte-colony stimulating factor
OC	ovarian carcinoma		
OD	daily	R-HuEPO	recombinant human erythropoietin
PAH	primary arterial pulmonary hypertension	SBECD	sulphobutylether beta cyclodextrin sodium
PCA	patient-controlled analgesia	SC	subcutaneous
PCP	*Pneumocystis carinii* pneumonia	SLE	systemic lupus erythematosus
PCR	polymerous chain reaction	SPC	Summary of Product Characteristics
PD	peritoneal dialysis	SR	sustained release
	Parkinson's disease	SSRI	selective serotonin reuptake inhibitor
PE	pulmonary embolism	SVT	symptomatic non-sustained ventricular tachyarrhythmias
	phenytoin equivalent		
PO	orally	$t_{1/2}$	elimination half-life
PR	rectally	T_3	tri-iodothyronine (liothyronine)
PRCA	pure red cell aplasia	T_4	thyroxine (levothyroxine)
prn	when required	TDM	therapeutic-drug monitoring
PTH	parathyroid hormone	TPN	total parenteral nutrition
PVC	polyvinyl chloride	UTI	urinary-tract infection
RA	rheumatoid arthritis	WM	Waldenström's macroglobinaemia
RBC	red blood cells		

Abacavir

Clinical use

Nucleoside reverse transcriptase inhibitor used for HIV infection in combination with other antiretroviral drugs

Dose in normal renal function

300 mg twice daily

Pharmacokinetics

Molecular weight (daltons)	670.7 (as sulphate)
% Protein binding	49
% Excreted unchanged in urine	2
Volume of distribution (L/kg)	0.8
Half-life – normal/ESRF (hrs)	1.5/unchanged

Dose in renal impairment GFR (mL/min)

20–50	Dose as in normal renal function
10–20	Dose as in normal renal function
<10	Dose as in normal renal function

Dose in patients undergoing renal replacement therapies

CAPD	Unknown dialysability. Dose as in normal renal function
HD	Unknown dialysability. Dose as in normal renal function
CAV/VVHD	Unknown dialysability. Dose as in normal renal function

Important drug interactions

POTENTIALLY HAZARDOUS INTERACTIONS WITH OTHER DRUGS

• None known

Administration

RECONSTITUTION

–

ROUTE

• Oral

RATE OF ADMINISTRATION

–

COMMENTS

–

Other information

–

Acarbose

Clinical use

Antidiabetic agent

Dose in normal renal function

50–200 mg three times a day

Pharmacokinetics

Molecular weight (daltons)	645.6
% Protein binding	15
% Excreted unchanged in urine	1.7 (35% including inactive metabolites)
Volume of distribution (L/kg)	0.39
Half-life – normal/ESRF (hrs)	3–9/prolonged

Dose in renal impairment GFR (mL/min)

25–50	Dose as in normal renal function
10–25	Avoid
<10	Avoid

Dose in patients undergoing renal replacement therapies

CAPD	Unknown dialysability. Avoid
HD	Unknown dialysability. Avoid. See 'Other information'
CAV/VVHD	Unknown dialysability. Avoid

Important drug interactions

POTENTIALLY HAZARDOUS INTERACTIONS WITH OTHER DRUGS

• None known

Administration

RECONSTITUTION

–

ROUTE

• Oral

RATE OF ADMINISTRATION

–

COMMENTS

–

Other information

• Only 1–2% of active drug is absorbed
• In renal impairment, peak concentrations are five times higher than in the general population and the AUC is six times higher
• There is one paper which used acarbose in a haemodialysis patient who had a total gastrectomy to treat oxyhyperglycaemia at a dose of 100 mg before meals. *Endocr J.* (2000) **47**(4): 437–42

Acebutolol (hydrochloride)

Clinical use

Beta-adrenoceptor blocker for hypertension, angina, arrhythmias

Dose in normal renal function

Hypertension: 400 mg once a day or 200 mg twice daily increased after 2 weeks to 400 mg twice daily if necessary

Angina: 400 mg once a day or 200 mg twice daily initially. Increase up to 300 mg three times daily (max 1200 mg)

Arrhythmias: 400–1200 mg/day (in 2–3 divided doses)

Pharmacokinetics

Molecular weight (daltons)	372.9 (as hydrochloride)
% Protein binding	20
% Excreted unchanged in urine	55
Volume of distribution (L/kg)	1.2
Half-life – normal/ESRF (hrs)	7–9/unchanged

Dose in renal impairment GFR (mL/min)

20–50	Dose as in normal renal function, but frequency should not exceed once daily in renal impairment
10–20	50% of normal dose, but frequency should not exceed once daily in renal impairment
<10	30–50% of normal dose, but frequency should not exceed once daily in renal impairment

Dose in patients undergoing renal replacement therapies

CAPD	Unknown dialysability. Dose as in GFR = <10 mL/min
HD	Dialysed. Dose as in GFR = <10 mL/min
CAV/VVHD	Dialysed. Dose as in GFR = 10–20 mL/min

Important drug interactions

POTENTIALLY HAZARDOUS INTERACTIONS WITH OTHER DRUGS

- Enhanced hypotensive effect with anaesthetics
- Increased risk of myocardial depression and bradycardia with anti-arrhythmics. With amiodarone increased risk of bradycardia and AV block
- Enhanced hypotensive effect with antihypertensives. Increased risk of first-dose hypotensive effect with post-synaptic alpha-blockers such as prazosin
- Increased risk of bradycardia and AV block with diltiazem. Severe hypotension and heart failure occasionally with nifedipine. Asystole, severe hypotension and heart failure with verapamil
- Severe hypertension with adrenaline and noradrenaline (especially with non-selective beta-blockers)
- Moxisylyte: possibly severe postural hypotension

Administration

RECONSTITUTION

–

ROUTE

- Oral

RATE OF ADMINISTRATION

–

COMMENTS

–

Other information

- Administration of high doses in severe renal failure cautioned due to accumulation
- Dose frequency should not exceed once daily in renal impairment

Aceclofenac

Clinical use

NSAID, used for pain and inflammation in osteoarthritis, rheumatoid arthritis and ankylosing spondylitis

Dose in normal renal function

100 mg twice daily

Pharmacokinetics

Molecular weight (daltons)	354.2
% Protein binding	>99
% Excreted unchanged in urine	66 (mainly as metabolites)
Volume of distribution (L/kg)	25 litres
Half-life – normal/ESRF (hrs)	4/–

Dose in renal impairment GFR (mL/min)

20–50	Dose as in normal renal function but use with caution
10–20	Dose as in normal renal function but avoid if possible
<10	Dose as in normal renal function but only if ESRD on dialysis

Dose in patients undergoing renal replacement therapies

CAPD	Not dialysed. Dose as in normal renal function
HD	Not dialysed. Dose as in normal renal function
CAV/VVHD	Not dialysed. Dose as in normal renal function

Important drug interactions

POTENTIALLY HAZARDOUS INTERACTIONS WITH OTHER DRUGS

- Anticoagulants: effects of acenocoumarol and warfarin enhanced
- Antidiabetic agents: effects of sulphonylureas enhanced
- ACE inhibitors and AT-II antagonists: antagonism of hypotensive effect, increased risk of renal damage and hyperkalaemia
- Ciclosporin: may potentiate nephrotoxicity
- Cytotoxic agents: reduced excretion of methotrexate
- Lithium: excretion decreased
- Other analgesics: avoid concomitant use of two or more NSAIDs, including aspirin (increased side-effects)
- Antibacterials: possibly increased risk of convulsions with quinolones
- Antivirals: increased risk of haematological toxicity with zidovudine; plasma concentration possibly increased by ritonavir
- Diuretics: increased risk of nephrotoxicity
- Tacrolimus: increased risk of nephrotoxicity

Administration

RECONSTITUTION

–

ROUTE

- Oral

RATE OF ADMINISTRATION

–

COMMENTS

–

Other information

- Use with caution in uraemic patients predisposed to GI bleeding or uraemic coagulopathies
- Inhibition of renal prostaglandin synthesis by NSAIDs may interfere with renal function, especially in the presence of existing renal disease. Avoid if possible. If not, check serum creatinine 48–72 hours after starting NSAID therapy. If raised, discontinue NSAID therapy
- Use normal dose in patients with ESRD on dialysis
- Use with great caution in renal transplant recipients: it can reduce intra-renal autocoid synthesis

Acenocoumarol (nicoumalone)

Clinical use

Anticoagulant

Dose in normal renal function

8–12 mg on first day; 4–8 mg on second day; maintenance dose usually 1–8 mg daily according to INR

Pharmacokinetics

Molecular weight (daltons)	353
% Protein binding	>98
% Excreted unchanged in urine	<0.2
Volume of distribution (L/kg)	0.16–0.18 R(+) enantiomer; 0.22–0.34 S(−) enantiomer
Half-life – normal/ESRF (hrs)	8–11/–

Dose in renal impairment GFR (mL/min)

20–50	Dose as in normal renal function
10–20	Dose as in normal renal function
<10	Dose as in normal renal function

Dose in patients undergoing renal replacement therapies

CAPD	Unknown dialysability. Dose as in normal renal function
HD	Unknown dialysability. Dose as in normal renal function
CAV/VVHD	Unknown dialysability. Dose as in normal renal function

Important drug interactions

POTENTIALLY HAZARDOUS INTERACTIONS WITH OTHER DRUGS

• Increased INR: alcohol, analgesics, anti-arrhythmics, colestyramine, antibacterials, antidepressants (SSRI), anti-epileptics (phenytoin, valproate), antifungals (imidazoles), proguanil, antiplatelet agents, cytotoxics (ifosfamide), disulfiram, hormone antagonists, lipid-lowering drugs, thyroxine, ulcer-healing drugs, uricosuric agents, anabolic steroids, antivirals

• Decreased INR: colestyramine, rifampicin, anti-epileptics (carbamazepine, phenobarbital, primidone, phenytoin), griseofulvin, aminoglutethimide, oestrogens and progestogens, retinoids, sucralfate, vitamin K

Administration

RECONSTITUTION

–

ROUTE

• Oral

RATE OF ADMINISTRATION

–

COMMENTS

–

Other information

• Acenocoumarol prolongs the thromboplastin time within approximately 36–72 hours

• Decreased protein binding in uraemia

• Titrate dose to end point INR

• Company advises avoid in severe renal disease due to risk of haemorrhage

Acetazolamide

Clinical use

Glaucoma, diuretic, epilepsy

Dose in normal renal function

Glaucoma/Epilepsy: 0.25–1 g daily in divided doses
Diuretic: 250–375 mg daily

Pharmacokinetics

Molecular weight (daltons)	222.2
% Protein binding	70–95
% Excreted unchanged in urine	100
Volume of distribution (L/kg)	0.2
Half-life – normal/ESRF (hrs)	1.7–8/34

Dose in renal impairment GFR (mL/min)

20–50	250 mg up to four times a day
10–20	250 mg up to twice a day
<10	250 mg daily

Dose in patients undergoing renal replacement therapies

CAPD	Not dialysed. Dose as in GFR = <10 mL/min
HD	Unlikely dialysability. Dose as in GFR = <10 mL/min
CAV/VVHD	Unknown dialysability. Dose as in GFR = 10–20 mL/min

Important drug interactions

POTENTIALLY HAZARDOUS INTERACTIONS WITH OTHER DRUGS

- Aspirin reduces excretion of acetazolamide (risk of toxicity)
- Increased toxicity of cardiac glycosides if hypokalaemia occurs
- Lithium excretion increased
- Anti-epileptics: increased risk of osteomalacia with phenytoin. Increased plasma concentrations of acetazolamide with carbamazepine

Administration

RECONSTITUTION

- Add at least 5 mL of water for injection

ROUTE

- Oral, IM, IV

RATE OF ADMINISTRATION

- Give slow IV

COMMENTS

- Avoid IM due to alkaline pH
- Monitor for signs of extravasation and skin necrosis during administration

Other information

- Use cautioned in severe renal failure
- Acetazolamide sodium (Diamox) parenteral contains 2.36 millimoles of sodium per vial
- Severe metabolic acidosis may occur in the elderly and in patients with reduced renal function

Acetylcysteine

Clinical use

Treatment of paracetamol overdose
Renal protection during radiological scans
involving contrast media (unlicensed)

Dose in normal renal function

IV infusion: initially 150 mg/kg in 200 mL glucose
5% over 15 minutes followed by 50 mg/kg in
500 mL glucose 5% over 4 hours, then 100 mg/kg
in 1000 mL over 16 hours

Renal protection – see 'Other information'

Pharmacokinetics

Molecular weight (daltons)	163
% Protein binding	50
% Excreted unchanged in urine	30
Volume of distribution (L/kg)	0.33–0.47
Half-life – normal/ESRF (hrs)	2.3–6/–

Dose in renal impairment
GFR (mL/min)

20–50	Dose as in normal renal function
10–20	Dose as in normal renal function
<10	Dose as in normal renal function. See 'Other information'

Dose in patients undergoing renal replacement therapies

CAPD	Likely dialysability. Dose as in normal renal function
HD	Likely dialysability. Dose as in normal renal function
CAV/VVHD	Likely dialysability. Dose as in normal renal function

Important drug interactions

POTENTIALLY HAZARDOUS INTERACTIONS WITH
OTHER DRUGS

• None known

Administration

RECONSTITUTION

• Glucose 5%

ROUTE

• IV, PO (PO route unlicensed in the UK)

RATE OF ADMINISTRATION

• See under 'Dose in normal renal function'

COMMENTS

• Children should be treated with the same doses
  and regimen as adults; however, the quantity of IV
  fluid should be modified to account for age and
  weight
• Acetylcysteine has been administered neat or in
  a 1 to 1 dilution using an infusion pump. These
  are unlicensed methods of administration

Other information

• Bennett recommends administering 75% of dose
  for patients with severe renal impairment,
  however, Evans Medical do not recommend a
  dose reduction and, from their records, neither
  do the National Poisons Centre
• There is some evidence that acetylcysteine may
  have a renoprotective effect during scans
  involving the use of contrast media, in patients
  with already impaired renal function
• Dose = 600 mg PO BD the day before the scan,
  repeated the day of the scan, together with IV or
  PO fluids. Injection may be taken orally, or tablets
  are available from IDIS
• Alternatively, give 1 g acetylcysteine IV in 500 mL
  sodium chloride 0.9% or glucose 5%, the day
  before the scan, repeated on the day of the scan

Aciclovir (IV)

Clinical use

Antiviral agent for herpes simplex and herpes zoster infection

Dose in normal renal function

Herpes simplex treatment: normal or immunocompromised 5 mg/kg every 8 hours

Recurrent varicella zoster infection: normal immune status 5 mg/kg every 8 hours

Primary and recurrent varicella zoster infection: immunocompromised 10 mg/kg every 8 hours

Herpes simplex encephalitis: normal or immunocompromised 10 mg/kg every 8 hours

Pharmacokinetics

Molecular weight (daltons)	225
% Protein binding	15–30
% Excreted unchanged in urine	40–70
Volume of distribution (L/kg)	0.7
Half-life – normal/ESRF (hrs)	2.1–3.8/20 (dialysis:6)

Dose in renal impairment GFR (mL/min)

25–50	5–10 mg/kg every 12 hours
10–25	5–10 mg/kg every 24 hours (some units use 3.5–7 mg/kg every 24 hours)
<10	2.5–5 mg/kg every 24 hours

Dose in patients undergoing renal replacement therapies

CAPD	Not dialysed. Dose as in GFR = <10 mL/min
HD	Dialysed. Dose as in GFR = <10 mL/min
CAV/VVHD	Dialysed. Dose as for GFR = 10–25 mL/min

Important drug interactions

POTENTIALLY HAZARDOUS INTERACTIONS WITH OTHER DRUGS

- Ciclosporin: reports of increased and decreased ciclosporin levels. Some editors report no experience of interaction locally
- Higher plasma levels of aciclovir and mycophenolate mofetil with concomitant administration

Administration

RECONSTITUTION

- Sodium chloride 0.9% or water for injection; 10 mL to each 250-mg vial; 20 mL to 500-mg vial (resulting solution contains 25 mg/mL)

ROUTE

- IV

RATE OF ADMINISTRATION

- 1 hour. Can worsen renal impairment if injected too rapidly!

COMMENTS

- Reconstituted solution may be further diluted to concentrations not greater than 5 mg/mL
- Compatible with sodium chloride 0.9% and glucose 5%
- *Do not refrigerate*
- Do not use turbid or crystal-containing solutions
- Reconstituted solution very alkaline (pH 11)

Other information

- Aciclovir clearance in CAVHD is approximately equivalent to urea clearance, i.e. lower clearance than in intermittent haemodialysis
- Monitor aciclovir levels in critically ill patients. **Reports of neurological toxicity at maximum recommended doses**
- Renal impairment developing during treatment with aciclovir usually responds rapidly to rehydration of the patient and/or dosage reduction or withdrawal of the drug. Adequate hydration of the patient should be maintained

Aciclovir (oral)

Clinical use

Antiviral agent for herpes simplex and herpes zoster infection

Dose in normal renal function

Simplex treatment: 200–400 mg five times daily (4-hourly omitting the nighttime dose)

Prophylaxis: 200–400 mg every 6 hours

Suppression: 200 mg every 6 hours, or 400 mg every 12 hours

Zoster: 800 mg five times a day for 7 days

Pharmacokinetics

Molecular weight (daltons)	225
% Protein binding	15–30
% Excreted unchanged in urine	40–70
Volume of distribution (L/kg)	0.7
Half-life – normal/ESRF (hrs)	2.1–3.8/20 (dialysis: 6)

Dose in renal impairment GFR (mL/min)

20–50	Dose as in normal renal function
10–20	Simplex: 200 mg 3–4 times daily Zoster: 400–800 mg every 8 hours
<10	Simplex: 200 mg every 12 hours Zoster: 400–800 mg every 12 hours

Dose in patients undergoing renal replacement therapies

CAPD	Not dialysed. Dose as in GFR = <10 mL/min
HD	Dialysed. Dose as in GFR = <10 mL/min. Give dose after dialysis
CAV/VVHD	Dialysed. Dose as in GFR = 10–20 mL/min

Important drug interactions

POTENTIALLY HAZARDOUS INTERACTIONS WITH OTHER DRUGS

- Ciclosporin: reports of increase and decrease in ciclosporin levels. Some editors report no experience of interaction locally
- Higher plasma levels of aciclovir and mycophenolate mofetil with concomitant administration

Administration

RECONSTITUTION

–

ROUTE

- Oral

RATE OF ADMINISTRATION

–

COMMENTS

- Dispersible tablets may be dispersed in a minimum of 50 mL of water or swallowed whole with a little water

Other information

- Consider IV therapy for zoster infection if patient severely immunocompromised
- Monitor aciclovir levels

Acitretin

Clinical use

Severe extensive psoriasis, palmoplantar pustular psoriasis, severe congenital ichthyosis, severe Darier's disease

Dose in normal renal function

Initially 25–30 mg daily (Darier's disease 10 mg daily) – for 2–4 weeks adjusted according to response. Usually 25–50 mg/day (maximum 75 mg) for further 6–8 weeks. (In Darier's disease and ichthyosis not more than 50 mg daily for up to 6 months.)

Pharmacokinetics

Molecular weight (daltons)	326.4
% Protein binding	Highly bound. Less than 0.1% present as unbound drug in pooled human plasma.
% Excreted unchanged in urine	Excreted as metabolites
Volume of distribution (L/kg)	9
Half-life – normal/ESRF (hrs)	47/–

Dose in renal impairment GFR (mL/min)

20–50	No data available. Assume dose as in normal renal function
10–20	No data available. Assume dose as in normal renal function
<10	No data available. Assume dose as in normal renal function

Dose in patients undergoing renal replacement therapies

CAPD	Unlikely dialysability. Dose as in normal renal function
HD	Not dialysed. Dose as in normal renal function
CAV/VVHD	Unknown dialysability. Dose as in normal renal function

Important drug interactions

POTENTIALLY HAZARDOUS INTERACTIONS WITH OTHER DRUGS

• Possible antagonism of the anticoagulant effect of warfarin
• Increased plasma concentration of methotrexate (also increased risk of hepatotoxicity) – avoid concomitant use
• Antibacterials: possibly increased risk of benign intracranial hypertension – avoid concomitant use

Administration

RECONSTITUTION

–

ROUTE

• Oral

RATE OF ADMINISTRATION

–

COMMENTS

• Take once daily with meals or with milk

Other information

• Manufacturer's literature contra-indicates the use of acitretin in renal failure

Acrivastine

Clinical use

Antihistamine – symptomatic relief of allergy such as hayfever, urticaria

Dose in normal renal function

8 mg three times a day

Pharmacokinetics

Molecular weight (daltons)	348.4
% Protein binding	50
% Excreted unchanged in urine	–
Volume of distribution (L/kg)	0.6–0.7
Half-life – normal/ESRF (hrs)	1.4–2.1/–

Dose in renal impairment GFR (mL/min)

20–50	8 mg twice a day
10–20	8 mg once – twice a day
<10	8 mg daily

Dose in patients undergoing renal replacement therapies

CAPD	Unknown dialysability. Dose as in GFR = <10 mL/min
HD	Unknown dialysability. Dose as in GFR = <10 mL/min
CAV/VVHD	Unknown dialysability. Dose as in GFR = 10–20 mL/min

Important drug interactions

POTENTIALLY HAZARDOUS INTERACTIONS WITH OTHER DRUGS

- MAOIs and tricyclics increase the antimuscarinic and sedative effects
- Concomitant use of terfenadine and mizolastine not recommended (risk of hazardous arrhythmias)
- Increased risk of ventricular arrhythmias with sotalol

Administration

RECONSTITUTION

–

ROUTE

- Oral

RATE OF ADMINISTRATION

–

COMMENTS

–

Other information

- Manufacturers do not recommend use in patients with significant renal impairment

Adenosine

Clinical use

Rapid reversion to sinus rhythm of paroxysmal supraventricular tachycardias. Diagnosis of broad or narrow complex supraventricular tachycardias

Dose in normal renal function

Initially: 3 mg over 2 seconds with cardiac monitoring followed, if necessary, by 6 mg after 1–2 minutes and then by 12 mg after a further 1–2 minutes

Pharmacokinetics

Molecular weight (daltons)	267.2
% Protein binding	0
% Excreted unchanged in urine	<5
Volume of distribution (L/kg)	–
Half-life – normal/ESRF (hrs)	<10 seconds/ unchanged

Dose in renal impairment GFR (mL/min)

20–50	Dose as in normal renal function
10–20	Dose as in normal renal function
<10	Dose as in normal renal function

Dose in patients undergoing renal replacement therapies

CAPD	Not dialysed. Dose as in normal renal function
HD	Not dialysed. Dose as in normal renal function
CAV/VVHD	Not dialysed. Dose as in normal renal function

Important drug interactions

POTENTIALLY HAZARDOUS INTERACTIONS WITH OTHER DRUGS

- Effect is enhanced and extended by dipyridamole therefore if use of adenosine is essential, dosage should be reduced by a factor of 4 (i.e. initial dosage of 0.5–1 mg)
- Theophylline and other xanthines are potent inhibitors of adenosine

Administration

RECONSTITUTION

–

ROUTE

- IV

RATE OF ADMINISTRATION

- Rapid IV bolus (see dose)

COMMENTS

- Do not refrigerate
- Administer into central vein, large peripheral vein, or into an IV line. If IV line used, follow dose by rapid sodium chloride 0.9% flush

Other information

- Neither the kidney nor the liver are involved in the degradation of exogenous adenosine, so dose adjustments are not required in hepatic or renal insufficiency
- Unlike verapamil, adenosine may be used in conjunction with a beta-blocker
- Common side-effects: facial flushing, chest pain, dyspnoea, bronchospasm, nausea and lightheadedness – the side-effects are short-lived

Adrenaline (epinephrine)

Clinical use

Sympathomimetic and inotropic agent

Dose in normal renal function

1–20 micrograms/minute

Pharmacokinetics

Molecular weight (daltons)	183.2
% Protein binding	50
% Excreted unchanged in urine	1
Volume of distribution (L/kg)	–
Half-life – normal/ESRF (hrs)	Phase 1: 3 minutes, Phase 2: 10 minutes

Dose in renal impairment GFR (mL/min)

20–50	Dose as in normal renal function
10–20	Dose as in normal renal function
<10	Dose as in normal renal function

Dose in patients undergoing renal replacement therapies

CAPD	Not dialysed. Dose as in normal renal function
HD	Not dialysed. Dose as in normal renal function
CAV/VVHD	Not dialysed. Dose as in normal renal function

Important drug interactions

POTENTIALLY HAZARDOUS INTERACTIONS WITH OTHER DRUGS

- Risk of arrhythmias if given with volatile anaesthetics
- Risk of arrhythmias and hypertension if given with tricyclic antidepressants
- Risk of severe hypertension if given with beta-blockers

Administration

RECONSTITUTION

- 1 mg in 100 mL glucose 5%
- 6 mL/hour = 1 microgram/minute – according to local protocol

ROUTE

- IV, IM, SC

RATE OF ADMINISTRATION

- Monitor blood pressure and adjust dose according to response

COMMENTS

–

Other information

- Catecholamines have a high non-renal systemic clearance, therefore the effect of any renal replacement therapy is unlikely to be relevant

Albendazole (unlicensed product)

Clinical use

Treatment of *Echinococcus granulosus*
(hydatid disease), in combination with surgery

Treatment of nematode infections

Dose in normal renal function

Echinococcus granulosus: >60 kg:
400 mg twice daily for 28 days

<60 kg: 15 mg/kg in two divided doses to a
maximum of 800 mg daily

Treatment of nematode infections:
400 mg as a single dose

Pharmacokinetics

Molecular weight (daltons)	265.3
% Protein binding	70
% Excreted unchanged in urine	<1
Volume of distribution (L/kg)	No data
Half-life – normal/ESRF (hrs)	8–12 (metabolite)

Dose in renal impairment
GFR (mL/min)

20–50	Dose as in normal renal function
10–20	Dose as in normal renal function
<10	Dose as in normal renal function

Dose in patients undergoing
renal replacement therapies

CAPD	Unlikely dialysability. Dose as in normal renal function
HD	Not dialysed. Dose as in normal renal function
CAV/VVHD	Unlikely dialysability. Dose as in normal renal function

Important drug interactions

POTENTIALLY HAZARDOUS INTERACTIONS WITH
OTHER DRUGS

• Dexamethasone: increased concentrations of
metabolite of albendazole

Administration

RECONSTITUTION

–

ROUTE

• Oral

RATE OF ADMINISTRATION

–

COMMENTS

–

Other information

• Available on a named patient basis from IDIS
(Zentel)

• Undergoes first-pass metabolism

Alemtuzumab (MabCampath)

Clinical use

Treatment of chronic lymphocytic leukaemia not totally responsive to other treatment, transplant rejection prophylaxis (unlicensed)

Dose in normal renal function

3–10 mg (increasing in first week to 30 mg if tolerated)

Maximum dose: 30 mg three times a week

Pharmacokinetics

Molecular weight (daltons)	150,000
% Protein binding	–
% Excreted unchanged in urine	–
Volume of distribution (L/kg)	–
Half-life – normal/ESRF (hrs)	23–30

Dose in renal impairment GFR (mL/min)

20–50	Use with extreme caution. See 'Other information'
10–20	Use with extreme caution. See 'Other information'
<10	Use with extreme caution. See 'Other information'

Dose in patients undergoing renal replacement therapies

CAPD	Unlikely dialysability. Dose as in GFR = <10 mL/min
HD	Unlikely dialysability. Dose as in GFR = <10 mL/min
CAV/VVHD	Unlikely dialysability. Dose as in GFR = 10–20 mL/min

Important drug interactions

POTENTIALLY HAZARDOUS INTERACTIONS WITH OTHER DRUGS

- Other chemotherapy: do not give within 3 weeks of each other
- Live vaccines: avoid for at least 12 months after treatment

Administration

RECONSTITUTION

–

ROUTE

- IV infusion

RATE OF ADMINISTRATION

- 2 hours

COMMENTS

- Add to 100 mL sodium chloride 0.9% or glucose 5%
- Once diluted protect from light and use within 8 hours
- Add dose through a low protein-binding 5-micron filter

Other information

- Patients should have a premedication of an antihistamine and paracetamol 30 minutes before treatment
- Patients should also receive anti-herpes and anti-infective prophylaxis against PCP during and up to 2 months after stopping treatment
- No studies have been done on renal patients
- More than 80% of patients will experience side-effects, usually during the first week of therapy
- There have been no studies using alemtuzumab in renal failure and there is no information on excretion, therefore if it must be used it should be with great care at the consultant's discretion

Alendronate sodium

Clinical use

Treatment and prophylaxis of osteoporosis

Dose in normal renal function

Treatment: 5–10 mg daily or 70 mg once weekly
Prophylaxis: 35 mg once weekly

Pharmacokinetics

Molecular weight (daltons)	325.1
% Protein binding	78 (influenced by pH, plasma calcium, circulating drug concentration)
% Excreted unchanged in urine	40–50
Volume of distribution (L/kg)	28 litres
Half-life – normal/ESRF (hrs)	10.9 years/ increased

Dose in renal impairment GFR (mL/min)

35–50	Dose as in normal renal function
<35	Avoid. See 'Other information'

Dose in patients undergoing renal replacement therapies

CAPD	Unlikely dialysability. Dose as in GFR < 35 mL/min
HD	Not dialysed. Dose as in GFR < 35 mL/min
CAV/VVHD	Unlikely dialysability. Dose as in GFR < 35 mL/min

Important drug interactions

POTENTIALLY HAZARDOUS INTERACTIONS WITH OTHER DRUGS

• Calcium salts: reduced absorption of alendronate

Administration

RECONSTITUTION

–

ROUTE

• Oral

RATE OF ADMINISTRATION

–

COMMENTS

–

Other information

• Swallow whole with a glass of water on an empty stomach, at least 30 minutes before breakfast and any other oral medication

• The patient should stand or sit upright for at least 30 minutes after taking tablets

• Combination therapy with alendronate and intravenous calcitriol for the treatment of secondary hyperparathyroidism in haemodialysis patients has been used at a dose of 10 mg alendronate plus IV calcitriol 2 micrograms post dialysis to reduce PTH levels. McCarthy JT et al. (1999) J Am Soc Nephrol. 10 (Program & Abstract suppl.): 81A–82A

• Manufacturers do not recommend use of alendronate in severe renal impairment due to lack of data

• Anecdotally, has been used in a patient with a serum creatinine of 300 micromol/L at a dose of 5 mg daily without any problems

• Other examples of use in different units are: 70 mg weekly
Standard doses of all preparations

Alfacalcidol

Clinical use

Vitamin D analogue. Increase serum calcium levels. Inhibition of parathyroid hormone release, and suppression of PTH production

Dose in normal renal function

0.25–1 microgram daily according to response. Alternatively, up to 4 micrograms PO/IV three times a week

Pharmacokinetics

Molecular weight (daltons)	400.6
% Protein binding	Extensive plasma protein binding
% Excreted unchanged in urine	19–41
Volume of distribution (L/kg)	–
Half-life – normal/ESRF (hrs)	<3/–

Dose in renal impairment GFR (mL/min)

20–50	Dose as in normal renal function
10–20	Dose as in normal renal function
<10	Dose as in normal renal function

Dose in patients undergoing renal replacement therapies

CAPD	Not dialysed. Dose as in normal renal function
HD	Not dialysed. Dose as in normal renal function
CAV/VVHD	Not Dialysed. Dose as in normal renal function

Important drug interactions

POTENTIALLY HAZARDOUS INTERACTIONS WITH OTHER DRUGS

• Carbamazepine, phenytoin, phenobarbital and primidone may increase metabolism of alfacalcidol necessitating larger doses than normal to produce the desired effect

Administration

RECONSTITUTION

–

ROUTE

• Oral, IV

RATE OF ADMINISTRATION

• IV over 30 seconds

COMMENTS

–

Other information

• Adjust dose according to response. Serum calcium ref range 2.1–2.6 mmol/L (total)

• An IV preparation (2 micrograms/mL) and an oral solution (2 micrograms/mL) are also available

• Doses of 1 microgram daily for 5 days may need to be given immediately prior to parathyroidectomy. Alternatively, 5 micrograms immediately prior to parathyroidectomy

• Capsules of One-Alfa (Leo) contain sesame oil

Alfentanil

Clinical use

Opioid analgesic – used for short surgical procedures or intensive care sedation

Dose in normal renal function

IV injection: spontaneous respiration – up to 500 micrograms over 30 seconds – supplemental dose = 250 micrograms. Assisted ventilation: 30–50 micrograms/kg – supplemental dose = 15 micrograms/kg

By IV infusion with assisted ventilation: loading dose 50–100 micrograms/kg as bolus or fast infusion over 10 minutes followed by 0.5–1 micrograms/kg/minute. Discontinue infusion 30 minutes before anticipated end of surgery

For analgesia and suppression of respiratory activity during intensive care with assisted ventilation: by IV infusion 30 micrograms/kg/hour – adjusted according to response (usual range 0.5–10 mg/hour)

For more rapid initial control give 5 mg IV in divided portions over 10 minutes (slower if hypotension or bradycardia develop) – additional doses of 0.5–1 mg may be given by IV injection during short painful procedures

Pharmacokinetics

Molecular weight (daltons)	453.0
% Protein binding	88–95
% Excreted unchanged in urine	<1
Volume of distribution (L/kg)	0.3–1.0
Half-life – normal/ESRF (hrs)	1–4/unchanged

Dose in renal impairment GFR (mL/min)

20–50	Dose as in normal renal function
10–20	Dose as in normal renal function
<10	Dose as in normal renal function

Dose in patients undergoing renal replacement therapies

CAPD	Not dialysed. Dose as in normal renal function
HD	Not dialysed. Dose as in normal renal function
CAV/VVHD	Not dialysed. Dose as in normal renal function

Important drug interactions

POTENTIALLY HAZARDOUS INTERACTIONS WITH OTHER DRUGS

- Anti-arrhythmics: delayed absorption of mexiletine
- Possible CNS excitation or depression (hypertension or hypotension) in patients also receiving MAOIs (including moclobemide)
- Antipsychotics: enhanced sedative and hypotensive effect
- Cimetidine or erythromycin can inhibit clearance of alfentanil. This may increase the risk of prolonged respiratory depression
- Beta-blockers and anaesthetics depressing the heart of increasing vagal tone may predispose to bradycardia or hypotension

Administration

RECONSTITUTION

–

ROUTE

- IV bolus, IV infusion

RATE OF ADMINISTRATION

- See dose

COMMENTS

- Alfentanil can be mixed with sodium chloride 0.9%, glucose 5% or compound sodium lactate injection (Hartmann's solution)

Other information

- There is an increase in free fraction of drug in renal failure, hence dose requirements may be reduced
- IV administration: 500 micrograms alfentanil has peak effect in 90 seconds, and provides analgesia for 5–10 minutes (in unpremedicated adults)
- Transient fall in BP and bradycardia may occur on administration
- Analgesic potency = $1/4$ of that of fentanyl
- Duration of action = $1/3$ of that of an equianalgesic dose of fentanyl
- Onset of action = 4 times more rapid than an equianalgesic dose of fentanyl

ALG – Imtix (Horse) (Lymphoglobuline) (unlicensed product)

Clinical use

Prophylaxis and/or treatment of acute or steroid-resistant transplant rejection

Dose in normal renal function

2.5–10 mg/kg/day for up to 10–14 days

Pharmacokinetics

Molecular weight (daltons)	–
% Protein binding	–
% Excreted unchanged in urine	–
Volume of distribution (L/kg)	–
Half-life – normal/ESRF (hrs)	48–72/–

Dose in renal impairment GFR (mL/min)

20–50	Dose as in normal renal function
10–20	Dose as in normal renal function
<10	Dose as in normal renal function

Dose in patients undergoing renal replacement therapies

CAPD	Not dialysed. Dose as in normal renal function
HD	Not dialysed. Dose as in normal renal function
CAV/VVHD	Not dialysed. Dose as in normal renal function

Important drug interactions

POTENTIALLY HAZARDOUS INTERACTIONS WITH OTHER DRUGS

• Ciclosporin: risk of over immunosuppression
• Do not give blood or blood derivatives concomitantly
• Avoid simultaneous infusion of glucose solutions in same line

Administration

RECONSTITUTION

• Dilute total dose in 250 mL sodium chloride 0.9% (maximum concentration 1 mg/mL)

ROUTE

• IV centrally: if there is no central access, via peripheral vein with good blood flow rates

RATE OF ADMINISTRATION

• 4–16 hours

COMMENTS

• To minimise risk of adverse effects, chlorphenamine (10 mg IV) and hydrocortisone (100 mg IV) may be given 15–60 minutes before administration of full ALG dose
• Chlorpheniramine, hydrocortisone and adrenaline should be immediately available in case of severe anaphylaxis

Other information

• Dose may be modified to optimise immunosuppression. Aim to keep Total Lymphocyte Count below 3% of Total White Cell Count or 50 cells/mm³. Alternatively, keep absolute T-cell count below 50 cells/microlitre, and only dose when above this
• Avoid simultaneous transfusions of blood or blood derivatives and infusions of other solutions, particularly lipids
• A test dose is advised in accordance with manufacturer's literature
• ALG should not be administered in presence of fluid overload, allergy to horse protein, pregnancy

Allopurinol

Clinical use

Gout prophylaxis, hyperuricaemia

Dose in normal renal function

100–900 mg/day (usually 300 mg/day)
Doses above 300 mg should be given in divided doses

Pharmacokinetics

Molecular weight (daltons)	136.1
% Protein binding	<5
% Excreted unchanged in urine	30
Volume of distribution (L/kg)	0.5
Half-life – normal/ESRF (hrs)	2–8/unchanged

Dose in renal impairment GFR (mL/min)

20–50	200–300 mg daily
10–20	100–200 mg daily
<10	100 mg daily/alternate days

Dose in patients undergoing renal replacement therapies

CAPD	Dialysed. Dose as in GFR = <10 mL/min
HD	Dialysed. Dose as in GFR = <10 mL/min
CAV/VVHD	Dialysed. Dose as in GFR = 10–20 mL/min

Important drug interactions

POTENTIALLY HAZARDOUS INTERACTIONS WITH OTHER DRUGS

• Ciclosporin: isolated reports of raised CyA levels (risk of nephrotoxicity)
• Effects of azathioprine, cyclophosphamide and mercaptopurine enhanced with increased toxicity
• Increased risk of toxicity with captopril

Administration

RECONSTITUTION

–

ROUTE

• Oral

RATE OF ADMINISTRATION

–

COMMENTS

• In all grades of renal impairment commence with 100 mg/day and increase if serum and/or urinary urate response is unsatisfactory. Doses less than 100 mg/day may be required in some patients
• Take as a single daily dose, preferably after food

Other information

• A parenteral preparation is available from Glaxo Wellcome on a 'named patient' basis
• HD patients may be given 300 mg post dialysis, i.e. on alternate days
• There is an increased incidence of skin rash in patients with renal impairment
• Efficient dialysis usually controls serum uric acid levels
• If a patient is prescribed azathioprine or 6-mercaptopurine concomitantly, reduce azathioprine or 6-mercaptopurine dose by 75%
• Used occasionally in patients with impaired renal function prescribed concomitantly with colchicine in severe acute gout episodes, who are unable to be prescribed NSAIDs
• Main active metabolite oxipurinol – renally excreted. % plasma protein binding – 17% Half-life – normal/ESRF = 13–18/>125 hours – 1 week

Alteplase (t-PA) (recombinant human tissue-type plasminogen activator)

Clinical use

Fibrinolytic drug used for acute myocardial infarction and pulmonary embolism; acute ischaemic stroke; to unblock dialysis lines (unlicensed indication)

Dose in normal renal function

Myocardial infarction: accelerated regimen (initiated within 6 hours) 15 mg IV bolus, 50 mg over 30 minutes, then 35 mg over 1 hour (total dose 100 mg); or (if initiated within 6–12 hours) 10 mg over 1–2 minutes followed by IV infusion of 50 mg over 1 hour, then 40 mg over subsequent 2 hours (total dose – 100 mg over 3 hours)

Pulmonary embolism: total dose of 100 mg should be administered in 2 hours. Total dose should not exceed 1.5 mg/kg in patients who weigh <65 kg

Acute ischaemic stroke: 0.9 mg/kg over 60 mins, 10% of dose as initial bolus. Maximum 90 mg. Start within 3 hours of symptoms

Pharmacokinetics

Molecular weight (daltons)	64,497.8 (non-glycosylated protein)
% Protein binding	–
% Excreted unchanged in urine	–
Volume of distribution (L/kg)	0.1
Half-life – normal/ESRF (hrs)	0.5/–

Dose in renal impairment GFR (mL/min)

20–50	Dose as in normal renal function
10–20	Dose as in normal renal function
<10	Dose as in normal renal function

Dose in patients undergoing renal replacement therapies

CAPD	Not dialysed. Dose as in normal renal function
HD	Not dialysed. Dose as in normal renal function
CAV/VVHD	Not dialysed. Dose as in normal renal function

Important drug interactions

POTENTIALLY HAZARDOUS INTERACTIONS WITH OTHER DRUGS

- Risk of haemorrhage can be increased by the use of coumarin derivatives, platelet aggregation inhibitors, heparin and other agents influencing coagulation

Administration

RECONSTITUTION

- 50-mg vial – dissolve in 50 mL water for injection
- 20-mg vial – dissolve in 20 mL water for injection
- The reconstituted solutions can be further diluted (minimum concentration 0.2 mg/mL) with sterile sodium chloride 0.9%

ROUTE

- IV

RATE OF ADMINISTRATION

- See under dose

COMMENTS

- Water or glucose solution must NOT be used for dilution
- 50-mg vial = 29 mega units/vial
- 20-mg vial = 11.6 mega units/vial

Other information

- Patients weighing less than 65 kg should receive a total dose of 1.5 mg/kg according to dose schedule
- Allergic reactions are less likely with alteplase than streptokinase and repeated administration is possible
- 1.7 g arginine in the 50-mg vial, 0.7 g arginine in 20-mg vial – may lead to hyperkalaemia in renal failure
- Pay attention to potential bleeding sites during treatment
- To unblock dialysis lines, use at a dose of 2 mg down each lumen and leave in for at least 60 minutes or until the next dialysis session
- Alternative regimens: an infusion of 20 mg over 20 hours or 50 mg over 12 hours

Aluminium hydroxide

Clinical use

Phosphate-binding agent, antacid

Dose in normal renal function

As Alu-Caps: 4–20 capsules daily in divided doses
As mixture: 20–100 mL daily in divided doses in
accordance with response

Pharmacokinetics

Molecular weight (daltons)	78
% Protein binding	70–90
% Excreted unchanged in urine	–
Volume of distribution (L/kg)	–
Half-life – normal/ESRF (hrs)	–

Dose in renal impairment GFR (mL/min)

20–50	Dose as in normal renal function
10–20	Dose as in normal renal function
<10	Dose as in normal renal function

Dose in patients undergoing renal replacement therapies

CAPD	Unknown dialysability. Dose as in normal renal function
HD	Unknown dialysability. Dose as in normal renal function
CAV/VVHD	Unknown dialysability. Dose as in normal renal function

Important drug interactions

POTENTIALLY HAZARDOUS INTERACTIONS WITH OTHER DRUGS

• None known

Administration

RECONSTITUTION

–

ROUTE

• Oral

RATE OF ADMINISTRATION

–

COMMENTS

–

Other information

• ESRF patients on chronic therapy may develop aluminium toxicity, therefore best avoided in all but short-term therapy (calcium carbonate, calcium acetate or sevelamer used in chronic therapy)

• Take/administer with or immediately before meals

• In patients undergoing chronic therapy with aluminium hydroxide: serum aluminium levels should be monitored using the Desferrioxamine Test (5 mg/kg), see local protocol

• Suspension available (not prescribable by GPs)

Amantadine

Clinical use

Parkinson's disease (but not drug-induced extrapyramidal symptoms), herpes zoster, prophylaxis and treatment of influenza A

Dose in normal renal function

Parkinson's disease: 100 mg once a day increased after 1 week to 100 mg twice a day

Herpes zoster: 100 mg twice a day for 14 days

Influenza A: treatment – 100 mg once a day for 4–5 days, prophylaxis – 100 mg once a day

Pharmacokinetics

Molecular weight (daltons)	187.7
% Protein binding	67
% Excreted unchanged in urine	90
Volume of distribution (L/kg)	4–5
Half-life – normal/ESRF (hrs)	12/500

Dose in renal impairment GFR (mL/min)

20–50	100 mg every 24–48 hours
10–20	100 mg every 48–72 hours
<10	100 mg every 7 days

Dose in patients undergoing renal replacement therapies

CAPD	Not dialysed. Dose as in GFR = <10 mL/min
HD	Not dialysed. Dose as in GFR = <10 mL/min
CAV/VVHD	Unknown dialysability. Dose as in GFR = 10–20 mL/min

Important drug interactions

POTENTIALLY HAZARDOUS INTERACTIONS WITH OTHER DRUGS

• None known

Administration

RECONSTITUTION

–

ROUTE

• Oral

RATE OF ADMINISTRATION

–

COMMENTS

–

Other information

• Peripheral oedema may occur in some patients, which should be considered when the drug is prescribed for those with congestive heart failure

• Side-effects are often mild and transient. They usually appear within 2–4 days of treatment and disappear 24–48 hours after discontinuation of the drug

• Due to extensive tissue binding, <5% of a dose is removed by a 4-hour haemodialysis session

• A reduction in creatinine clearance to 40 mL/min may result in a 5-fold increase in elimination half-life

Amifostine

Clinical use

Reduction of neutropenia in patients on cisplatin or cyclophosphamide
Reduce risk of nephrotoxicity with cisplatin
Protects against xerostoma during head and neck radiotherapy

Dose in normal renal function

Cisplatin and cyclophosphamide therapy:
740–910 mg/m^2
Xerostoma: 200 mg/m^2 once daily, as a 3-minute infusion

Pharmacokinetics

Molecular weight (daltons)	214.2
% Protein binding	0
% Excreted unchanged in urine	0.7–1
Volume of distribution (L/kg)	7 litres
Half-life – normal/ESRF (hrs)	<10 minutes

Dose in renal impairment GFR (mL/min)

20–50	Dose as in normal renal function
10–20	Dose as in normal renal function
<10	Avoid – see 'Other information'

Dose in patients undergoing renal replacement therapies

CAPD	Avoid
HD	Avoid
CAV/VVHD	Dose as in GFR = 10–20 ml/min

Important drug interactions

POTENTIALLY HAZARDOUS INTERACTIONS WITH OTHER DRUGS

• Antihypertensives: enhanced effect

Administration

RECONSTITUTION

• Sodium chloride 0.9%

ROUTE

• IV

RATE OF ADMINISTRATION

• Over 15 minutes
• Once reconstituted, stable for 24 hours at 2–8°C

COMMENTS

–

Other information

• Give no more than 30 minutes before chemotherapy or radiotherapy
• Can decrease blood pressure – discontinue antihypertensives and ensure adequate rehydration
• 15-minute infusion better tolerated than longer infusion times
• Increased risk of nephrotoxicity with other nephrotoxic agents, dehydration, and hypotension

Amikacin

Clinical use

Antibacterial agent

Dose in normal renal function

15 mg/kg/day in two divided doses (maximum dose: 1.5 g/day, maximum total dose: 15 g)

Pharmacokinetics

Molecular weight (daltons)	585.6
% Protein binding	<5
% Excreted unchanged in urine	95
Volume of distribution (L/kg)	0.22–0.29
Half-life – normal/ESRF (hrs)	1.4–2.3/17–150

Dose in renal impairment
GFR (mL/min)

20–50	5–6 mg/kg every 12 hours
10–20	3–4 mg/kg every 24 hours
<10	2 mg/kg every 24–48 hours

Dose in patients undergoing renal replacement therapies

CAPD	Dialysed. Dose as in GFR = <10 mL/min
HD	Dialysed. Give 5 mg/kg after dialysis
CAV/VVHD	Dialysed. Dose as in GFR = 10–20 mL/min and monitor levels

Important drug interactions

POTENTIALLY HAZARDOUS INTERACTIONS WITH OTHER DRUGS

• Botulinum toxin: neuromuscular block enhanced – risk of toxicity
• Cholinergics: antagonism of effect of neostigmine and pyridostigmine
• Ciclosporin: increased risk of nephrotoxicity
• Cytotoxics: increased risk of nephrotoxicity and possibly of ototoxicity with cisplatin
• Diuretics: increased risk of ototoxicity with loop diuretics
• Muscle relaxants: effects of non-depolarising muscle relaxants such as tubocurarine enhanced

Administration

RECONSTITUTION

–

ROUTE

• IM/IV

RATE OF ADMINISTRATION

• IV bolus – slow over 2–3 minutes
• Infusion – at concentration 2.5 mg/mL over 30 minutes (Diluents: sodium chloride 0.9%, glucose 5% and others)

COMMENTS

• May be used intraperitoneally
• Do not mix physically with any other antibacterial agents

Other information

• Nephrotoxic and ototoxic. Toxicity no worse when hyperbilirubinaemic
• Serum levels must be measured for efficacy and toxicity
• Peritoneal absorption increases with presence of inflammation
• Vd increases with oedema, obesity and ascites
• Peak serum concentration should not exceed 30 mg/L
• Trough serum concentration should be less than 2.5 mg/L
• Amikacin affects auditory function to a greater extent than gentamicin

Amiloride

Clinical use

Potassium-sparing diuretic

Dose in normal renal function

2.5–20 mg daily

Pharmacokinetics

Molecular weight (daltons)	302.1
% Protein binding	30–40
% Excreted unchanged in urine	50
Volume of distribution (L/kg)	5–5.2
Half-life – normal/ESRF (hrs)	6–9/10–144

Dose in renal impairment GFR (mL/min)

20–50	50% of normal dose
10–20	50% of normal dose
<10	Avoid

Dose in patients undergoing renal replacement therapies

CAPD	Avoid
HD	Avoid
CAV/VVHD	Avoid

Important drug interactions

POTENTIALLY HAZARDOUS INTERACTIONS WITH OTHER DRUGS

- ACE inhibitors & AT-II antagonists: enhanced hypotensive effect; risk of severe hyperkalaemia
- Analgesics: increased risk of nephrotoxicity with NSAIDs; increased risk of hyperkalaemia, especially with indometacin
- Antihypertensives: enhanced hypotensive effect; increased risk of first-dose hypotensive effect of post-synaptic alpha-blockers, e.g. prazosin
- Ciclosporin: increased risk of hyperkalaemia
- Lithium: reduced excretion of lithium therefore risk of lithium toxicity
- Potassium salts: increased risk of hyperkalaemia
- Tacrolimus: increased risk of hyperkalaemia

Administration

RECONSTITUTION

–

ROUTE

- Oral

RATE OF ADMINISTRATION

–

COMMENTS

–

Other information

- Hyperkalaemia occurs with a GFR < 30 mL/min, especially in diabetics. Can lead to hyperchloraemic metabolic acidosis

Aminophylline

Clinical use

Reversible airways obstruction, acute severe asthma

Dose in normal renal function

Oral: 100–300 mg 3–4 times daily, maximum 900 mg daily

IV loading dose: 5 mg/kg

Maintenance dose: 0.5 mg/kg/hour

Modified release: 225–450 mg twice daily

Pharmacokinetics

Molecular weight (daltons)	420.4
% Protein binding	40–60 (theophylline)
% Excreted unchanged in urine	<10
Volume of distribution (L/kg)	0.4–0.7 (theophylline)
Half-life – normal/ESRF (hrs)	4–12/unchanged (theophylline)

Dose in renal impairment GFR (mL/min)

20–50	200–400 mg every 12 hours
10–20	200–300 mg every 12 hours and adjust in accordance with blood levels
<10	200–300 mg every 12 hours and adjust in accordance with blood levels

Dose in patients undergoing renal replacement therapies

CAPD	Not dialysed. Dose as in GFR = <10 mL/min. Monitor blood levels
HD	Not dialysed. Dose as in GFR = <10 mL/min. Monitor blood levels
CAV/VVHD	Not dialysed. Dose as in GFR = 10–20 mL/min. Monitor blood levels

Important drug interactions

POTENTIALLY HAZARDOUS INTERACTIONS WITH OTHER DRUGS

• Plasma concentration increased by ciprofloxacin, erythromycin, clarithromycin and norfloxacin. Also by diltiazem, verapamil, cimetidine, combined oral contraceptives, fluvoxamine and ticlopidine

• Plasma concentrations reduced by carbamazepine, phenobarbital, phenytoin, primidone, ritonavir, St John's Wort and rifampicin

• Antagonism of anti-arrhythmic effect of adenosine

Administration

RECONSTITUTION

–

ROUTE

• IV, oral

RATE OF ADMINISTRATION

• Loading dose over 20 minutes by slow IV injection

COMMENTS

• Can be added to glucose 5%, sodium chloride 0.9% and compound sodium lactate

Other information

• Optimum response obtained at plasma theophylline levels of 10–20 mg/L (55–110 micromol/L)

• Increased incidence of GI and neurological side-effects in renal impairment at plasma levels above optimum range

• Aminophylline: 80% theophylline + 20% ethylenediamine

Amiodarone

Clinical use

Cardiac arrhythmias

Dose in normal renal function

Oral: 200 mg three times a day for 1 week, then twice a day for 1 week, then 200 mg daily maintenance dose or minimum required to control arrhythmia

IV: via central catheter: 5 mg/kg (maximum 1.2 g in 24 hours)

Pharmacokinetics

Molecular weight (daltons)	645.3
% Protein binding	96
% Excreted unchanged in urine	<5
Volume of distribution (L/kg)	70–140
Half-life – normal/ESRF (hrs)	14–120 days/ unchanged

Dose in renal impairment GFR (mL/min)

20–50	Dose as in normal renal function
10–20	Dose as in normal renal function
<10	Dose as in normal renal function

Dose in patients undergoing renal replacement therapies

CAPD	Not dialysed. Dose as in normal renal function
HD	Not dialysed. Dose as in normal renal function
CAV/VVHD	Not dialysed. Dose as in normal renal function

Important drug interactions

POTENTIALLY HAZARDOUS INTERACTIONS WITH OTHER DRUGS

- Other anti-arrhythmics: additive effect and increased risk of myocardial depression
- Antibacterials: increased risk of ventricular arrhythmias with parenteral erythromycin and co-trimoxazole – avoid concomitant use
- Warfarin: metabolism inhibited (increased anticoagulant effect)
- Antidepressants: increased risk of ventricular arrhythmias with tricyclic antidepressants – avoid concomitant use
- Phenytoin: metabolism inhibited (increased plasma concentration)
- Anti-malarials: increased risk of ventricular arrhythmias with chloroquine, hydroxychloroquine, mefloquine and quinine – avoid concomitant use
- Antivirals: increased risk of ventricular arrhythmias with nelfinavir and ritonavir – avoid concomitant use
- Beta-blockers and calcium-channel blockers: increased risk of bradycardia, AV block and myocardial depression
- Ciclosporin: increased levels of CyA possible
- Digoxin: increased plasma concentration (halve digoxin maintenance dose)
- Pentamidine: increased risk of ventricular arrhythmias – avoid concomitant use
- Terfenadine and mizolastine: increased risk of ventricular arrythmias
- Phenothiazines: increased risk of ventricular arrythmias

Administration

RECONSTITUTION

–

ROUTE

- Oral
- IV via central catheter or peripherally in veins with good blood flow

RATE OF ADMINISTRATION

- 20–120 minutes (max 1.2 g in up to 500 mL glucose 5% in 24 hours)

COMMENTS

- Add dose to 250 mL glucose 5%
- Solutions containing less than 300 mg in 500 mL glucose 5% should not be used as unstable
- Volumetric pump should be used as amiodarone can reduce drop size

Other information

- Amiodarone and desethylamiodarone levels can be monitored to assess compliance
- In extreme clinical emergency may be given by slow IV bolus using 150–300 mg in 10–20 mL glucose 5% over a minimum of 3 minutes with close patient monitoring. This should not be repeated for at least 15 minutes
- Incompatible with sodium chloride 0.9%
- Rapid IV administration has been associated with anaphylactic shock, hot flushes, sweating, and nausea

Amisulpride

Clinical use

Treatment of acute and chronic schizophrenia

Dose in normal renal function

50–1200 mg daily (in divided doses if >300 mg)
varies according to indication

Pharmacokinetics

Molecular weight (daltons)	369.5
% Protein binding	16
% Excreted unchanged in urine	50
Volume of distribution (L/kg)	5.8
Half-life – normal/ESRF (hrs)	12/unchanged

Dose in renal impairment
GFR (mL/min)

30–60	Reduce dose by 50%
10–30	Use a third of the dose (see 'Other information')
<10	Use with caution. Start with minimum dose and increase according to patient's response

Dose in patients undergoing renal replacement therapies

CAPD	Not dialysed. Dose as in GFR < 10 mL/min
HD	Poorly dialysed. Dose as in GFR < 10 mL/min
CAV/VVHD	Poorly dialysed. Dose as in GFR = 10–30 mL/min

Important drug interactions

POTENTIALLY HAZARDOUS INTERACTIONS WITH
OTHER DRUGS

- Anaesthetics: enhanced hypotensive effect
- Alcohol: may enhance CNS effects of alcohol
- Antihypertensives: increased risk of hypotension
- Analgesics: enhanced sedative and hypotensive effect with opioid analgesics
- Sibutramine: increased risk of CNS toxicity (avoid concomitant use)
- Anti-arrhythmics and other drugs which may prolong the QT interval, e.g. cisapride, thioridazine: avoid concomitant use due to risk of torsades de pointes

Administration

RECONSTITUTION

–

ROUTE

- Oral

RATE OF ADMINISTRATION

–

COMMENTS

–

Other information

The elimination half-life is unchanged in patients with renal insufficiency while systemic clearance is reduced by a factor of 2.5–3. The AUC of amisulpride in mild renal failure is increased 2-fold, and almost 10-fold in moderate renal failure. Experience is limited and there are no data with doses >50 mg

Eliminated by renal route, therefore, in severe renal impairment, intermittent treatment should be prescribed at a reduced dose

Amitriptyline

Clinical use

Tricyclic antidepressant used especially where sedation is required

Dose in normal renal function

Oral: initially 75 mg/day – increased gradually to maximum 200 mg. Usual maintenance: 50–100 mg daily

Pharmacokinetics

Molecular weight (daltons)	277.4
% Protein binding	96
% Excreted unchanged in urine	<10
Volume of distribution (L/kg)	6–36
Half-life – normal/ESRF (hrs)	24–40/unchanged

Dose in renal impairment GFR (mL/min)

20–50	Dose as in normal renal function
10–20	Dose as in normal renal function
<10	Dose as in normal renal function

Dose in patients undergoing renal replacement therapies

CAPD	Not dialysed. Dose as in normal renal function
HD	Not dialysed. Dose as in normal renal function
CAV/VVHD	Not dialysed. Dose as in normal renal function

Important drug interactions

POTENTIALLY HAZARDOUS INTERACTIONS WITH OTHER DRUGS

• Anaesthetics: risk of arrhythmias and hypotension increased

• Antihypertensives: hypotensive effect enhanced
• Antipsychotics: increased risk of ventricular arrhythmias
• Interaction with anti-arrhythmics – increased risk of ventricular arrhythmias with drugs which prolong QT interval
• MAOI: CNS excitation and hypertension
• Antagonism with anti-epileptics – convulsive threshold lowered. Also anti-epileptics may lower plasma concentration of some tricyclics
• Antihistamines: increased antimuscarinic and sedative effects – increased risk of ventricular arrhythmias with terfenadine
• Beta-blockers: increased risk of ventricular arrhythmias with sotalol
• Dopaminergics: avoid use with entacapone; CNS toxicity reported with selegiline
• Hypertension and arrhythmias with adrenaline
• Hypertension with noradrenaline
• Sibutramine: increased risk of CNS toxicity – avoid concomitant use

Administration

RECONSTITUTION

–

ROUTE

• Oral

RATE OF ADMINISTRATION

–

COMMENTS

–

Other information

• Introduce treatment gradually in renal impairment due to dizziness and postural hypotension
• Withdraw treatment gradually
• Anticholinergic side-effects – causes urinary retention, drowsiness, dry mouth, blurred vision and constipation

Amlodipine

Clinical use

Calcium-channel blocker for: hypertension, angina prophylaxis

Dose in normal renal function

5–10 mg daily

Pharmacokinetics

Molecular weight (daltons)	567.1
% Protein binding	>95
% Excreted unchanged in urine	<10
Volume of distribution (L/kg)	21
Half-life – normal/ESRF (hrs)	35–50/50

Dose in renal impairment GFR (mL/min)

20–50	Dose as in normal renal function
10–20	Dose as in normal renal function
<10	Dose as in normal renal function

Dose in patients undergoing renal replacement therapies

CAPD	Not dialysed. Dose as in normal renal function
HD	Not dialysed. Dose as in normal renal function
CAV/VVHD	Not dialysed. Dose as in normal renal function

Important drug interactions

POTENTIALLY HAZARDOUS INTERACTIONS WITH OTHER DRUGS

• Antihypertensives: enhanced hypotensive effect, increased risk of first-dose hypotensive effect of pre-synaptic alpha-blockers

Administration

RECONSTITUTION

–

ROUTE

• Oral

RATE OF ADMINISTRATION

–

COMMENTS

–

Other information

• Amlodipine is extensively metabolised to inactive metabolites

Amoxicillin

Clinical use

Antibacterial agent

Dose in normal renal function

250–500 mg every 8 hours (maximum 6 g per day)

Pharmacokinetics

Molecular weight (daltons)	365.4
% Protein binding	15–25
% Excreted unchanged in urine	50–70
Volume of distribution (L/kg)	0.26
Half-life – normal/ESRF (hrs)	0.9–2.3/5–20

Dose in renal impairment GFR (mL/min)

20–50	Dose as in normal renal function
10–20	Dose as in normal renal function
<10	250 mg every 8 hours

Dose in patients undergoing renal replacement therapies

CAPD	Dialysed. Dose as in GFR = <10 mL/min
HD	Dialysed. Dose as in GFR = <10 mL/min
CAV/VVHD	Dialysed. Dose as in normal renal function

Important drug interactions

POTENTIALLY HAZARDOUS INTERACTIONS WITH OTHER DRUGS

• Amoxicillin can reduce the excretion of methotrexate (increased risk of toxicity)

Administration

RECONSTITUTION

• IV: dissolve each 250 mg in 5 mL water for injection
• IV infusion: dilute in 100 mL glucose 5% or sodium chloride 0.9%
• IM: dissolve:
    • 250 mg in 1.5 mL water for injection
    • 500 mg in 2.5 mL water for injection
    • 1 g in 2.5 mL water for injection or 1% sterile lidocaine hydrochloride

ROUTE

• Oral, IV, IM

RATE OF ADMINISTRATION

• Slow bolus IV over 3–4 minutes
• Infusion over 30–60 minutes

COMMENTS

• Stability in infusion depends upon diluent

Other information

• Sodium – 3.3 mmol/g vial of Amoxil
• Do not mix with aminoglycosides

Amphotericin (IV) – Abelcet (lipid complex)

Clinical use

Antifungal agent for systemic fungal infections (yeasts and yeast-like fungi including *Candida albicans*)

Dose in normal renal function

5 mg/kg/day for at least 14 days (see individual product data sheet)

Pharmacokinetics

Molecular weight (daltons)	924
% Protein binding	90–97
% Excreted unchanged in urine	2–5
Volume of distribution (L/kg)	2286
Half-life – normal/ESRF (hrs)	173.4/unchanged

Dose in renal impairment GFR (mL/min)

20–50	Dose as in normal renal function
10–20	Dose as in normal renal function
<10	Dose as in normal renal function

Dose in patients undergoing renal replacement therapies

CAPD	Not dialysed. Dose as in normal renal function
HD	Not dialysed. Dose as in normal renal function
CAV/VVHD	Not dialysed. Dose as in normal renal function

Important drug interactions

POTENTIALLY HAZARDOUS INTERACTIONS WITH OTHER DRUGS

- Ciclosporin: increased nephrotoxicity
- Tacrolimus: increased nephrotoxicity
- Increased risk of nephrotoxicity with aminoglycosides and other nephrotoxic agents and cytotoxics
- Cardiac glycosides: increased toxicity if hypokalaemia occurs
- Corticosteroids: increased risk of hypokalaemia (avoid concomitant use unless corticosteroids are required to control reactions)
- Flucytosine: enhanced toxicity in combination with amphotericin

Administration

RECONSTITUTION

- See individual data sheet. Prepare intermittent infusion in glucose 5% (incompatible with sodium chloride 0.9%, electrolytes or other drugs)
- Dilute to a concentration of 1–2 mg/ml

ROUTE

- IV infusion

RATE OF ADMINISTRATION

- 2.5 mg/kg/hour

COMMENTS

- Paracetamol and parenteral pethidine may alleviate rigors associated with amphotericin administration. Can also use antihistamines to control reactions
- Flush existing IV line with glucose 5% before and after infusion administration
- For patients on CAV/VVHD, amphotericin should be given into the venous return of the dialysis circuit
- Should be given post dialysis

Other information

- **AMPHOTERICIN IS HIGHLY NEPHROTOXIC**
- Can cause distal tubular acidosis
- May cause polyurea, hypovolaemia, hypokalaemia and acidosis
- Amphotericin and flucytosine act synergistically when co-administered enabling lower doses to be used effectively
- A test dose of amphotericin is recommended at the beginning of a new course
- Monitor renal function, full blood count, potassium, magnesium and calcium levels
- Liposomal amphotericin is considerably less nephrotoxic compared with conventional amphotericin B, but is considerably more expensive

Amphotericin (IV) – Ambisome (liposomal)

Clinical use

Antifungal agent for systemic fungal infections (yeasts and yeast-like fungi including *Candida albicans*)

Treatment of visceral leishmaniasis

Dose in normal renal function

1–3 mg/kg/day (see individual product data sheet)

V. leishmaniasis: total dose of 21–30 mg/kg given over 10–21 days

Pharmacokinetics

Molecular weight (daltons)	924
% Protein binding	90–97
% Excreted unchanged in urine	2–5
Volume of distribution (L/kg)	0.1–0.44
Half-life – normal/ESRF (hrs)	6.3–10.7/ unchanged

Dose in renal impairment GFR (mL/min)

20–50	Dose as in normal renal function
10–20	Dose as in normal renal function
<10	Dose as in normal renal function

Dose in patients undergoing renal replacement therapies

CAPD	Not dialysed. Dose as in normal renal function
HD	Not dialysed. Dose as in normal renal function
CAV/VVHD	Not dialysed. Dose as in normal renal function

Important drug interactions

POTENTIALLY HAZARDOUS INTERACTIONS WITH OTHER DRUGS

- Ciclosporin: increased nephrotoxicity
- Tacrolimus: increased nephrotoxicity
- Increased risk of nephrotoxicity with aminoglycosides and other nephrotoxic agents and cytotoxics
- Cardiac glycosides: increased toxicity if hypokalaemia occurs
- Corticosteroids: increased risk of hypokalaemia (avoid concomitant use unless corticosteroids are required to control reactions)
- Flucytosine: enhanced toxicity in combination with amphotericin

Administration

RECONSTITUTION

- See individual data sheet. Prepare intermittent infusion in glucose 5% (incompatible with sodium chloride 0.9%, electrolytes or other drugs). Reconstitute vial contents with water for injection
- Dilute to a concentration of 0.2–2 mg/ml

ROUTE

- IV infusion

RATE OF ADMINISTRATION

- 30–60 minutes

COMMENTS

- Paracetamol and parenteral pethidine may alleviate rigors associated with amphotericin administration. Antihistamines can also be administered to control reactions
- Flush existing IV line with glucose 5% before and after infusion administration
- For patients on CAV/VVHD, amphotericin should be given into the venous return of the dialysis circuit
- Should be given post dialysis

Other information

- **AMPHOTERICIN IS HIGHLY NEPHROTOXIC**
- Can cause distal tubular acidosis
- May cause polyurea, hypovolaemia, hypokalaemia and acidosis
- Amphotericin and flucytosine act synergistically when co-administered enabling lower doses to be used effectively
- A test dose of amphotericin is recommended at the beginning of a new course. (1 mg over 10 minutes then stop and observe for next 30 minutes)
- Monitor renal function, full blood count, potassium, magnesium and calcium levels
- Liposomal amphotericin is considerably less nephrotoxic compared with amphotericin, but is considerably more expensive

Amphotericin (IV) – Amphocil (complex with sodium cholesteryl sulphate)

Clinical use

Antifungal agent for systemic fungal infections (yeasts and yeast-like fungi including *Candida albicans*)

Dose in normal renal function

1–6 mg/kg/day (see individual product data sheet)

Pharmacokinetics

Molecular weight (daltons)	924
% Protein binding	90–97
% Excreted unchanged in urine	2–5
Volume of distribution (L/kg)	2.25–3.61
Half-life – normal/ESRF (hrs)	22.1–27.2/ unchanged

Dose in renal impairment GFR (mL/min)

20–50	Dose as in normal renal function
10–20	Dose as in normal renal function
<10	Dose as in normal renal function

Dose in patients undergoing renal replacement therapies

CAPD	Not dialysed. Dose as in normal renal function
HD	Not dialysed. Dose as in normal renal function
CAV/VVHD	Not dialysed. Dose as in normal renal function

Important drug interactions

- Ciclosporin: increased nephrotoxicity
- Tacrolimus: increased nephrotoxicity
- Increased risk of nephrotoxicity with aminoglycosides and other nephrotoxic agents and cytotoxics
- Cardiac glycosides: increased toxicity if hypokalaemia occurs
- Corticosteroids: increased risk of hypokalaemia (avoid concomitant use unless corticosteroids are required to control reactions)
- Flucytosine: enhanced toxicity in combination with amphotericin

Administration

RECONSTITUTION

- See individual data sheet. Prepare intermittent infusion in glucose 5% (incompatible with sodium chloride 0.9%, electrolytes or other drugs). Reconstitute vial contents with water for injection

ROUTE

- IV infusion

RATE OF ADMINISTRATION

- 1–2 mg/kg/hour

COMMENTS

- Paracetamol and parenteral pethidine may alleviate rigors associated with amphotericin administration. Antihistamines can also be administered to control reactions
- Flush existing IV line with glucose 5% before and after infusion administration
- For patients on CAV/VVHD, amphotericin should be given into the venous return of the dialysis circuit
- Should be given post dialysis

Other information

- **AMPHOTERICIN IS HIGHLY NEPHROTOXIC**
- Can cause distal tubular acidosis
- May cause polyurea, hypovolaemia, hypokalaemia and acidosis
- Amphotericin and flucytosine act synergistically when co-administered enabling lower doses to be used effectively
- A test dose of amphotericin is recommended at the beginning of a new course
- Monitor renal function, full blood count, potassium, magnesium and calcium levels
- Less nephrotoxic than conventional amphotericin B

Amphotericin (IV) – Fungizone

Clinical use

Antifungal agent for systemic fungal infections (yeasts and yeast-like fungi including *Candida albicans*)

Dose in normal renal function

250 micrograms – 1.5 mg/kg/day
(see individual product data sheet)
Can be given on alternate days if using a higher dose

Pharmacokinetics

Molecular weight (daltons)	924
% Protein binding	>90
% Excreted unchanged in urine	2–5
Volume of distribution (L/kg)	4
Half-life – normal/ESRF (hrs)	24–48/unchanged

Dose in renal impairment GFR (mL/min)

20–50	Dose as in normal renal function
10–20	Dose as in normal renal function
<10	250 micrograms – 1.5 mg/kg every 24–36 hours

Dose in patients undergoing renal replacement therapies

CAPD	Not dialysed. Dose as in GFR = <10 mL/min
HD	Not dialysed. Dose as in GFR = <10 mL/min
CAV/VVHD	Not dialysed. Dose as in GFR = 10–20 mL/min

Important drug interactions

POTENTIALLY HAZARDOUS INTERACTIONS WITH OTHER DRUGS

• Ciclosporin: increased nephrotoxicity
• Tacrolimus: increased nephrotoxicity
• Increased risk of nephrotoxicity with aminoglycosides and other nephrotoxic agents and cytotoxics
• Cardiac glycosides: increased toxicity if hypokalaemia occurs
• Corticosteroids: increased risk of hypokalaemia (avoid concomitant use unless corticosteroids are required to control reactions)
• Flucytosine: enhanced toxicity in combination with amphotericin

Administration

RECONSTITUTION

• See individual data sheet. Prepare intermittent infusion in glucose 5% (incompatible with sodium chloride 0.9%, electrolytes or other drugs). Reconstitute vial contents with water for injection. pH should be adjusted to >4.2
• Dilute to a concentration of 10 mg in 100 mL

ROUTE

• IV infusion

RATE OF ADMINISTRATION

• 2–6 hours
• If given over 12–24 hours there is a reduced incidence of side-effects

COMMENTS

• Higher rates of infusion are associated with greater risk of adverse reactions. Administration over less than 1 hour particularly in renal failure has been associated with hyperkalaemia and arrhythmias
• Paracetamol and parenteral pethidine may alleviate rigors associated with amphotericin administration. Can also give antihistamines and corticosteroids to control reactions
• Flush existing IV line with glucose 5% before and after infusion administration
• For patients on CAV/VVHD, amphotericin should be given into the venous return of the dialysis circuit

Other information

• **AMPHOTERICIN IS HIGHLY NEPHROTOXIC**
• Permanent renal impairment may occur, particularly in patients receiving conventional amphotericin B at doses >1 mg/kg/day, or with pre-existing renal impairment, prolonged therapy, sodium depletion or concurrent nephrotoxic drugs
• Nephrotoxicity may be reduced by giving an IV infusion of sodium chloride 0.9% 250–500 mL over 30–45 minutes immediately before administering amphotericin B

- Can cause distal tubular acidosis
- May cause polyurea, hypovolaemia, hypokalaemia and acidosis
- Amphotericin and flucytosine act synergistically when co-administered enabling lower doses to be used effectively
- A test dose of amphotericin is recommended at the beginning of a new course (1 mg over 20–30 minutes then stop and observe for 30 minutes)

- Monitor renal function, full blood count, potassium, magnesium and calcium levels
- Liposomal amphotericin is considerably less nephrotoxic compared with conventional amphotericin B, but is considerably more expensive
- There are reports of the use of amphotericin in 20% lipid solution being as well tolerated as liposomal amphotericin

Ampicillin

Clinical use

Antibacterial agent

Dose in normal renal function

Oral: 250 mg – 1 g every 6 hours
IM/IV: 500 mg – 2 g every 4–6 hours

Pharmacokinetics

Molecular weight (daltons)	349
% Protein binding	20
% Excreted unchanged in urine	30–90
Volume of distribution (L/kg)	0.17–0.31
Half-life – normal/ESRF (hrs)	0.8–1.5/7–20

Dose in renal impairment GFR (mL/min)

20–50	Dose as in normal renal function
10–20	250–500 mg every 6 hours
<10	250 mg every 6 hours

Dose in patients undergoing renal replacement therapies

CAPD	Dialysed. Dose as in GFR = <10 mL/min
HD	Dialysed. Dose as in GFR = <10 mL/min
CAV/VVHD	Dialysed. Dose as in GFR = 10–20 mL/min

Important drug interactions

POTENTIALLY HAZARDOUS INTERACTIONS WITH OTHER DRUGS

• Ciclosporin: may increase ciclosporin levels
• Reduces excretion of methotrexate (increased risk of toxicity)

Administration

RECONSTITUTION

• Use water for injection: 5 mL for each 250 mg (1.5 mL for 250 mg or 500 mg for IM administration)

ROUTE

• Oral, IV, IM

RATE OF ADMINISTRATION

• Slow IV bolus over 3–4 minutes. Doses greater than 500 mg should be given by infusion at a rate not exceeding 500 mg/minute

COMMENTS

• Can be diluted in glucose 5% or sodium chloride 0.9%

Other information

• Rashes more common in patients with renal impairment
• Can cause nephrotoxicity if dose not reduced in renal impairment
• Sodium content of injection 1.47 mmol/500-mg vial
• Ampicillin may be used in peritoneal dialysis fluids for treatment of peritonitis
• Do not mix with aminoglycosides

Anastrozole

Clinical use

Treatment of breast cancer in post-menopausal women

Dose in normal renal function

1 mg daily

Pharmacokinetics

Molecular weight (daltons)	293.4
% Protein binding	40
% Excreted unchanged in urine	<10
Volume of distribution (L/kg)	No data
Half-life – normal/ESRF (hrs)	40–50/–

Dose in renal impairment GFR (mL/min)

20–50	Dose as in normal renal function
10–20	Dose as in normal renal function
<10	0.5–1 mg daily

Dose in patients undergoing renal replacement therapies

CAPD	Dialysed. Dose as in GFR < 10 mL/min
HD	Dialysed. Dose as in GFR < 10 mL/min
CAV/VVHD	Dialysed. Dose as in GFR = 10–20 mL/min

Important drug interactions

POTENTIALLY HAZARDOUS INTERACTIONS WITH OTHER DRUGS

- Oestrogen-containing therapies: avoid concomitant administration as would negate pharmacological action
- Tamoxifen: avoid concomitant administration

Administration

RECONSTITUTION

–

ROUTE

- Oral

RATE OF ADMINISTRATION

–

COMMENTS

–

Other information

- Anastrozole is extensively metabolised in the liver only 10% of unchanged drug and 60% of metabolites (largely inactive) are excreted in the urine
- Although renal clearance of anastrozole decreases proportionally with creatinine clearance, the reduction in renal clearance does not affect total body clearance of anastrozole. Therefore, adjustment of dosage in patients with renal impairment is not usually required. (AHFS 2000)
- The manufacturer recommends avoiding the use of anastrozole in patients with GFR <20 ml/min

Apomorphine

Clinical use

Treatment of erectile dysfunction (ED);
Parkinson's disease (PD)

Dose in normal renal function

ED: 2–3 mg administered approximately
20 minutes before sexual activity

PD: 3–30 mg daily in divided doses, infusion:
1–4 mg/hour during waking hours. Maximum dose
100 mg daily

Pharmacokinetics

Molecular weight (daltons)	303.79
% Protein binding	90
% Excreted unchanged in urine	<2
Volume of distribution (L/kg)	2–19
Half-life – normal/ESRF (hrs)	• sublingual: 2–3/increases by 0.24 hrs with each 10 mL/min/1.73m^2 decrease in creatinine clearance
	• subcutaneous: 33 minutes

Dose in renal impairment
GFR (mL/min)

20–50	Dose as in normal renal function
10–20	Dose as in normal renal function (ED). Use with caution if using for Parkinson's disease
<10	2 mg (ED). Use with caution if using for Parkinson's disease

Dose in patients undergoing renal replacement therapies

CAPD	N/A. Dose as in GFR = <10 mL/min
HD	N/A. Dose as in GFR = <10 mL/min
CAV/VVHD	N/A. Dose as in GFR = 10–20 mL/min

Important drug interactions

POTENTIALLY HAZARDOUS INTERACTIONS WITH
OTHER DRUGS

• Nitrates: enhanced hypotensive effect
• Antihypertensives: enhance hypotensive effect

Administration

RECONSTITUTION

–

ROUTE

• ED: sublingual; Parkinson's disease: SC

RATE OF ADMINISTRATION

• 1–4 mg/hour

COMMENTS

• Change site every 4 hours for SC administration

Other information

• For Parkinson's disease, pretreatment with
domperidone is required for at least 2 days
before and at least 3 days after treatment
• Bioavailability by subcutaneous administration is
17–18%
• Undergoes extensive first-pass metabolism when
given orally and has a low bioavailability
• Most of dose is excreted in the urine as active
metabolites

Aprotinin

Clinical use

Treatment of patients at risk of major blood loss during and following open heart surgery with extra-corporeal circulation. Also for treatment of life-threatening haemorrhage due to hyperplasminaemia

Dose in normal renal function

Cardiac surgery:

Loading dose – 200 ml (2,000,000 KIU)

Maintenance dose – continuous infusion of 50 ml (500,000 KIU) per hour

Hyperplasminaemia:

Initially 50–100 ml (500,000–1,000,000 KIU) by slow IV injection or infusion (maximum rate 10 ml/min). If necessary, follow by 20 ml/hr until bleeding stops

Pharmacokinetics

Molecular weight (daltons)	6512
% Protein binding	–
% Excreted unchanged in urine	<5
Volume of distribution (L/kg)	–
Half-life – normal/ESRF (hrs)	2–7/13.3–14.9

Dose in renal impairment GFR (mL/min)

20–50	100% dose
10–20	75–100 % dose
<10	50% dose – see 'Other information'

Dose in patients undergoing renal replacement therapies

CAPD	Unknown dialysability. Dose as in GFR < 10 ml/min
HD	Unknown dialysability. Dose as in GFR < 10 ml/min
CAV/VVHD	Unknown dialysability. Dose as in GFR = 10–20 ml/min

Important drug interactions

POTENTIALLY HAZARDOUS INTERACTIONS WITH OTHER DRUGS

• Aprotinin has a dose-dependent inhibitory effect on the action of thrombolytic agents, e.g. streptokinase, urokinase, alteplase, etc

Administration

RECONSTITUTION

–

ROUTE

• IV

RATE OF ADMINISTRATION

–

COMMENTS

–

Other information

• Aprotinin is degraded by lysosomal activity in the kidney, and the resulting products are excreted renally. Aprotinin is not excreted unchanged in the urine

• Abnormal kidney function has been observed in clinical studies. Only single cases of reversible kidney failure have been reported in post-marketing surveillance

• The pharmacokinetics of aprotinin were studied in two patients with chronic renal impairment undergoing hysterectomy. Both patients received 1,000,000 KIU over 30 minutes following the first incision. There was a substantial decrease in aprotinin clearance and an increase in elimination half-life and AUC of aprotinin compared to normal. (Muuler FO et al. (1996) Br J Clin Pharmacol. **41**: 619–20)

• In a study of 16 dialysis patients undergoing cardiac surgery, seven received aprotinin (2,000,000 KIU pump prime, 500,000 KIU/hr infusion maintenance dose), whilst the other nine acted as controls. Aprotinin administration was associated with a decrease in bleeding and blood transfusions. No complications were seen related to the drug. (Lemmer JH et al. (1998) J Thorac Cardiovasc Surg. **112**: 192–4)

• Another study looked at 26 cardiopulmonary bypass surgical patients with normal and abnormal renal function. Patients received 2,000,000 KIU loading dose, followed by 250,000 KIU/hr maintenance infusion, with no aprotinin pump prime. Aprotinin clearance was reduced and half-life increased in patients with renal insufficiency. The authors suggest omitting the pump prime, and reducing the maintenance dose to 250,000 KIU/hr, as in this study

Ascorbic acid

Clinical use

Acidification of urine, vitamin C deficiency

Dose in normal renal function

Up to 4 g daily in divided doses
Prophylaxis: 25–75 mg daily
Therapeutic: 250 mg daily in divided doses
IV: 0.5–1 g daily
Preventative therapy: 200–500 mg daily

Pharmacokinetics

Molecular weight (daltons)	176
% Protein binding	24
% Excreted unchanged in urine	<10
Volume of distribution (L/kg)	–
Half-life – normal/ESRF (hrs)	3–4/unchanged

Dose in renal impairment
GFR (mL/min)

20–50	Dose as in normal renal function
10–20	Dose as in normal renal function
<10	Dose as in normal renal function

Dose in patients undergoing renal replacement therapies

CAPD	Dialysed. Dose as in normal renal function
HD	Dialysed. Dose as in normal renal function
CAV/VVHD	Dialysed. Dose as in normal renal function

Important drug interactions

POTENTIALLY HAZARDOUS INTERACTIONS WITH OTHER DRUGS

• None known

Administration

RECONSTITUTION
–

ROUTE
• Oral, IV

RATE OF ADMINISTRATION
–

COMMENTS
–

Other information

• No scientific evidence in clinical trial of efficacy in reducing UTI via acidification of urine

Aspirin

Clinical use

NSAID, used for mild–moderate pain, pyrexia

Prophylaxis of cerebrovascular disease or myocardial infarction

Dose in normal renal function

Analgesia: 300–900 mg every 4–6 hours. Maximum 4 g daily

Prophylaxis of cerebrovascular disease or myocardial infarction: 75–300 mg daily

Pharmacokinetics

Molecular weight (daltons)	180
% Protein binding	72–95
% Excreted unchanged in urine	5 (acidic urine); 85 (alkaline urine)
Volume of distribution (L/kg)	0.1–0.2
Half-life – normal/ESRF (hrs)	2–3/unchanged

Dose in renal impairment GFR (mL/min)

20–50	Dose as in normal renal function. See 'Other information'
10–20	Dose as in normal renal function. See 'Other information'
<10	Dose as in normal renal function. See 'Other information'

Dose in patients undergoing renal replacement therapies

CAPD	Dialysed. Dose as in normal renal function
HD	Dialysed. Dose as in normal renal function
CAV/VVHD	Dialysed. Dose as in normal renal function

Important drug interactions

POTENTIALLY HAZARDOUS INTERACTIONS WITH OTHER DRUGS

• Anticoagulants: increased risk of bleeding due to antiplatelet effect

• Cytotoxics: reduced excretion of methotrexate. Risk of increased toxicity

• Other analgesics: avoid concomitant use with other NSAIDs due to increased risk of side-effects

Administration

RECONSTITUTION

–

ROUTE

• Oral

RATE OF ADMINISTRATION

–

COMMENTS

–

Other information

• Aspirin at analgesic/antipyretic dose is best avoided in patients with renal impairment, especially if severe

• Antiplatelet effect may add to uraemic, GI and haematologic symptoms

• Degree of protein binding reduced in ESRD

Atenolol

Clinical use

Beta-adrenoceptor blocker – for hypertension, angina, arrhythmias

Dose in normal renal function

Oral: 50–100 mg daily

IV: arrhythmias – 2.5 mg at a rate of 1 mg/min repeated at 5-minute intervals to a maximum of 10 mg

Infusion: 150 micrograms/kg, repeat every 12 hours if required

Pharmacokinetics

Molecular weight (daltons)	266.3
% Protein binding	3
% Excreted unchanged in urine	>90
Volume of distribution (L/kg)	0.5–1.5
Half-life – normal/ESRF (hrs)	6.7/15–35

Dose in renal impairment GFR (mL/min)

20–50	Dose as in normal renal function
10–20	Dose as in normal renal function
<10	50 mg once a day

Dose in patients undergoing renal replacement therapies

CAPD	Not dialysed. Dose as in GFR = <10 mL/min
HD	Dialysed. Dose as in GFR = <10 mL/min
CAV/VVHD	Dialysed. Dose as in normal renal function

Important drug interactions

POTENTIALLY HAZARDOUS INTERACTIONS WITH OTHER DRUGS

• Anaesthetics: enhanced hypotensive effect
• Anti-arrhythmics: increased risk of myocardial depression and bradycardia; increased risk of bradycardia and AV block with amiodarone
• Antihypertensives: enhanced hypotensive effect; increased risk of first-dose hypotensive effect with post-synaptic alpha-blockers like prazosin
• Calcium-channel blockers: increased risk of bradycardia and AV block with diltiazem. Hypotension and heart failure possible with nifedipine. Asystole, severe hypotension and heart failure with verapamil
• Sympathomimetics: severe hypertension with adrenaline and noradrenaline
• Moxisylyte: possibly severe postural hypotension

Administration

RECONSTITUTION

–

ROUTE

• Oral, IV

RATE OF ADMINISTRATION

• Infusion: 20 minutes
• IV injection: 1 mg/minute

COMMENTS

• Dilute with glucose 5% or sodium chloride 0.9%

Other information

• CSM advise that beta-blockers are contra-indicated in patients with asthma or history of obstructive airway disease

ATG – Imtix (Rabbit) (Thymoglobuline) (unlicensed product)

Clinical use

Prophylaxis and treatment of acute (or steroid-resistant) transplant rejection

Dose in normal renal function

1.25–5 mg/kg/day for up to 10–14 days

Pharmacokinetics

Molecular weight (daltons)	–
% Protein binding	–
% Excreted unchanged in urine	–
Volume of distribution (L/kg)	–
Half-life – normal/ESRF (hrs)	48–72/–

Dose in renal impairment GFR (mL/min)

20–50	Dose as in normal renal function
10–20	Dose as in normal renal function
<10	Dose as in normal renal function

Dose in patients undergoing renal replacement therapies

CAPD	Not dialysed. Dose as in normal renal function
HD	Not dialysed. Dose as in normal renal function
CAV/VVHD	Not dialysed. Dose as in normal renal function

Important drug interactions

POTENTIALLY HAZARDOUS INTERACTIONS WITH OTHER DRUGS

• Risk of over immunosuppression

Administration

RECONSTITUTION

• Dilute dose in 250 mL sodium chloride 0.9%, maximum concentration 5 mg/mL (for peripheral administration)

ROUTE

• IV via central line or via peripheral vein with good blood flow rates

RATE OF ADMINISTRATION

• 4–16 hours

COMMENTS

• To minimise risk of adverse effects, chlorphenamine (10 mg IV) and hydrocortisone (100 mg IV) may be given 15–60 minutes before administration of full dose ATG

• Chlorphenamine, hydrocortisone and adrenaline should be immediately available in case of severe anaphylaxis

Other information

• Dosage may be modified to optimise immunosuppression. Aim to keep Total Lymphocyte Count below 3% of Total White Cell Count or 50 cells/mm³. Alternatively, keep absolute T-cell count below 50 cells/µl and only dose when above this

• Avoid simultaneous transfusions of blood or blood derivatives and infusions of other solutions, particularly lipids

• A test dose is advised in accordance with manufacturer's literature

• ATG should not be administered in presence of: fluid overload, allergy to rabbit protein, pregnancy, acute viral illness

• Local experience at Oxford: ATG is always given centrally and the maximum concentration (1 mg/2 mL) recommended by the company has often been exceeded. Concentrations of 1 mg/mL have been given over 8 hours with no problems. In addition, local in-house data is available to support a 28-day expiry of drug when reconstituted in Pharmacy CIVAS

Atorvastatin

Clinical use

Hyperlipidaemia and hypercholesterolaemia

Dose in normal renal function

10–80 mg daily

Pharmacokinetics

Molecular weight (daltons)	558.6 (1209.4 as calcium salt)
% Protein binding	>98
% Excreted unchanged in urine	Negligible
Volume of distribution (L/kg)	381 litres
Half-life – normal/ESRF (hrs)	14 (active metabolite 20–30)/ unchanged

Dose in renal impairment GFR (mL/min)

20–50	Dose as in normal renal function
10–20	Dose as in normal renal function
<10	Dose as in normal renal function

Dose in patients undergoing renal replacement therapies

CAPD	Not dialysed. Dose as in normal renal function
HD	Not dialysed. Dose as in normal renal function
CAV/VVHD	Not dialysed. Dose as in normal renal function

Important drug interactions

POTENTIALLY HAZARDOUS INTERACTIONS WITH OTHER DRUGS

- Antifungals: increased risk of myopathy with itraconazole and possibly other imidazoles and triazoles – avoid concomitant use
- Antivirals: increased risk of myopathy with indinavir, amprenavir, nelfinavir
- Ciclosporin: increased risk of myopathy
- Lipid-lowering agents: increased risk of myopathy with fibrates and nicotinic acid
- Antibacterials: erythromycin and clarithromycin possibly increase risk of myopathy; clarithromycin increases plasma atorvastatin concentration

Administration

RECONSTITUTION

–

ROUTE

- Oral

RATE OF ADMINISTRATION

–

COMMENTS

–

Other information

- Rhabdomyolysis with renal dysfunction secondary to myoglobinaemia has been reported with other statins

Atovaquone

Clinical use

Treatment of PCP if intolerant to co-trimoxazole

Dose in normal renal function

750 mg twice daily for 21 days

Pharmacokinetics

Molecular weight (daltons)	366.8
% Protein binding	99.9
% Excreted unchanged in urine	<1
Volume of distribution (L/kg)	0.62 ± 0.19
Half-life – normal/ESRF (hrs)	2–3 days/no data

Dose in renal impairment
GFR (mL/min)

20–50	Dose as in normal renal function
10–20	Dose as in normal renal function
<10	Dose as in normal renal function – use with caution

Dose in patients undergoing renal replacement therapies

CAPD	Not dialysed. Dose as in normal renal function
HD	Not dialysed. Dose as in normal renal function
CAV/VVHD	Unlikely to be dialysed. Dose as in normal renal function

Important drug interactions

POTENTIALLY HAZARDOUS INTERACTIONS WITH OTHER DRUGS

• Rifampicin and tetracycline: reduce atovaquone levels by 50%

• Metoclopramide: significant reduction in plasma atovaquone levels

Administration

RECONSTITUTION

–

ROUTE

• Oral

RATE OF ADMINISTRATION

–

COMMENTS

–

Other information

• Administer with food. The presence of food, particularly high fat food, increases bioavailability by 2–3-fold

• The most commonly reported abnormalities in laboratory parameters are increased liver function tests and amylase levels and hyponatraemia

Atracurium

Clinical use

A non-depolarising muscle relaxant of short to medium duration

Dose in normal renal function

0.3–0.6 mg/kg – depending on duration of full block required. Full block can be prolonged with supplementary doses of 0.1–0.2 mg/kg as required

Pharmacokinetics

Molecular weight (daltons)	1243.5
% Protein binding	82
% Excreted unchanged in urine	0
Volume of distribution (L/kg)	0.15–0.18
Half-life – normal/ESRF (hrs)	0.3–0.4/ unchanged

Dose in renal impairment GFR (mL/min)

20–50	Dose as in normal renal function
10–20	Dose as in normal renal function
<10	Dose as in normal renal function

Dose in patients undergoing renal replacement therapies

CAPD	Unlikely dialysability. Dose as in normal renal function
HD	Unlikely dialysability. Dose as in normal renal function
CAV/VVHD	Unlikely dialysability. Dose as in normal renal function

Important drug interactions

POTENTIALLY HAZARDOUS INTERACTIONS WITH OTHER DRUGS

• Procainamide and quinidine enhance muscle relaxant effect
• Aminoglycosides, azlocillin, clindamycin, colistin, piperacillin enhance effect of atracurium
• Atracurium enhances the neuromuscular block produced by botulinum toxin (risk of toxicity)

Administration

RECONSTITUTION

–

ROUTE

• IV bolus, IV infusion

RATE OF ADMINISTRATION

• IV infusion: initial bolus dose of 0.3–0.6 mg/kg over 60 seconds, then administer as a continuous infusion at rates of 0.3–0.6 mg/kg/hour

COMMENTS

• Stable in sodium chloride 0.9% for 24 hours, and glucose 5% for 8 hours when diluted to concentrations of 0.5 mg/mL or above

Other information

–

Auranofin

Clinical use

Active progressive rheumatoid arthritis in adults when NSAIDs inadequate alone

Dose in normal renal function

6 mg daily (maximum 9 mg)

Pharmacokinetics

Molecular weight (daltons)	678.5
% Protein binding	60–80
% Excreted unchanged in urine	50
Volume of distribution (L/kg)	–
Half-life – normal/ESRF (hrs)	70–80 days/–

Dose in renal impairment GFR (mL/min)

20–50	3–6 mg daily
10–20	3 mg daily
<10	Avoid

Dose in patients undergoing renal replacement therapies

CAPD	Unknown dialysability. Dose as in GFR = <10 mL/min
HD	Not dialysed. Dose as in GFR = <10 mL/min
CAV/VVHD	Not dialysed. Dose as in GFR = 10–20 mL/min

Important drug interactions

POTENTIALLY HAZARDOUS INTERACTIONS WITH OTHER DRUGS

• None known

Administration

RECONSTITUTION

–

ROUTE

• Oral

RATE OF ADMINISTRATION

–

COMMENTS

• Take with or after food
• Start initially with morning and evening dose – if well tolerated, can take dose once a day

Other information

• Warn patients to tell the doctor immediately if sore throat, mouth ulcers, bruising, fever, malaise, rash, diarrhoea or non-specific illness develops
• Blood tests should be carried out monthly, and treatment should be withdrawn if the platelets fall below 100,000/mm³, or if signs and symptoms suggestive of thrombocytopenia appear
• Gold can produce nephrotic syndrome or less severe glomerular disease with proteinuria and haematuria, which are usually mild and transient. If persistent or clinically significant proteinuria develops, treatment with gold should be discontinued. Minor transient changes in renal function may also occur
• Urine tests should be carried out monthly to test for proteinuria and haematuria

Azathioprine

Clinical use

Immunosuppression for prophylaxis of transplant rejection and treatment of various autoimmune conditions

Dose in normal renal function

Oral and IV: 1–5 mg/kg/day

Pharmacokinetics

Molecular weight (daltons)	277.3
% Protein binding	20–30
% Excreted unchanged in urine	<2
Volume of distribution (L/kg)	0.55–0.8
Half-life – normal/ESRF (hrs)	0.16–1/increased

Dose in renal impairment GFR (mL/min)

20–50	Dose as in normal renal function
10–20	75–100%
<10	50–75%

Dose in patients undergoing renal replacement therapies

CAPD	Dialysed. Dose as in GFR = <10 mL/min
HD	Dialysed. 40–50% removed. Dose as for normal renal function
CAV/VVHD	Dialysed. Dose as in GFR = 10–20 mL/min

Important drug interactions

POTENTIALLY HAZARDOUS INTERACTIONS WITH OTHER DRUGS

• Allopurinol enhances effect with increased toxicity. Reduce azathioprine dose by 50–75% if administered concomitantly

• Ciclosporin: ? decreased ciclosporin absorption and bioavailability

• Cytotoxic agents may be additive or synergistic in producing toxicity, particularly on the bone marrow

Administration

RECONSTITUTION

• Add 5 mL water for injection to each vial (50 mg)

ROUTE

• Oral, IV

RATE OF ADMINISTRATION

• Over not less than 1 minute

COMMENTS

• IV bolus peripherally, preferably in the side arm of a fast-running infusion

• **Very irritant to veins.** Flush with 50 mL sodium chloride 0.9% after administration

• Take tablets with or after food

Other information

• Extensively metabolised to mercaptopurine

• 1 mg by IV injection is equivalent to 1 mg by oral route

• 6-mercaptopurine levels can be monitored in patients with low urate clearance

• Monitor white cell and platelet counts

• **Cytotoxic drug – do not handle**

• Can be given as an intermittent infusion (up to 250 mg in 100 mL)

Azithromycin

Clinical use

Antibacterial agent

Dose in normal renal function

Genital chlamydial infections: 1 g as single dose
All other indications: 500 mg daily for 3 days

Pharmacokinetics

Molecular weight (daltons)	785
% Protein binding	8–50
% Excreted unchanged in urine	6–12
Volume of distribution (L/kg)	18
Half-life – normal/ESRF (hrs)	10–60/–

Dose in renal impairment
GFR (mL/min)

20–50	Dose as in normal renal function
10–20	Dose as in normal renal function
<10	Dose as in normal renal function

Dose in patients undergoing renal replacement therapies

CAPD	Unknown dialysability. Dose as in normal renal function
HD	Unknown dialysability. Dose as in normal renal function
CAV/VVHD	Unknown dialysability. Dose as in normal renal function

Important drug interactions

POTENTIALLY HAZARDOUS INTERACTIONS WITH OTHER DRUGS

- Ciclosporin: may inhibit the metabolism of ciclosporin (increased plasma ciclosporin levels)
- Antidepressants: the manufacturer of reboxetine advises avoid concomitant use
- The effect of digoxin may be enhanced
- Azithromycin and ergot derivatives should not be co-administered due to possibility of ergotism
- Effect of acenocoumarol and warfarin may be enhanced
- May inhibit the metabolism of mizolastine and terfenadine (risk of hazardous arrhythmias)

Administration

RECONSTITUTION

- Powder for oral suspension to be reconstituted with water (200 mg/5 mL strength)

ROUTE

- Oral

RATE OF ADMINISTRATION

–

COMMENTS

- Administer as a once-daily dose one hour before food or two hours after food

Other information

- ESRD dosing based on extrapolation as no data yet available

Aztreonam

Clinical use

Antibacterial agent

Dose in normal renal function

1–8 g daily (usually 3–4 g daily) in divided doses, i.e. 0.5–2.0 g every 6–12 hours

Pharmacokinetics

Molecular weight (daltons)	435.4
% Protein binding	55
% Excreted unchanged in urine	75
Volume of distribution (L/kg)	0.1–2.0
Half-life – normal/ESRF (hrs)	1.7–2.9/6–8

Dose in renal impairment GFR (mL/min)

30–50	Dose as in normal renal function
10–30	50% of appropriate normal dose
<10	25% of appropriate normal dose

Dose in patients undergoing renal replacement therapies

CAPD	Dialysed. Dose as in GFR = <10 mL/min
HD	Dialysed. Dose as in GFR = <10 mL/min
CAV/VVHD	Dialysed. Dose as in GFR = 10–20 mL/min

Important drug interactions

POTENTIALLY HAZARDOUS INTERACTIONS WITH OTHER DRUGS

• Possibly enhanced anticoagulant effect of acenocoumarol and warfarin

Administration

RECONSTITUTION

• 3 mL of water for injection per 1-g vial

ROUTE

• IM, IV bolus, IV infusion

RATE OF ADMINISTRATION

• IM injection: give by deep injection into a large muscle mass
• IV: slowly inject directly into the vein over a period of 3–5 minutes
• IV infusion: give over 20–60 minutes

COMMENTS

• Suitable infusion solutions: glucose 5%, sodium chloride 0.9%, compound sodium lactate
• Dilute to a concentration of not less than 20 mg/ml
• Once reconstituted aztreonam can be stored in a refrigerator for 24 hours
• IV route recommended for single doses >1 g

Other information

• Manufacturers recommend that patients with renal impairment be given the usual initial dose followed by a maintenance dose adjusted according to creatinine clearance. The normal dose interval should not be altered

Baclofen

Clinical use

Chronic severe spasticity of voluntary muscles

Dose in normal renal function

5 mg three times a day – increase oral dose gradually up to 100 mg/day

Pharmacokinetics

Molecular weight (daltons)	213.7
% Protein binding	30
% Excreted unchanged in urine	70
Volume of distribution (L/kg)	0.7
Half-life – normal/ESRF (hrs)	3–4/–

Dose in renal impairment GFR (mL/min)

20–50	5 mg three times a day and titrate according to response
10–20	5 mg twice a day and titrate according to response
<10	5 mg/day

Dose in patients undergoing renal replacement therapies

CAPD	Unknown dialysability. Dose as in GFR = <10 mL/min
HD	Unknown dialysability. Dose as in GFR = <10 mL/min
CAV/VVHD	Unknown dialysability. Dose as in GFR = 10–20 mL/min

Important drug interactions

POTENTIALLY HAZARDOUS INTERACTIONS WITH OTHER DRUGS

• Procainamide, quinidine and tricyclic antidepressants enhance muscle relaxant effect
• Antihypertensives and ACE inhibitors enhance hypotensive effect

Administration

RECONSTITUTION

–

ROUTE

• Oral – tablets/liquid
• Intrathecal injection

RATE OF ADMINISTRATION

–

COMMENTS

• Take with or after food
• Baclofen can be given intrathecally (at doses greatly reduced compared with oral dose) by bolus injection or continuous infusion. Individual titration of dosage is essential due to variability in response. Test doses must be given. Maintenance dose: 10–1200 micrograms/day

Other information

• Withdraw treatment gradually over 1–2 weeks to avoid anxiety and confusional state, etc
• Drowsiness and nausea frequent at the start of therapy

Balsalazide

Clinical use

Treatment, and maintenance of remission in mild to moderate ulcerative colitis

Dose in normal renal function

Acute treatment: 2.25 g three times a day
Maintenance: 1.5 g twice daily. Max 6 g/day

Pharmacokinetics

Molecular weight (daltons)	357.3 (437.3 as dihydrate)
% Protein binding	40 (similar to mesalazine)
% Excreted unchanged in urine	25 (as metabolites NASA and NABA)
Volume of distribution (L/kg)	No data
Half-life – normal/ESRF (hrs)	No data ($t_{1/2}$ NASA = 6–9)

Dose in renal impairment GFR (mL/min)

20–50	Dose as in normal renal function
10–20	Use with caution only if necessary
<10	Start with low doses and monitor closely

Dose in patients undergoing renal replacement therapies

CAPD	Removal unlikely. Dose as in GFR < 10 mL/min
HD	Removal unlikely. Dose as in GFR < 10 mL/min
CAV/VVHD	Unknown dialysability. Dose as in GFR = 10–20 mL/min

Important drug interactions

POTENTIALLY HAZARDOUS INTERACTIONS WITH OTHER DRUGS

• None known

Administration

RECONSTITUTION

–

ROUTE

• Oral

RATE OF ADMINISTRATION

–

COMMENTS

–

Other information

• Balsalazide is a pro-drug of mesalazine (5-ASA)

• Mesalazine is best avoided in patients with established renal impairment, but if necessary should be used with caution and the patient carefully monitored

• Serious blood dyscrasias have been reported with mesalazine, monitor full blood count closely

Basiliximab

Clinical use

Chimeric murine/human monoclonal anti-CD25 antibody for the prophylaxis of acute allograft rejection, in combination with maintenance immunosuppression

Dose in normal renal function

20 mg 2 hours before transplant and 20 mg 4 days after transplant

Pharmacokinetics

Molecular weight (daltons)	Approx 156 kDa
% Protein binding	See 'Other information'
% Excreted unchanged in urine	No data
Volume of distribution (L/kg)	8.6 ± 4.1 litres
Half-life – normal/ESRF (hrs)	7.2 ± 3.2 days/ unchanged

Dose in renal impairment GFR (mL/min)

20–50	Dose as in normal renal function
10–20	Dose as in normal renal function
<10	Dose as in normal renal function

Dose in patients undergoing renal replacement therapies

CAPD	Not dialysed. Dose as in normal renal function
HD	Not dialysed. Dose as in normal renal function
CAV/VVHD	Not dialysed. Dose as in normal renal function

Important drug interactions

POTENTIALLY HAZARDOUS INTERACTIONS WITH OTHER DRUGS

• None known

Administration

RECONSTITUTION

• Reconstitute each vial with 5 mL water for injection then dilute to 50 mL or greater with sodium chloride 0.9% or glucose 5%

ROUTE

• IV infusion

RATE OF ADMINISTRATION

• 20–30 minutes

COMMENTS

–

Other information

• In vitro studies indicate that basiliximab binds only to activated lymphocytes and macrophages/monocytes
• Basiliximab is detectable in serum for up to 3 months after 15–25 mg doses

Benzatropine (benztropine mesylate)

Clinical use

Parkinson's disease, drug-induced extrapyramidal side-effects

Dose in normal renal function

Oral: 0.5–6 mg daily at bedtime or in up to four divided doses

IV/IM (emergency use): 1–2 mg

Pharmacokinetics

Molecular weight (daltons)	403.5
% Protein binding	See 'Other information'
% Excreted unchanged in urine	See 'Other information'
Volume of distribution (L/kg)	See 'Other information'
Half-life – normal/ESRF (hrs)	See 'Other information'

Dose in renal impairment GFR (mL/min)

20–50	Start with low doses and adjust according to response
10–20	Start with low doses and adjust according to response
<10	Start with low doses and adjust according to response

Dose in patients undergoing renal replacement therapies

CAPD	Unknown dialysability. Dose as in GFR < 10 mL/min
HD	Unknown dialysability. Dose as in GFR < 10 mL/min
CAV/VVHD	Unknown dialysability. Dose as in GFR = 10–20 mL/min

Important drug interactions

POTENTIALLY HAZARDOUS INTERACTIONS WITH OTHER DRUGS

• Phenothiazines and tricyclic antidepressants: may cause paralytic ileus, which can be fatal

Administration

RECONSTITUTION

–

ROUTE

• Oral, IV, IM

RATE OF ADMINISTRATION

–

COMMENTS

–

Other information

• Benzatropine pharmacokinetics are not well studied, but the drug apparently is hepatically metabolised to conjugates and may undergo entero-hepatic recycling

• Benzatropine has a cumulative effect and a prolonged duration of action, therefore treatment should commence with the lowest possible dosage and titrated according to response

Benzbromarone (unlicensed product)

Clinical use

Treatment of hyperuricaemia, chronic gout and tophaceous gout

Dose in normal renal function

50–300 mg daily

(Usual dose 50–100 mg daily)

Pharmacokinetics

Molecular weight (daltons)	424.1
% Protein binding	Highly
% Excreted unchanged in urine	6
Volume of distribution (L/kg)	19 litres
Half-life – normal/ESRF (hrs)	2.77 ± 1.07

Dose in renal impairment GFR (mL/min)

20–50	100 mg – 200 mg daily *
15–20	100 mg daily *
<15	Avoid. Ineffective

Dose in patients undergoing renal replacement therapies

CAPD	Avoid. Ineffective
HD	Avoid. Ineffective
CAV/VVHD	Use with caution. Dose as in GFR = 15–20 mL/min

Important drug interactions

POTENTIALLY HAZARDOUS INTERACTIONS WITH OTHER DRUGS

• Aspirin and salicylates: antagonise effects of benzbromarone

• Anticoagulants: may enhance effect of coumarin oral anticoagulants

• Pyrazinamide: reduced effect of benzbromarone

• Hepatotoxic agents: enhanced hepatotoxicity

Administration

RECONSTITUTION

–

ROUTE

• Oral

RATE OF ADMINISTRATION

–

COMMENTS

–

Other information

• Similar to other uricosurics, treatment with benzbromarone should not be started during an acute attack of gout

• Maintain an adequate fluid intake to reduce the risk of uric acid renal calculi

• Biological effect of 100 mg benzbromarone is equivalent to 1.5 g probenecid or 300 mg of allopurinol. (Masbernard A et al. (1981) Ten years experience with benzbromarone in the management of gout and hyperuricaemia. SA Medical Journal. 9 May: 701–6)

• Benzbromarone is considered unsafe in patients with acute porphyria
* (J Clin Rheumatol. (1999) 5: 49–55)

Benzylpenicillin

Clinical use

Antibacterial agent

Dose in normal renal function

600 mg – 14.4 g daily in 2–4 divided doses

Pharmacokinetics

Molecular weight (daltons)	334
% Protein binding	50
% Excreted unchanged in urine	60–85
Volume of distribution (L/kg)	0.3–0.42
Half-life – normal/ESRF (hrs)	0.5/6–20

Dose in renal impairment GFR (mL/min)

20–50	Dose as in normal renal function
10–20	75%
<10	20–50%

Dose in patients undergoing renal replacement therapies

CAPD	Dialysed. Dose as in GFR < 10 mL/min
HD	Dialysed. Dose as in GFR < 10 mL/min
CAV/VVHD	Dialysed. Dose as in GFR = 10–20 mL/min

Important drug interactions

POTENTIALLY HAZARDOUS INTERACTIONS WITH OTHER DRUGS

• Reduced excretion of methotrexate

Administration

RECONSTITUTION

• IV bolus: 600 mg in 5 mL water for injection
• IV infusion: 600 mg in at least 10 mL sodium chloride 0.9%
• IM: 600 mg in 1.6 mL water for injection; 600 mg displaces 0.4 mL

ROUTE

• IV bolus, IV infusion, IM

RATE OF ADMINISTRATION

• IV bolus: over 3–4 minutes
• IV infusion: over 30–60 minutes

COMMENTS

• IV doses in excess of 1.2 g must be given slowly at minimum rate of 300 mg/minute

Other information

• Dose in *normal* renal function: meningitis up to 14.4 g daily, bacterial endocarditis 4.8 g daily
• Maximum dose in severe renal impairment: 2.4–3.6 g per day
• 600 mg of benzylpenicillin sodium (1 mega unit) contains 1.68 mmol of sodium and 600 mg of benzylpenicillin potassium contains 1.7 mmol potassium
• Increased incidence of neurotoxicity in renal impairment (seizures)
• False positive urinary protein reactions may be caused by benzylpenicillin therapy

Betahistine

Clinical use

Treatment of vertigo, tinnitus and hearing loss associated with Ménière's syndrome

Dose in normal renal function

24–48 mg daily in three divided doses

Pharmacokinetics

Molecular weight (daltons)	209.1
% Protein binding	Negligible
% Excreted unchanged in urine	90
Volume of distribution (L/kg)	No data
Half-life – normal/ESRF (hrs)	3.5/no data

Dose in renal impairment GFR (mL/min)

20–50	Dose as in normal renal function
10–20	8 mg three times a day
<10	8 mg two to three times a day

Dose in patients undergoing renal replacement therapies

CAPD	Likely to be dialysed. Dose as in GFR < 10 mL/min
HD	Likely to be dialysed. Dose as in GFR < 10 mL/min
CAV/VVHD	Likely to be dialysed. Dose as in GFR = 10–20 mL/min

Important drug interactions

POTENTIALLY HAZARDOUS INTERACTIONS WITH OTHER DRUGS

• None known

Administration

RECONSTITUTION

–

ROUTE

• Oral

RATE OF ADMINISTRATION

–

COMMENTS

–

Other information

• Betahistine is rapidly and completely absorbed after oral administration

• It is excreted almost exclusively in the urine as 2-pyridylacetic acid within 24 hours of administration

Betamethasone

Clinical use

Corticosteroid, used for suppression of inflammatory and allergic disorders

Dose in normal renal function

Oral: 0.5–5 mg daily

Injection: 4–20 mg repeated up to four times in 24 hours

Pharmacokinetics

Molecular weight (daltons)	392.5
% Protein binding	65
% Excreted unchanged in urine	5
Volume of distribution (L/kg)	1.4
Half-life – normal/ESRF (hrs)	5.5/–

Dose in renal impairment GFR (mL/min)

20–50	Dose as in normal renal function
10–20	Dose as in normal renal function
<10	Dose as in normal renal function

Dose in patients undergoing renal replacement therapies

CAPD	Unknown dialysability. Dose as in normal renal function
HD	Unknown dialysability. Dose as in normal renal function
CAV/VVHD	Unknown dialysability. Dose as in normal renal function

Important drug interactions

POTENTIALLY HAZARDOUS INTERACTIONS WITH OTHER DRUGS

- Antifungals: increased risk of hypokalaemia with amphotericin – avoid concomitant use
- Ciclosporin: rare reports of convulsions in patients on ciclosporin and high-dose corticosteroids
- Metabolism accelerated by rifampicin, carbamazepine, phenobarbital, phenytoin, primidone
- Enhanced hypokalaemic effects of acetazolamide, loop diuretics and thiazide diuretics
- Efficacy of coumarin anticoagulants may be enhanced

Administration

RECONSTITUTION

–

ROUTE

- Orally, IV, IM, topically

RATE OF ADMINISTRATION

- IV bolus: over half to one minute

COMMENTS

- Can be added to glucose 5% or sodium chloride 0.9%

Other information

- 750 micrograms betamethasone ≡ 5 mg prednisolone
- Even when applied topically, sufficient corticosteroid may be absorbed to give a systemic effect
- The effects of betamethasone on sodium and water retention are less than those of prednisolone and approximately equal to those of dexamethasone

Betaxolol

Clinical use

Beta-adrenoceptor blocker – for hypertension
Glaucoma: topical use

Dose in normal renal function

20–40 mg daily (elderly: 10 mg)

Pharmacokinetics

Molecular weight (daltons)	307.4
% Protein binding	45–60
% Excreted unchanged in urine	80–90
Volume of distribution (L/kg)	5–10
Half-life – normal/ESRF (hrs)	15–20/30–35

Dose in renal impairment GFR (mL/min)

20–50	Dose as in normal renal function
10–20	Dose as in normal renal function
<10	10–20 mg daily

Dose in patients undergoing renal replacement therapies

CAPD	Unlikely dialysability. Dose as in GFR = <10 mL/min
HD	Unlikely dialysability. Dose as in GFR = <10 mL/min
CAV/VVHD	Unknown dialysability. Dose as in normal renal function

Important drug interactions

POTENTIALLY HAZARDOUS INTERACTIONS WITH OTHER DRUGS

• Enhanced hypotensive effect with anaesthetics
• Increased risk of myocardial depression and bradycardia with anti-arrhythmics; with amiodarone increased risk of bradycardia and AV block
• Enhanced hypotensive effect with antihypertensives. Increased risk of first-dose hypotensive effect with post-synaptic alpha-blockers such as prazosin
• Increased risk of bradycardia and AV block with diltiazem. Severe hypotension and heart failure occasionally with nifedipine. Asystole, severe hypotension and heart failure with verapamil
• Severe hypertension with adrenaline and noradrenaline (especially with non-selective beta-blockers)
• Moxisylyte: possibly severe postural hypotension

Administration

RECONSTITUTION

–

ROUTE

• Oral (topically for glaucoma)

RATE OF ADMINISTRATION

–

COMMENTS

–

Other information

• Use with caution in patients with asthma, or a history of obstructive airways disease or diabetes
• Systemic absorption may follow topical administration to the eye

Bezafibrate

Clinical use

Hyperlipidaemia

Dose in normal renal function

200 mg three times a day (200 mg twice a day in hypertriglyceridaemia)

Modified release: 400 mg daily

Pharmacokinetics

Molecular weight (daltons)	361.8
% Protein binding	95
% Excreted unchanged in urine	35–40
Volume of distribution (L/kg)	0.24–0.35
Half-life – normal/ESRF (hrs)	2.1/7.8

Dose in renal impairment GFR (mL/min)

40–60	400 mg daily
15–40	200 mg every 24–48 hours
<15	Avoid

Dose in patients undergoing renal replacement therapies

CAPD	Unlikely dialysability. 200 mg every 72 hours
HD	Unlikely dialysability. 200 mg every 72 hours
CAV/VVHD	Unknown dialysability. Dose as in GFR = 15–40 mL/min

Important drug interactions

POTENTIALLY HAZARDOUS INTERACTIONS WITH OTHER DRUGS

• Enhances effect of acenocoumarol, phenindione, and warfarin. (Dosage of anticoagulant should be reduced by up to 50% and readjusted by monitoring INR.)

• Increased risk of myopathy with combination therapy with HMG CoA reductase inhibition

Administration

RECONSTITUTION

–

ROUTE

• Oral

RATE OF ADMINISTRATION

–

COMMENTS

–

Other information

• Take dose with or after food

• Contra-indicated in nephrotic syndrome

• There should be an interval of 2 hours between intake of ion exchange resin and bezafibrate

• Modified release is not appropriate in renal impairment

Bicalutamide

Clinical use

Treatment of prostate cancer

Dose in normal renal function

50–150 mg daily
(with orchidectomy or gonadorelin therapy)

Pharmacokinetics

Molecular weight (daltons)	430.4
% Protein binding	96
% Excreted unchanged in urine	Approx 50
Volume of distribution (L/kg)	No data
Half-life – normal/ESRF (hrs)	5.8 days

Dose in renal impairment GFR (mL/min)

20–50	Dose as in normal renal function
10–20	Dose as in normal renal function
<10	Dose as in normal renal function

Dose in patients undergoing renal replacement therapies

CAPD	Unlikely to be dialysed. Dose as in normal renal function
HD	Unlikely to be dialysed. Dose as in normal renal function
CAV/VVHD	Unlikely to be dialysed. Dose as in normal renal function

Important drug interactions

POTENTIALLY HAZARDOUS INTERACTIONS WITH OTHER DRUGS

• Antihistamines: avoid concomitant use with terfenadine and mizolastine
• Cisapride: avoid concomitant use

Administration

RECONSTITUTION

–

ROUTE

• Oral

RATE OF ADMINISTRATION

–

COMMENTS

–

Other information

• In vitro studies have shown that bicalutamide is an inhibitor of CYP450 3A4. For drugs eliminated by this route, e.g. ciclosporin, tacrolimus, sirolimus, it is recommended that plasma concentrations and clinical condition be monitored following initiation or cessation of bicalutamide therapy

Bisacodyl

Clinical use

Laxative

Dose in normal renal function

Oral: 5–10 mg at night, maximum 15–20 mg

Rectal: 10 mg in the morning

Pharmacokinetics

Molecular weight (daltons)	361.4
% Protein binding	Negligible
% Excreted unchanged in urine	10–34
Volume of distribution (L/kg)	See 'Other information'
Half-life – normal/ESRF (hrs)	See 'Other information'

Dose in renal impairment GFR (mL/min)

20–50	Dose as in normal renal function
10–20	Dose as in normal renal function
<10	Dose as in normal renal function

Dose in patients undergoing renal replacement therapies

CAPD	Unknown dialysability – dose as in normal renal function
HD	Unknown dialysability – dose as in normal renal function
CAV/VVHD	Unknown dialysability – dose as in normal renal function

Important drug interactions

POTENTIALLY HAZARDOUS INTERACTIONS WITH OTHER DRUGS

• None known

Administration

RECONSTITUTION

–

ROUTE

• Oral, rectal

RATE OF ADMINISTRATION

–

COMMENTS

–

Other information

• Absorption is <5% orally or rectally

• It is rapidly converted in the gut by intestinal and bacterial enzymes to its active, but non-absorbed, desacetyl metabolite

Bisoprolol

Clinical use

Beta$_1$-adrenoceptor blocker – for hypertension, angina, adjunctive treatment for heart failure

Dose in normal renal function

5–10 mg daily (maximum 20 mg daily)
Heart failure: 1.25 mg daily increasing to 10 mg daily

Pharmacokinetics

Molecular weight (daltons)	767
% Protein binding	30
% Excreted unchanged in urine	50
Volume of distribution (L/kg)	3.2
Half-life – normal/ESRF (hrs)	10–12/18.5–24

Dose in renal impairment GFR (mL/min)

20–50	Dose as in normal renal function
10–20	Dose as in normal renal function
<10	1.25–10 mg daily

Dose in patients undergoing renal replacement therapies

CAPD	Unlikely dialysability. Dose as in GFR = <10 mL/min
HD	Not dialysed. Dose as in GFR = <10 mL/min
CAV/VVHD	Unknown dialysability. Dose as in GFR = 10–20 mL/min

Important drug interactions

POTENTIALLY HAZARDOUS INTERACTIONS WITH OTHER DRUGS

• Enhanced hypotensive effect with anaesthetics
• Increased risk of myocardial depression and bradycardia with anti-arrhythmics; with amiodarone increased risk of bradycardia and AV block
• Enhanced hypotensive effect with antihypertensives. Increased risk of first-dose hypotensive effect with post-synaptic alpha-blockers such as prazosin
• Increased risk of bradycardia and AV block with diltiazem. Severe hypotension and heart failure occasionally with nifedipine. Asystole, severe hypotension and heart failure with verapamil
• Severe hypertension with adrenaline and noradrenaline (especially with non-selective beta-blockers)
• Moxisylyte: possibly severe postural hypotension

Administration

RECONSTITUTION

–

ROUTE

• Oral

RATE OF ADMINISTRATION

–

COMMENTS

–

Other information

• Use with caution in patients with chronic obstructive airways disease, asthma or diabetes

Bleomycin

Clinical use

Antineoplastic agent

Dose in normal renal function

- Squamous cell carcinoma and testicular
  teratoma: range 45–60 x 10³ IU per week IM/IV
  (total cumulative dose up to 500 x 10³ IU) or
  continuous IV infusion 15 x 10³ IU/24 hours for
  up to 10 days, or 30 x 10³ IU/24 hours for up
  to 5 days
- Malignant lymphomas: 15–30 x 10³ IU/week IM
  to total dose of 225 x 10³ IU. Lower doses
  required in combination chemotherapy
- Malignant effusions: 60 x 10³ IU in 100 mL
  sodium chloride 0.9% introduced intrapleural
  (total cumulative dose of 500 x 10³ IU)

Pharmacokinetics

Molecular weight (daltons)	Approx 1500
% Protein binding	1
% Excreted unchanged in urine	60
Volume of distribution (L/kg)	0.3
Half-life – normal/ESRF (hrs)	9/20

Dose in renal impairment
GFR (mL/min)

20–50	Dose as in normal renal function
10–20	75% of normal dose (100% for malignant effusions)
<10	50% of normal dose (100% for malignant effusions)

Dose in patients undergoing renal replacement therapies

CAPD	Not dialysed. Dose as in GFR = <10 mL/min
HD	Not dialysed. Dose as in GFR = <10 mL/min
CAV/VVHD	Unknown dialysability. Dose as in GFR = 10–20 mL/min

Important drug interactions

POTENTIALLY HAZARDOUS INTERACTIONS WITH OTHER DRUGS

- Bleomycin plus vinca alkaloids can lead to
  morbus Raynaud's syndrome and peripheral
  ischaemia

Administration

RECONSTITUTION

- IM: dissolve required dose in up to 5 mL sodium
  chloride 0.9% (or 1% solution of lidocaine if pain
  on injection)
- IV: dissolve dose in 5–200 mL sodium chloride
  0.9%
- Intra-cavitary: 60 x 10³ IU in 100 mL sodium
  chloride 0.9%
- Locally: dissolve in sodium chloride 0.9% to make
  a 1–3 x10³ IU/mL solution

ROUTE

- IM, IV, also intra-arterially, intrapleurally,
  intraperitoneally, locally into tumour

RATE OF ADMINISTRATION

- Give by slow IV injection, or add to reservoir of
  a running IV infusion

COMMENTS

- Avoid direct contact with the skin

Other information

- Lesions of skin and oral mucosa common after
  full course of bleomycin
- Pulmonary toxicity: interstitial pneumonia and
  fibrosis – most serious delayed effect

Bosentan

Clinical use

Treatment of primary arterial pulmonary hypertension (PAH), and PAH secondary to scleroderma without significant interstitial pulmonary disease

Dose in normal renal function

62.5–500 mg twice daily

Pharmacokinetics

Molecular weight (daltons)	569.64
% Protein binding	>98
% Excreted unchanged in urine	<3
Volume of distribution (L/kg)	18 litres
Half-life – normal/ESRF (hrs)	5.4/unchanged

Dose in renal impairment GFR (mL/min)

20–50	Dose as in normal renal function
10–20	Dose as in normal renal function
<10	Dose as in normal renal function

Dose in patients undergoing renal replacement therapies

CAPD	Not dialysed. Dose as in normal renal function
HD	Not dialysed. Dose as in normal renal function
CAV/VVHD	Not dialysed. Dose as in normal renal function

Important drug interactions

POTENTIALLY HAZARDOUS INTERACTIONS WITH OTHER DRUGS

• Ciclosporin: co-administration of ciclosporin and bosentan is contra-indicated. When ciclosporin and bosentan are co-administered, initial trough concentrations of bosentan are 30 times higher than normal. At steady state, trough levels are 3–4 times higher than normal. Blood concentrations of ciclosporin decreased by 50%

• Antifungals: fluconazole, ketoconazole and itraconazole cause large increases in plasma concentrations of bosentan – avoid concomitant use

• Antivirals: ritonavir causes greatly increased bosentan levels – avoid concomitant use

• Contraceptive pill: may be failure of contraception – use alternative method

• Glibenclamide: bosentan decreases plasma glibenclamide levels by 40% – significant decrease of hypoglycaemic effect

• Simvastatin: bosentan decreases plasma simvastatin levels by 45% – monitor cholesterol levels and adjust dose of statin

Administration

RECONSTITUTION

–

ROUTE

• Oral

RATE OF ADMINISTRATION

–

COMMENTS

–

Other information

• Bosentan should only be used if the systemic systolic blood pressure is >85 mm/Hg

• Treatment with bosentan is associated with a dose-related, modest decrease in haemoglobin concentration

• Bosentan is an inducer of CYP 3A4 and CYP 2C9

• Bosentan has been associated with dose-related elevations in liver aminotransferases

• Side-effects include leg oedema and hypotension

Bretylium

Clinical use

Ventricular arrhythmias resistant to other treatment

Dose in normal renal function

IV bolus: 5 mg/kg – if no response after 5 minutes repeat dose or increase to 10 mg/kg

IV infusion: 5–10 mg/kg over 15–30 minutes repeated at 1–2 hour intervals. Once arrhythmias controlled, give this dose every 6 hours or continuously infuse at 1–2 mg/minute

IM: 5–10 mg/kg given every 6–8 hours

Pharmacokinetics

Molecular weight (daltons)	414.4
% Protein binding	6
% Excreted unchanged in urine	75
Volume of distribution (L/kg)	8.2
Half-life – normal/ESRF (hrs)	6–13.6/16–32

Dose in renal impairment GFR (mL/min)

20–50	Dose as in normal renal function
10–20	25–50%
<10	25%

Dose in patients undergoing renal replacement therapies

CAPD	Dialysed. Dose as in GFR = <10 mL/min
HD	Dialysed. Dose as in GFR = <10 mL/min
CAV/VVHD	Dialysed. Dose as in GFR = 10–20 mL/min

Important drug interactions

POTENTIALLY HAZARDOUS INTERACTIONS WITH OTHER DRUGS

- Anaesthetics: enhanced hypotensive effect
- Analgesics: NSAIDs antagonise hypotensive effect
- Bretylium may exacerbate arrhythmias caused by digoxin toxicity

Administration

RECONSTITUTION

- For IV infusion can be diluted with glucose 5% or sodium chloride 0.9% to give a final concentration of not more than 10 mg/mL

ROUTE

- IV, IM

RATE OF ADMINISTRATION

- IV bolus: undiluted by rapid injection
- IV infusion: infuse diluted dose over at least 8 minutes (preferably 15–30 minutes)
- IV continuous maintenance: infuse at rate of 1–2 mg/minute

COMMENTS

- If bretylium is to be used for less serious ventricular rhythm disturbances, give more slowly and in diluted form to reduce the risk of vomiting

Other information

- Orthostatic hypotension may occur 20–30 minutes after acute administration

Bromocriptine

Clinical use

Parkinsonism (but not drug-induced extrapyramidal symptoms), endocrine disorders

Dose in normal renal function

- Parkinson's disease: Week 1: 1–1.25 mg at night. Week 2: 2–2.5 mg at night. Week 3: 2.5 mg twice daily. Week 4: 2.5 mg three times daily. Then increasing by 2.5 mg every 3–14 days according to response – usual range 10–40 mg daily
- Hypogonadism/galactorrhoea, infertility: 1–1.25 mg at night, increased gradually; usual dose 7.5 mg daily in divided doses (maximum 30 mg daily)
- Infertility without hyperprolactinaemia: 2.5 mg twice daily
- Cyclical benign breast disease and cyclical menstrual disorders: 1–1.25 mg at night increased gradually; usual dose 2.5 mg twice daily
- Acromegaly: 1–1.25 mg at night increased gradually to 5 mg every 6 hours
- Prolactinoma: 1–1.25 mg at night increased gradually to 5 mg every 6 hours (maximum 30 mg daily)

Pharmacokinetics

Molecular weight (daltons)	750.7
% Protein binding	90–96
% Excreted unchanged in urine	2
Volume of distribution (L/kg)	1–3
Half-life – normal/ESRF (hrs)	2–12/–

Dose in renal impairment GFR (mL/min)

20–50	Dose as in normal renal function
10–20	Dose as in normal renal function
<10	Dose as in normal renal function

Dose for patients undergoing renal replacement therapies

CAPD	Not dialysed. Dose as in normal renal function
HD	Not dialysed. Dose as in normal renal function
CAV/VVHD	Not dialysed. Dose as in normal renal function

Important drug interactions

POTENTIALLY HAZARDOUS INTERACTIONS WITH OTHER DRUGS

- Increased risk of toxicity with bromocriptine and isometheptene or phenylpropanolamine

Administration

RECONSTITUTION

–

ROUTE

- Oral

RATE OF ADMINISTRATION

–

COMMENTS

- Take with food

Other information

- Hypotensive reactions may occur during the first few days of treatment. Tolerance may be reduced by alcohol
- Digital vasospasm can occur
- Concomitant administration of macrolide antibiotics may elevate bromocriptine levels

Brompheniramine

Clinical use

Symptomatic relief of allergy, such as hayfever, urticaria

Dose in normal renal function

4–8 mg 3–4 times daily

Pharmacokinetics

Molecular weight (daltons)	435.3
% Protein binding	72
% Excreted unchanged in urine	3
Volume of distribution (L/kg)	2.5–10
Half-life – normal/ESRF (hrs)	6/–

Dose in renal impairment GFR (mL/min)

20–50	Dose as in normal renal function
10–20	Dose as in normal renal function
<10	Dose as in normal renal function

Dose in patients undergoing renal replacement therapies

CAPD	Unknown dialysability. Dose as in normal renal function
HD	Unknown dialysability. Dose as in normal renal function
CAV/VVHD	Unknown dialysability. Dose as in normal renal function

Important drug interactions

POTENTIALLY HAZARDOUS INTERACTIONS WITH OTHER DRUGS

• None known

Administration

RECONSTITUTION

–

ROUTE

• Oral

RATE OF ADMINISTRATION

–

COMMENTS

–

Other information

• Use with care in epileptiform patients
• Drowsiness may occur
• Predominantly hepatically metabolised with renal elimination of metabolites

Budesonide

Clinical use

Asthma, allergic and vasomotor rhinitis, inflammatory skin disorders

Dose in normal renal function

• Inhaler/Turbohaler: 200–1600 micrograms daily in divided doses

• Respules: 1–2 mg twice daily. Half doses for maintenance

• Nasal spray: 100 micrograms each nostril twice daily or 200 micrograms each nostril once daily. Reduce to 100 micrograms each nostril once daily when symptoms controlled

• Topical preparations: apply 1–2 times daily

• Capsules: 3 mg three times a day

Pharmacokinetics

Molecular weight (daltons)	430.5
% Protein binding	88
% Excreted unchanged in urine	0
Volume of distribution (L/kg)	4.3
Half-life – normal/ESRF (hrs)	2–2.7/–

Dose in renal impairment GFR (mL/min)

20–50	Dose as in normal renal function
10–20	Dose as in normal renal function
<10	Dose as in normal renal function

Dose in patients undergoing renal replacement therapies

CAPD	Unknown dialysability. Dose as in normal renal function
HD	Unknown dialysability. Dose as in normal renal function
CAV/VVHD	Unknown dialysability. Dose as in normal renal function

Important drug interactions

POTENTIALLY HAZARDOUS INTERACTIONS WITH OTHER DRUGS

• None known

Administration

RECONSTITUTION

• Respules: may be diluted up to 50% with sterile sodium chloride 0.9%

ROUTE

• Inhalation, topical, oral

RATE OF ADMINISTRATION

–

COMMENTS

–

Other information

• Special care is needed in patients with quiescent lung tuberculosis, fungal and viral infections in the airways

Bumetanide

Clinical use

Loop diuretic

Dose in normal renal function

Oral: 1 mg in the morning repeated after 6–8 hours if necessary, severe cases 5 mg or more daily

Injection: IV 1–2 mg repeated after 20 minutes; IM, if necessary, 1 mg then adjust according to response

IV infusion: 2–5 mg over 30–60 minutes

Pharmacokinetics

Molecular weight (daltons)	364.4
% Protein binding	99
% Excreted unchanged in urine	42–82
Volume of distribution (L/kg)	0.2–0.5
Half-life – normal/ESRF (hrs)	1.2–1.5/1.5

Dose in renal impairment GFR (mL/min)

20–50	Dose as in normal renal function
10–20	Dose as in normal renal function
<10	Dose as in normal renal function

Dose in patients undergoing renal replacement therapies

CAPD	Not dialysed. Dose as in normal renal function
HD	Not dialysed. Dose as in normal renal function
CAV/VVHD	Not dialysed. Dose as in normal renal function

Important drug interactions

POTENTIALLY HAZARDOUS INTERACTIONS WITH OTHER DRUGS

- Risk of cardiac toxicity with anti-arrhythmics if hypokalaemia occurs

- Increased risk of ototoxicity with aminoglycosides, colistin and vancomycin
- Antihistamines: hypokalaemia increases risk of ventricular arrhythmias with mizolastine and terfenadine
- Antihypertensives: enhanced hypotensive effect – increased risk of first-dose hypotensive effect with alpha-blockers – increased risk of hypokalaemia with indapamide
- Cardiac glycosides: increased toxicity if hypokalaemia occurs with bumetanide
- Lithium: risk of toxicity

Administration

RECONSTITUTION

–

ROUTE

- Oral, IV, IM

RATE OF ADMINISTRATION

- IV infusion: 2–5 mg in 500 mL of infusion fluid over 30–60 minutes

COMMENTS

- Compatible with glucose 5% or sodium chloride 0.9%

Other information

- 1 mg bumetanide ≡ 40 mg frusemide at low doses, but avoid direct substitution at high doses
- In patients with severe chronic renal failure given high doses of bumetanide there are reports of musculoskeletal pain and muscle spasm
- Orally: diuresis begins within 30 minutes, peaks after 1–2 hours, lasts 3 hours
- IV: diuresis begins within few minutes and ceases in about 2 hours
- Use with caution in patients receiving nephrotoxic or ototoxic drugs
- Smaller doses may be sufficient in the elderly and cirrhotics – 500 micrograms
- Use twice daily for higher doses

Bupropion (amfebutamone)

Clinical use

Adjunct to smoking cessation

Dose in normal renal function

150 mg once daily for 6 days, then twice daily

Pharmacokinetics

Molecular weight (daltons)	276.2
% Protein binding	84
% Excreted unchanged in urine	0.5
Volume of distribution (L/kg)	2000 litres
Half-life – normal/ESRF (hrs)	14–20/–

Dose in renal impairment GFR (mL/min)

20–50	150 mg daily
10–20	150 mg daily
<10	150 mg daily

Dose in patients undergoing renal replacement therapies

CAPD	Not dialysed. Dose as in GFR = <10 ml/min
HD	Not dialysed. Dose as in GFR = <10 ml/min
CAV/VVHD	Unlikely dialysability. Dose as in GFR = 10–20 ml/min

Important drug interactions

POTENTIALLY HAZARDOUS INTERACTIONS WITH OTHER DRUGS

• Antidepressants: avoid MAOIs and linezolid with and for 2 weeks before starting treatment. Avoid concomitant treatment with moclobemide
• Antivirals: ritonavir can increase bupropion concentrations – risk of toxicity, avoid concomitant use

Administration

RECONSTITUTION
–

ROUTE
• Oral

RATE OF ADMINISTRATION
–

COMMENTS
–

Other information

• Bupropion and metabolites may accumulate in renal failure

Buspirone

Clinical use

Anxiolytic

Dose in normal renal function

Initially 5 mg 2–3 times daily. Usual range 15–30 mg daily in divided doses (maximum 45 mg daily)

Pharmacokinetics

Molecular weight (daltons)	422.0
% Protein binding	95
% Excreted unchanged in urine	0
Volume of distribution (L/kg)	5
Half-life – normal/ESRF (hrs)	2–3/5.8

Dose in renal impairment GFR (mL/min)

20–50	Dose as in normal renal function
10–20	Dose as in normal renal function
<10	Reduce by 25–50% if patient is anuric

Dose in patients undergoing renal replacement therapies

CAPD	Not dialysed. Dose as in GFR = <10 mL/min
HD	Not dialysed. Dose as in GFR = <10 mL/min
CAV/VVHD	Not dialysed. Dose as in normal renal function

Important drug interactions

POTENTIALLY HAZARDOUS INTERACTIONS WITH OTHER DRUGS

- MAOIs: risk of severe hypertension
- CYP 3A4 inhibitors, e.g. erythromycin, itraconazole, nefazodone, grapefruit juice, diltiazem, verapamil: reduce dose of buspirone to 2.5 mg twice daily
- Rifampicin: significantly reduces plasma buspirone concentration

Administration

RECONSTITUTION

–

ROUTE

- Oral

RATE OF ADMINISTRATION

–

COMMENTS

–

Other information

- Peak plasma levels occur 60–90 minutes after dosing
- Steady-state plasma concentrations achieved within 2 days, although response to treatment may take 2 weeks
- Non-sedative
- Do not use in patients with severe hepatic disease
- Use in severe renal impairment not recommended; risk of accumulation of active metabolites
- Dose reduction in anuric patients is from Mahmood I et al. (1999) Clin Pharmacokinet. **36**(4): 277–87

Cabergoline

Clinical use

Endocrine disorders; adjunct to levodopa (with a decarboxylase inhibitor) in Parkinson's disease
Inhibition/suppression of lactation

Dose in normal renal function

Parkinson's disease: 2–6 mg daily

Hyperprolactinaemic disorders: 0.25–2 mg weekly

Inhibition of lactation: single 1 mg dose during first day postpartum

Suppression of lactation: 0.25 mg twice a day for 2 days

Pharmacokinetics

Molecular weight (daltons)	451.6
% Protein binding	41–42
% Excreted unchanged in urine	2–3
Volume of distribution (L/kg)	–
Half-life – normal/ESRF (hrs)	63–68 (healthy individuals), 79–115 (hyper-prolactinaemic individuals)/–

Dose in renal impairment GFR (mL/min)

20–50	Dose as in normal renal function
10–20	Dose as in normal renal function
<10	Dose as in normal renal function

Dose in patients undergoing renal replacement therapies

CAPD	Removal unlikely. Dose as in normal renal function
HD	Removal unlikely. Dose as in normal renal function
CAV/VVHD	Unknown dialysability. Dose as in normal renal function

Important drug interactions

POTENTIALLY HAZARDOUS INTERACTIONS WITH OTHER DRUGS

• None known

Administration

RECONSTITUTION

–

ROUTE

• Oral

RATE OF ADMINISTRATION

–

COMMENTS

–

Other information

• 18% of radiolabelled dose is excreted as inactive metabolites in urine
• 72% of dose is excreted in faeces

Calcitriol

Clinical use

Vitamin D analogue. Promotes intestinal calcium absorption; suppresses PTH production and release

Dose in normal renal function

Orally: 250 nanograms daily or on alternate days, increased if necessary in steps of 250 nanograms at intervals of 2–4 weeks. Usual dose 0.5–1 microgram daily

IV: treatment of hyperparathyroidism in haemodialysis patients: initially 500 nanograms three times a week, increased if necessary in steps of 250–500 nanograms at intervals of 2–4 weeks. Usual dose 0.5–3 micrograms three times a week after dialysis

Pharmacokinetics

Molecular weight (daltons)	416.6
% Protein binding	>90
% Excreted unchanged in urine	Minimal
Volume of distribution (L/kg)	–
Half-life – normal/ESRF (hrs)	3.5/–

Dose in renal impairment
GFR (mL/min)

20–50	Dose as in normal renal function. Titrate to response
10–20	Dose as in normal renal function. Titrate to response
<10	Dose as in normal renal function. Titrate to response

Dose in patients undergoing renal replacement therapies

CAPD	Unlikley dialysability. Dose as in normal renal function
HD	Not dialysed. Dose as in normal renal function
CAV/VVHD	Unknown dialysability. Dose as in normal renal function

Important drug interactions

POTENTIALLY HAZARDOUS INTERACTIONS WITH OTHER DRUGS

• The effects of vitamin D may be reduced in patients taking barbiturates or anticonvulsants
• Increased risk of hypercalcaemia if thiazides given with vitamin D

Administration

RECONSTITUTION
–

ROUTE
• Oral, IV

RATE OF ADMINISTRATION
• Bolus

COMMENTS
–

Other information

• Check plasma calcium concentrations at regular intervals (initially weekly)
• Dose of phosphate-binding agent may need to be modified as phosphate transport in the gut and bone may be affected
• Hypercalcaemia and hypercalciuria are the major side-effects, and indicate excessive dosage

Calcium acetate

Clinical use

Phosphate-binding agent

Dose in normal renal function

–

Pharmacokinetics

Molecular weight (daltons)	158.2
% Protein binding	–
% Excreted unchanged in urine	–
Volume of distribution (L/kg)	–
Half-life – normal/ESRF (hrs)	–

Dose in renal impairment GFR (mL/min)

20–50	Dose as in normal renal function. Titrate to response
10–20	Dose as in normal renal function. Titrate to response
<10	Dose as in normal renal function. Titrate to response

Dose in patients undergoing renal replacement therapies

CAPD	Unknown dialysability. Dose as in normal renal function
HD	Unknown dialysability. Dose as in normal renal function
CAV/VVHD	Unknown dialysability. Dose as in normal renal function

Important drug interactions

POTENTIALLY HAZARDOUS INTERACTIONS WITH OTHER DRUGS

• None known

Administration

RECONSTITUTION

–

ROUTE

• Oral

RATE OF ADMINISTRATION

–

COMMENTS

• Take tablets with meals

Other information

• Calcium actetate (anhydrous): calcium content per gram = 250 mg (6.2 mmol)

Calcium carbonate

Clinical use

Phosphate-binding agent

Dose in normal renal function

420–2500 mg three times a day with meals. Dose adjusted according to serum phosphate and calcium levels

Pharmacokinetics

Molecular weight (daltons)	100
% Protein binding	45
% Excreted unchanged in urine	–
Volume of distribution (L/kg)	–
Half-life – normal/ESRF (hrs)	–

Dose in renal impairment GFR (mL/min)

20–50	Dose as in normal renal function. Titrate to response
10–20	Dose as in normal renal function. Titrate to response
<10	Dose as in normal renal function. Titrate to response

Dose in patients undergoing renal replacement therapies

CAPD	Unknown dialysability. Dose as in normal renal function
HD	Unknown dialysability. Dose as in normal renal function
CAV/VVHD	Unknown dialysability. Dose as in normal renal function

Important drug interactions

POTENTIALLY HAZARDOUS INTERACTIONS WITH OTHER DRUGS

• None known

Administration

RECONSTITUTION

–

ROUTE

• Oral

RATE OF ADMINISTRATION

–

COMMENTS

• Take with or immediately before meals

Other information

• Monitor for hypercalcaemia particularly if patient is also taking alfacalcidol
• Calcium carbonate impairs absorption of some drugs, e.g. iron, ciprofloxacin
• Titralac contains 420 mg calcium carbonate per tablet (168 mg elemental calcium)
• Calcichew contains 1250 mg calcium carbonate (500 mg elemental calcium)
• Calcium-500 contains 1250 mg calcium carbonate (500 mg elemental calcium)

Calcium gluconate (effervescent)

Clinical use

Hypocalcaemia

Dose in normal renal function

Depending on medication

Pharmacokinetics

Molecular weight (daltons)	448.4
% Protein binding	–
% Excreted unchanged in urine	–
Volume of distribution (L/kg)	–
Half-life – normal/ESRF (hrs)	–

Dose in renal impairment GFR (mL/min)

20–50	Dose as in normal renal function. Titrate to response
10–20	Dose as in normal renal function. Titrate to response
<10	Dose as in normal renal function. Titrate to response

Dose in patients undergoing renal replacement therapies

CAPD	Dialysed. Dose as in normal renal function
HD	Dialysed. Dose as in normal renal function
CAV/VVHD	Dialysed. Dose as in normal renal function

Important drug interactions

POTENTIALLY HAZARDOUS INTERACTIONS WITH OTHER DRUGS

• None known

Administration

RECONSTITUTION

–

ROUTE

• Oral, IV, IM

RATE OF ADMINISTRATION

• IV: slow 3–4 minutes for each 10 mL (2.25 mmol calcium)

COMMENTS

• Acute hypocalcaemia: give 10–20 mL calcium gluconate (2.25–4.5 mmol calcium) slow IV injection over 3–10 minutes

Other information

• Check patient's magnesium levels
• Monitor calcium and phosphate serum levels
• Calcium Sandoz 400: 10 mmol calcium per tablet
• Calcium Sandoz 1000: 25 mmol calcium per tablet
• Calcium levels cannot be corrected until magnesium levels are normal

Calcium Resonium

Clinical use

Hyperkalaemia (not for emergency treatment)

Dose in normal renal function

Oral: 15 g 3–4 times daily in water

PR: 30 g in methylcellulose solution retained for 9 hours

Pharmacokinetics

Molecular weight (daltons)   –
% Protein binding   –
% Excreted unchanged in urine   0
Volume of distribution (L/kg)   –
Half-life – normal/ESRF (hrs)   –

Dose in renal impairment GFR (mL/min)

20–50   Dose as in normal renal function. Titrate to response

10–20   Dose as in normal renal function. Titrate to response

<10   Dose as in normal renal function. Titrate to response

Dose in patients undergoing renal replacement therapies

CAPD   Not dialysed. Dose as in normal renal function

HD   Not dialysed. Dose as in normal renal function

CAV/VVHD Not dialysed. Dose as in normal renal function

Important drug interactions

POTENTIALLY HAZARDOUS INTERACTIONS WITH OTHER DRUGS

• None known

Administration

RECONSTITUTION

• PR: mix with methylcellulose solution 2%

• Oral: mix with a little water, sweetened if preferred

ROUTE

• Oral or PR

RATE OF ADMINISTRATION

–

COMMENTS

–

Other information

• Ensure a regular laxative is prescribed – can mix Calcium Resonium powder with lactulose to be taken orally

• Some units mix dose with a little water and give PR 4 times/day. Not retained for so long, but still effective

Candesartan

Clinical use

AT-II antagonist, antihypertensive agent

Dose in normal renal function

4–16 mg daily

Pharmacokinetics

Molecular weight (daltons)	610.7
% Protein binding	>99
% Excreted unchanged in urine	26
Volume of distribution (L/kg)	0.1
Half-life – normal/ESRF (hrs)	9/18

Dose in renal impairment GFR (mL/min)

20–50	Dose as in normal renal function
10–20	Initial dose 2 mg and increase according to response
<10	Initial dose 2 mg and increase according to response

Dose in patients undergoing renal replacement therapies

CAPD	Unlikely to be dialysed. Dose as for GFR = <10 mL/min
HD	Not dialysed. Dose as for GFR = <10 mL/min
CAV/VVHD	Unlikely to be dialysed. Dose as for GFR = 10–20 mL/min

Important drug interactions

POTENTIALLY HAZARDOUS INTERACTIONS WITH OTHER DRUGS

• Anaesthetics: enhanced hypotensive effect
• Ciclosporin: increased risk of hyperkalaemia and nephrotoxicity

• Diuretics: enhanced hypotensive effect, hyperkalaemia with potassium-sparing diuretics
• Lithium: reduced excretion. Possibility of enhanced lithium toxicity
• Potassium salts: hyperkalaemia
• NSAIDs: antagonism of hypotensive effect and increased risk of renal impairment and hyperkalaemia
• Tacrolimus: increased risk of nephrotoxicity and hyperkalaemia

Administration

RECONSTITUTION

–

ROUTE

• Oral

RATE OF ADMINISTRATION

–

COMMENTS

–

Other information

• Company does not recommended candesartan if GFR < 15 mL/min
• In patients with mild–moderate renal impairment C_{max} and AUC are increased by 50% and 70% respectively. Corresponding changes in patients with severe renal impairment were 50% and 110% respectively
• Adverse reactions, especially hyperkalaemia, are more common in patients with renal impairment
• Renal failure has been reported in association with AT-II antagonists in patients with renal artery stenosis, post renal transplant, or in those with congestive heart failure
• Close monitoring of renal function during therapy is necessary in those with renal insufficiency

Capreomycin

Clinical use

Antibacterial agent in combination with other drugs: tuberculosis resistant to first-line drugs

Dose in normal renal function

Deep IM injection: 1 g daily (not more than 20 mg/kg) for 2–4 months, then 1 g 2–3 times each week

Pharmacokinetics

Molecular weight (daltons)	652.7
% Protein binding	–
% Excreted unchanged in urine	50
Volume of distribution (L/kg)	–
Half-life – normal/ESRF (hrs)	2/doubled

Dose in renal impairment GFR (mL/min)

20–50	Dose as in normal renal function
10–20	Dose as in normal renal function
<10	1 g every 48 hours

Dose in patients undergoing renal replacement therapies

CAPD	Not dialysed. Dose as in GFR = <10 mL/min
HD	Not dialysed. Dose as in GFR = <10 mL/min
CAV/VVHD	Not dialysed. Dose as in normal renal function

Important drug interactions

POTENTIALLY HAZARDOUS INTERACTIONS WITH OTHER DRUGS

• Increased risk of nephrotoxicity and ototoxicity with aminoglycosides and vancomycin

Administration

RECONSTITUTION

• Dissolve in 2 mL of sodium chloride 0.9% or water for injection. 2–3 minutes should be allowed for complete solution

ROUTE

• Deep IM injection

RATE OF ADMINISTRATION

–

COMMENTS

–

Other information

• Nephrotoxic
• Check potassium levels as hypokalaemia may occur
• Desired steady-state serum capreomycin level is 10 micrograms/mL
• Dose should not exceed 1 g/day in renal failure
• Capreomycin sulphate 1,000,000 units approximately equivalent to capreomycin base 1 g

Captopril

Clinical use

ACE inhibitor: hypertension, heart failure, diabetic nephropathy

Dose in normal renal function

6.25–50 mg 2–3 times daily

Pharmacokinetics

Molecular weight (daltons)	217
% Protein binding	25–30
% Excreted unchanged in urine	30–40
Volume of distribution (L/kg)	0.7–3
Half-life – normal/ESRF (hrs)	1.9/21–32

Dose in renal impairment GFR (mL/min)

20–50	Start low – adjust according to response
10–20	Start low – adjust according to response
<10	Start low – adjust according to response

Dose in patients undergoing renal replacement therapies

CAPD	Not dialysed. Dose as in GFR = <10 mL/min
HD	Dialysed. Dose as in GFR = <10 mL/min
CAV/VVHD	Dialysed. Dose as in GFR = 10–20 mL/min

Important drug interactions

POTENTIALLY HAZARDOUS INTERACTIONS WITH OTHER DRUGS

• Anaesthetics: enhanced hypotensive effect
• Ciclosporin: increased risk of nephrotoxicity and hyperkalaemia
• Diuretics: enhanced hypotensive effect, hyperkalaemia with potassium-sparing diuretics
• Lithium: reduced excretion. Possibility of enhanced lithium toxicity
• NSAIDs: antagonism of hypotensive effect and increased risk of renal impairment and hyperkalaemia
• Potassium salts: hyperkalaemia
• Tacrolimus: increased risk of nephrotoxicity and hyperkalaemia

Administration

RECONSTITUTION

–

ROUTE

• Oral

RATE OF ADMINISTRATION

–

COMMENTS

• Tablets may be dispersed in water

Other information

• Adverse reactions, especially hyperkalaemia, are more common in patients with renal impairment
• Once-daily dosing in severe renal impairment is effective
• Effective sublingually in emergencies
• As renal function declines a hepatic elimination route for captopril becomes increasingly more significant
• 2 mg tablets are available on a 'named patient' basis
• Renal failure has been reported in association with ACE inhibitors in patients with renal artery stenosis, post renal transplant, or in those with congestive heart failure
• A high incidence of anaphylactoid reactions has been reported in patients dialysed with high-flux polyacrylonitrile membranes and treated concomitantly with an ACE inhibitor – this combination should therefore be avoided
• Close monitoring of renal function during therapy is necessary in those with renal insufficiency

Carbamazepine

Clinical use

All forms of epilepsy except absence seizures; trigeminal neuralgia, prophylaxis in manic depressive illness

Dose in normal renal function

- Epilepsy: oral – initially 100–200 mg 1–2 times daily, increased slowly to a usual dose of 0.8–1.2 g daily in divided doses. Maximum 1.6–2 g daily may be needed. Rectal – maximum 1 g daily in four divided doses for up to 7 days' use
- Trigeminal neuralgia: generally start with 100 mg 1–2 times daily. Usual dose 200 mg 3–4 times daily – up to 1600 mg/day. Reduce dose gradually as pain goes into remission
- Prophylaxis in manic depressive illness: initially 400 mg daily in divided doses – maximum 1600 mg/day. Usually 400–600 mg daily in divided doses

Pharmacokinetics

Molecular weight (daltons)	236.3
% Protein binding	75
% Excreted unchanged in urine	2–3
Volume of distribution (L/kg)	0.8–1.6
Half-life – normal/ESRF (hrs)	4–6/–

Dose in renal impairment GFR (mL/min)

20–50	Dose as in normal renal function
10–20	Dose as in normal renal function
<10	Dose as in normal renal function

Dose in patients undergoing renal replacement therapies

CAPD	Not dialysed. Dose as in normal renal function
HD	Not dialysed. Dose as in normal renal function
CAV/VVHD	Not dialysed. Dose as in normal renal function

Important drug interactions

POTENTIALLY HAZARDOUS INTERACTIONS WITH OTHER DRUGS

- Ciclosporin: metabolism accelerated (reduced plasma ciclosporin concentration)
- Analgesics: dextropropoxyphene enhances effect of carbamazepine. Carbamazepine decreases effect of tramadol and methadone
- Antibacterials: reduced effect of doxycycline, plasma carbamazepine concentration increased by clarithromycin, erythromycin and isoniazid. Increased risk of isoniazid hepatotoxicity. Carbamazepine concentration reduced by rifabutin
- Anticoagulants: metabolism of acenocoumarol and warfarin accelerated (reduced anticoagulant effect)
- Antidepressants: antagonism of anticonvulsant effect. Plasma concentration of carbamazepine increased by fluoxetine, fluvoxamine, viloxazine and nefazodone and plasma levels of nefazodone reduced by carbamazepine. Metabolism of mianserin and tricyclics accelerated. Avoid with MAOIs or within 2 weeks of MAOIs
- Other anti-epileptics: concomitant administration of two or more anti-epileptics can enhance toxicity without a corresponding increase in anti-epileptic effect
- Ulcer-healing drugs: cimetidine causes an increase in plasma carbamazepine concentration
- Antipsychotics: antagonism of anticonvulsant effect. Also reduces haloperidol, clozapine, olanzapine and risperidone concentrations
- Antivirals: plasma concentration of indinavir, lopinavir, nelfinavir and saquinavir reduced. Levels of carbamazepine increased by amprenavir
- Calcium-channel blockers: diltiazem and verapamil enhance effect of carbamazepine. Effect of felodipine, isradipine, nicardipine and nifedipine reduced
- Corticosteroids: reduced effect
- Diuretics: increased risk of hyponatraemia. Acetazolamide increases carbamazepine concentration
- Hormone antagonists: danazol inhibits metabolism of carbamazepine
- Oestrogens and progestogens: carbamazepine accelerates metabolism of oral contraceptives, gestrinone and tibolone
- Anti-malarials: chloroquine and mefloquine antagonise anticonvulsant effect

Administration

RECONSTITUTION

–

ROUTE

• Oral, rectal

RATE OF ADMINISTRATION

–

COMMENTS

• When switching a patient from tablets to liquid the same total dose may be used, but given in smaller more frequent doses

• Oral → rectal: increase the dose by approx 25%

Other information

• Important to initiate carbamazepine therapy at a low dose and build this up over 1–2 weeks, as it autoinduces its metabolism

• May cause inappropriate antidiuretic hormone secretion

• The therapeutic plasma concentration range = 4–12 micrograms/mL (17–50 micromol/L at steady state)

Carbimazole

Clinical use

Treatment of hyperthyroidism

Dose in normal renal function

5–60 mg daily

Pharmacokinetics

Molecular weight (daltons)	186.2
% Protein binding	Unbound (methimazole is 5%)
% Excreted unchanged in urine	7–12 (methimazole)
Volume of distribution (L/kg)	0.3–0.6 (methimazole)
Half-life – normal/ESRF (hrs)	3–6.4 (methimazole)/ increased

Dose in renal impairment GFR (mL/min)

20–50	Dose as in normal renal function
10–20	Dose as in normal renal function
<10	Dose as in normal renal function

Dose in patients undergoing renal replacement therapies

CAPD	Not dialysed. Dose as in normal renal function
HD	Not dialysed. Dose as in normal renal function
CAV/VVHD	Unknown dialysability. Dose as in normal renal function

Important drug interactions

POTENTIALLY HAZARDOUS INTERACTIONS WITH OTHER DRUGS

• None known

Administration

RECONSTITUTION

–

ROUTE

• Oral

RATE OF ADMINISTRATION

–

COMMENTS

–

Other information

• Carbimazole is a pro-drug which is rapidly and completely metabolised to methimazole, the active moiety

• There have been reports of glomerulonephritis associated with the development of antineutrophil cytoplasmic antibodies in patients receiving thiourea anti-thyroid drugs

Carboplatin

Clinical use

Antineoplastic agent. Ovarian carcinoma of epithelial origin; small-cell carcinoma of the lung

Dose in normal renal function

Dose = Target AUC x [GFR (mL/min) + 25] where AUC is commonly 5 or 6 depending on protocol used

Pharmacokinetics

Molecular weight (daltons)	371.2
% Protein binding	15–24
% Excreted unchanged in urine	50–75
Volume of distribution (L/kg)	0.23–0.28
Half-life – normal/ESRF (hrs)	6/increased

Dose in renal impairment GFR (mL/min)

20–50	Dose as in normal renal function
10–20	Dose as in normal renal function
<10	Dose as in normal renal function

Dose in patients undergoing renal replacement therapies

CAPD	Unknown dialysability. Dose as in GFR = <10 mL/min
HD	Dialysed. Dose as in GFR = <10 mL/min
CAV/VVHD	Unknown dialysability. Dose as in GFR = 10–20 mL/min

Important drug interactions

POTENTIALLY HAZARDOUS INTERACTIONS WITH OTHER DRUGS

• Concurrent therapy with nephrotoxic drugs may increase toxicity due to carboplatin-induced changes of renal clearance

Administration

RECONSTITUTION

–

ROUTE

• IV

RATE OF ADMINISTRATION

• IV infusion over 15–60 minutes

COMMENTS

• Therapy should not be repeated until 4 weeks after the previous carboplatin course
• The product may be diluted with glucose 5% or sodium chloride 0.9% to concentrations as low as 0.5 mg/mL

Other information

• Patients with abnormal kidney function or receiving concomitant therapy with nephrotoxic drugs are likely to experience more severe and prolonged myelotoxicity
• Blood counts and renal function should be monitored closely
• Some units still use a dose in normal renal function of 400 mg/m². In this instance, the dose should be reduced to 50% of normal for a GFR of 10–20 mL/min, and to 25% of normal for a GFR of <10 mL/min

Carmustine

Clinical use

Myeloma, lymphoma and brain tumours

Dose in normal renal function

200 mg/m^2 every 6 weeks (given as single dose or divided into daily injections)

Pharmacokinetics

Molecular weight (daltons)	214.1
% Protein binding	Negligible
% Excreted unchanged in urine	–
Volume of distribution (L/kg)	3.3
Half-life – normal/ESRF (hrs)	1.5/–

Dose in renal impairment GFR (mL/min)

20–50	Dose as in normal renal function
10–20	Dose as in normal renal function
<10	Dose as in normal renal function

Dose in patients undergoing renal replacement therapies

CAPD	Not dialysed. Dose as in normal renal function
HD	Not dialysed. Dose as in normal renal function
CAV/VVHD	Not dialysed. Dose as in normal renal function

Important drug interactions

POTENTIALLY HAZARDOUS INTERACTIONS WITH OTHER DRUGS

• None known

Administration

RECONSTITUTION

• Dissolve carmustine with 3 mL of the supplied diluent (absolute ethanol) then add 27 mL of sterile water for injection
• This solution may be further diluted with sodium chloride 0.9% for injection or glucose 5% for injection

ROUTE

• IV

RATE OF ADMINISTRATION

• Administer by IV drip over a period of 1–2 hours

COMMENTS

• Therapy should not be repeated before 6 weeks
• Can further dilute the reconstituted solution with 500 mL of sodium chloride 0.9% or glucose 5%

Other information

• Renal abnormalities, e.g. a decrease in kidney size, progressive azotaemia and renal failure have been reported in patients receiving large cumulative doses after prolonged therapy
• Carmustine is rapidly metabolised; some metabolites are active and are rapidly excreted in the urine, with approximately 30% of a dose being renally excreted after 24 hours

Carvedilol

Clinical use

Beta-adrenoceptor blocker with alpha$_1$-blocking action, used for hypertension, angina and heart failure

Dose in normal renal function

6.25–100 mg daily in one or two divided doses depending on indication and patient weight

Pharmacokinetics

Molecular weight (daltons)	406.5
% Protein binding	>98
% Excreted unchanged in urine	0–3
Volume of distribution (L/kg)	2
Half-life – normal/ESRF (hrs)	6–10/unchanged

Dose in renal impairment GFR (mL/min)

20–50	Dose as in normal renal function
10–20	Dose as in normal renal function
<10	Dose as in normal renal function

Dose in patients undergoing renal replacement therapies

CAPD	Unlikely dialysability. Dose as in normal renal function. Start with low doses and titrate according to response
HD	Not dialysed. Dose as in normal renal function. Start with low doses and titrate according to response
CAV/VVHD	Unlikely dialysability. Dose as in normal renal function. Start with low doses and titrate according to response

Important drug interactions

POTENTIALLY HAZARDOUS INTERACTIONS WITH OTHER DRUGS

• Ciclosporin: increased trough concentration, reduce dose by 20% in affected patients

• Anaesthetics: enhanced hypotensive effect
• Analgesics: NSAIDs antagonise hypotensive effect
• Anti-arrhythmics: increased risk of myocardial depression and bradycardia; increased risk of bradycardia and AV block with amiodarone
• Antidepressants: enhanced hypotensive effect with MAOIs
• Antihypertensives: enhanced hypotensive effect; increased risk of withdrawal hypertension with clonidine; increased risk of first-dose hypotensive effect with post-synaptic alpha-blockers such as prazosin
• Anti-malarials: increased risk of bradycardia with mefloquine
• Calcium-channel blockers: increased risk of bradycardia and AV block with diltiazem; hypotension and heart failure possible with nifedipine; asystole, severe hypotension and heart failure with verapamil
• Moxisylyte: possible severe postural hypotension
• Rifampicin: may reduce levels of carvedilol
• Sympathomimetics: severe hypertension with adrenaline and noradrenaline and possibly with dobutamine

Administration

RECONSTITUTION

–

ROUTE

• Oral

RATE OF ADMINISTRATION

–

COMMENTS

–

Other information

• First-pass elimination of 60–75% following oral administration

Caspofungin

Clinical use

Treatment of invasive aspergillosis in adult patients who are refractory to or intolerant of amphotericin B and/or itraconazole

Dose in normal renal function

70 mg loading dose on day 1 followed by 50 mg daily, thereafter

If patient weighs >80 kg use 70 mg daily

Pharmacokinetics

Molecular weight (daltons)	1213.4
% Protein binding	97
% Excreted unchanged in urine	1.4
Volume of distribution (L/kg)	No data
Half-life – normal/ESRF (hrs)	12–15 days/ increased but not significantly (see 'Other information')

Dose in renal impairment GFR (mL/min)

20–50	Dose as in normal renal function
10–20	Dose as in normal renal function
<10	Dose as in normal renal function

Dose in patients undergoing renal replacement therapies

CAPD	Not dialysed. Dose as in normal renal function
HD	Not dialysed. Dose as in normal renal function
CAV/VVHD	Not dialysed. Dose as in normal renal function

Important drug interactions

POTENTIALLY HAZARDOUS INTERACTIONS WITH OTHER DRUGS

- Ciclosporin: monitor liver enzymes as transient increases in ALT and AST have been reported with concomitant administration. Avoid co-administration if possible. Increases AUC of caspofungin by 35%
- Tacrolimus: reduces tacrolimus trough concentration by 26%
- Enzyme inducers, e.g. rifampicin, efavirenz, nevirapine, dexamethasone, phenytoin and carbamazepine: initial increase but subsequent reduction in AUC of caspofungin

Administration

RECONSTITUTION

- 10.5 mL water for injection

ROUTE

- IV infusion

RATE OF ADMINISTRATION

- Approximately 1 hour

COMMENTS

- Caspofungin is unstable in fluids containing glucose
- Add to 250 mL sodium chloride 0.9% or compound sodium lactate solution
- If patient is fluid restricted, doses of 35 or 50 mg may be added to 100 mL infusion fluid

Other information

- In ESRF the AUC is increased by 30–49% but a change in dosage schedule is not required
- Plasma concentrations of caspofungin decline in a polyphasic manner. A short α-phase occurs immediately post infusion, followed by a β-phase with a half-life of 9–11 hours. An additional γ-phase also occurs with a half-life of 45 hours. Distribution rather than excretion or biotransformation is the dominant mechanism influencing plasma clearance

Cefaclor

Clinical use

Antibacterial agent

Dose in normal renal function

250 mg every 8 hours (dose may be doubled for more severe infections – maximum 4 g daily)

Pharmacokinetics

Molecular weight (daltons)	385.8
% Protein binding	25
% Excreted unchanged in urine	70
Volume of distribution (L/kg)	0.24–0.35
Half-life – normal/ESRF (hrs)	1/3

Dose in renal impairment GFR (mL/min)

20–50	Dose as in normal renal function
10–20	Dose as in normal renal function
<10	125–250 mg every 8 hours

Dose in patients undergoing renal replacement therapies

CAPD	Unknown dialysability. 250 mg every 8–12 hours
HD	Dialysed. 250–500 mg every 8 hours
CAV/VVHD	Unknown dialysability. Dose as in normal renal function

Important drug interactions

POTENTIALLY HAZARDOUS INTERACTIONS WITH OTHER DRUGS

• Anticoagulants: effects of warfarin and acenocoumarol may be enhanced

Administration

RECONSTITUTION

–

ROUTE

• Oral

RATE OF ADMINISTRATION

–

COMMENTS

–

Other information

• Cefaclor is associated with protracted skin reactions

Cefadroxil

Clinical use

Antibacterial agent

Dose in normal renal function

500 mg – 1 g every 12–24 hours

Pharmacokinetics

Molecular weight (daltons)	381.4
% Protein binding	20
% Excreted unchanged in urine	70–90
Volume of distribution (L/kg)	0.31
Half-life – normal/ESRF (hrs)	1.4–22/–

Dose in renal impairment GFR (mL/min)

20–50	Dose as in normal renal function
10–20	Dose as in normal renal function
<10	500 mg – 1 g every 24–48 hours

Dose in patients undergoing renal replacement therapies

CAPD	Unknown dialysability. Dose as in GFR = <10 mL/min
HD	Dialysed. Dose as in GFR = <10 mL/min
CAV/VVHD	Unknown dialysability. Dose as in normal renal function

Important drug interactions

POTENTIALLY HAZARDOUS INTERACTIONS WITH OTHER DRUGS

• Anticoagulants: effects of warfarin and acenocoumarol may be enhanced

Administration

RECONSTITUTION

–

ROUTE

• Oral

RATE OF ADMINISTRATION

–

COMMENTS

–

Other information

–

Cefalexin

Clinical use

Antibacterial agent

Dose in normal renal function

250 mg every 6 hours or 500 mg every 8–12 hours – maximum 6 g daily

Recurrent UTI prophylaxis: 125 mg at night

Pharmacokinetics

Molecular weight (daltons)	365.4
% Protein binding	20
% Excreted unchanged in urine	98
Volume of distribution (L/kg)	0.35
Half-life – normal/ESRF (hrs)	0.7/16

Dose in renal impairment GFR (mL/min)

20–50	Dose as in normal renal function
10–20	500 mg every 8–12 hours
<10	250–500 mg every 12 hours

Dose in patients undergoing renal replacement therapies

CAPD	Dialysed. Dose as in GFR = <10 mL/min
HD	Dialysed. Dose as in GFR = <10 mL/min
CAV/VVHD	Dialysed. Dose as in GFR = 10–20 mL/min

Important drug interactions

POTENTIALLY HAZARDOUS INTERACTIONS WITH OTHER DRUGS

• Anticoagulants: effects of warfarin and acenocoumarol may be enhanced

Administration

RECONSTITUTION

–

ROUTE

• Oral

RATE OF ADMINISTRATION

–

COMMENTS

–

Other information

• Use dose for normal renal function to treat UTI in ESRF

• High doses, together with the use of nephrotoxic drugs, such as aminoglycosides or potent diuretics, may adversely affect renal function

Cefamandole

Clinical use

Antibacterial agent

Dose in normal renal function

500 mg – 2 g every 4–8 hours

Pharmacokinetics

Molecular weight (daltons)	462.5
% Protein binding	75
% Excreted unchanged in urine	50–100
Volume of distribution (L/kg)	0.16–0.25
Half-life – normal/ESRF (hrs)	1/6–11

Dose in renal impairment GFR (mL/min)

20–50	500 mg – 2 g every 6 hours
10–20	500 mg – 2 g every 6–8 hours
<10	500 mg – 2 g every 12 hours

Dose in patients undergoing renal replacement therapies

CAPD	Unknown dialysability. 500 mg – 1 g every 12 hours
HD	Dialysed. 500 mg – 1 g every 12 hours
CAV/VVHD	Unknown dialysability. Dose as in GFR = 10–20 mL/min

Important drug interactions

POTENTIALLY HAZARDOUS INTERACTIONS WITH OTHER DRUGS

• Anticoagulants: effects of warfarin and acenocoumarol may be enhanced

Administration

RECONSTITUTION

• IM: each gram of cefamandole should be reconstituted with 3 mL of water for injection or sodium chloride 0.9%
• IV: each gram of cefamandole should be reconstituted with 10 mL of water for injection, glucose 5% or sodium chloride 0.9%

ROUTE

• IV or deep IM injection

RATE OF ADMINISTRATION

• IV bolus: 1 g over 3–5 minutes
• IV infusion: over 15–30 minutes

COMMENTS

• For intermittent IV infusion: 100 mL of diluent should be added to 2 g of cefamandole. If water for injection is used, reconstitute with approx 20 mL/g to avoid a hypotonic solution
• For continuous IV infusion: add reconstituted solution to appropriate infusion solution
• Give aminoglycoside at separate site to cefamandole

Other information

• Nephrotoxicity has been reported following concomitant administration of aminoglycoside antibiotics and cephalosporins
• Kefadol contains 3.35 mmol/g sodium

Cefixime

Clinical use

Antibacterial agent

Dose in normal renal function

200–400 mg/day (given as a single dose or in two divided doses)

Pharmacokinetics

Molecular weight (daltons)	507.5
% Protein binding	50
% Excreted unchanged in urine	18–50
Volume of distribution (L/kg)	0.6–1.1
Half-life – normal/ESRF (hrs)	3.1/12

Dose in renal impairment GFR (mL/min)

20–50	Dose as in normal renal function
10–20	150–300 mg/day
<10	100–200 mg/day

Dose in patients undergoing renal replacement therapies

CAPD	Removal unlikely. Dose as in GFR = <10 mL/min
HD	Not dialysed. Dose as in GFR = <10 mL/min
CAV/VVHD	Dialysed. Dose as in GFR = 10–20 mL/min

Important drug interactions

POTENTIALLY HAZARDOUS INTERACTIONS WITH OTHER DRUGS

• Anticoagulants: effects of warfarin and acenocoumarol may be enhanced

Administration

RECONSTITUTION

–

ROUTE

• Oral

RATE OF ADMINISTRATION

–

COMMENTS

–

Other information

• Manufacturer recommends that patients having chronic CAPD or HD should not have dose greater than 200 mg/day

Cefotaxime

Clinical use

Antibacterial agent

Dose in normal renal function

Mild infection: 1 g every 12 hours

Moderate infection: 1 g every 8 hours

Severe infection: 2 g every 8 hours

Life-threatening infection: up to 12 g daily in 3–4 divided doses

Pharmacokinetics

Molecular weight (daltons)	478.5
% Protein binding	13–37
% Excreted unchanged in urine	60
Volume of distribution (L/kg)	0.15–0.55
Half-life – normal/ESRF (hrs)	1/15

Dose in renal impairment GFR (mL/min)

20–50	Dose as in normal renal function
10–20	Dose as in normal renal function
<10	0.5–1 g every 8–12 hours

Dose in patients undergoing renal replacement therapies

CAPD	Dialysed. Dose as in GFR = <10 mL/min
HD	Dialysed. Dose as in GFR = <10 mL/min
CAV/VVHD	Not dialysed. 1 g every 12 hours

Important drug interactions

POTENTIALLY HAZARDOUS INTERACTIONS WITH OTHER DRUGS

• Anticoagulants: effects of warfarin and acenocoumarol may be enhanced

Administration

RECONSTITUTION

• IV bolus/IM: 4 mL water for injection to 1 g
• IV infusion: 1 g in 50 mL sodium chloride 0.9%

ROUTE

• IV, IM

RATE OF ADMINISTRATION

• Bolus over 3–4 minutes, infusion over 20–60 minutes

COMMENTS

–

Other information

• 1 g contains 2.09 mmol sodium
• Reduce dose further if concurrent hepatic and renal failure

Cefoxitin

Clinical use

Antibacterial agent

Dose in normal renal function

1–2 g every 6–8 hours (1 g every 12 hours for uncomplicated UTI). Maximum 12 g/day

Pharmacokinetics

Molecular weight (daltons)	449.4
% Protein binding	41–75
% Excreted unchanged in urine	80
Volume of distribution (L/kg)	0.2
Half-life – normal/ESRF (hrs)	1/13–23

Dose in renal impairment GFR (mL/min)

20–50	1–2 g every 8 hours
10–20	1–2 g every 8–12 hours
<10	1–2 g every 24–48 hours

Dose in patients undergoing renal replacement therapies

CAPD	Unknown dialysability. Dose as in GFR = <10 mL/min
HD	Dialysed. Dose as in GFR = <10 mL/min
CAV/VVHD	Unknown dialysability. Dose as in GFR = 10–20 mL/min

Important drug interactions

POTENTIALLY HAZARDOUS INTERACTIONS WITH OTHER DRUGS

• Anticoagulants: effects of warfarin and acenocoumarol may be enhanced

Administration

RECONSTITUTION

• IV: reconstitute with water for injection. 10 mL to 1-g or 2-g vials
• IM: 2 mL water for injection to 1 g (or 0.5% or 1% lidocaine hydrochloride without adrenaline)

ROUTE

• IV, IM

RATE OF ADMINISTRATION

• IV bolus: 1–2 g over 3–5 minutes

COMMENTS

• IM: give by deep injection into a large muscle mass
• Cefoxitin is stable with aminoglycosides mixed in 200 mL of sodium chloride 0.9% or glucose 5%

Other information

• May falsely increase serum creatinine by interference with assay
• 1 gram contains 2.3 mmol sodium
• Active against anaerobic bacteria especially *Bacteroides fragilis*, so may be used for abdominal sepsis such as peritonitis

Cefpirome

Clinical use

Antibacterial agent

Dose in normal renal function

1–2 g twice daily

Dose depends on severity of infection

Pharmacokinetics

Molecular weight (daltons)	612.7
% Protein binding	<10
% Excreted unchanged in urine	80–90
Volume of distribution (L/kg)	0.26–0.29
Half-life – normal/ESRF (hrs)	2/14.5

Dose in renal impairment
GFR (mL/min)

20–50	1–2 g loading dose then 0.5–1 g twice daily
5–20	1–2 g loading dose then 0.5–1 g once daily
<5	1–2 g loading dose followed by 0.5–1 g daily

Dose in patients undergoing renal replacement therapies

CAPD	Not dialysed. Dose as in GFR = <5 mL/min
HD	Dialysed. Dose as in GFR = <5 mL/min
CAV/VVHD	Dialysed. 2 g stat then 1 g twice daily

Important drug interactions

POTENTIALLY HAZARDOUS INTERACTIONS WITH OTHER DRUGS

• Anticoagulants: effect of warfarin and acenocoumarol enhanced

Administration

RECONSTITUTION

• Water for injection

ROUTE

• IV

RATE OF ADMINISTRATION

• Bolus over 3–5 minutes
• Infusion over 20–30 minutes

COMMENTS

• Can use sodium chloride 0.9%, glucose 5% or 10%, or Ringer's solution as infusion fluids

Other information

• 48% of dose is removed after 4 hours of haemodialysis
• 62% of dose is removed with high-flux dialysis in a 3.5 hour session
• Some papers suggest a higher dose of 2 g three times a day may be required for CVVH using polysulfone high-flux haemofilters
• Bioavailability of 84% after IP administration
• Only 12.4% of the dose is removed by CAPD
• Cefpirome gives a strong creatinine-like reaction in creatinine assays based on the picrate method. The use of an enzyme method is recommended to avoid falsely high levels of serum creatinine

Cefpodoxime

Clinical use

Antibacterial agent

Dose in normal renal function

100–200 mg every 12 hours

Pharmacokinetics

Molecular weight (daltons)	557.6
% Protein binding	26
% Excreted unchanged in urine	30
Volume of distribution (L/kg)	0.6–1.2
Half-life – normal/ESRF (hrs)	2.5/26

Dose in renal impairment GFR (mL/min)

20–50	Dose as in normal renal function
10–20	Dose as in normal renal function
<10	100–200 mg every 24–48 hours

Dose in patients undergoing renal replacement therapies

CAPD	Unknown dialysability. Dose as in GFR = <10 mL/min
HD	Dialysed. Dose as in GFR = <10 mL/min
CAV/VVHD	Unknown dialysability. Dose as in normal renal function

Important drug interactions

POTENTIALLY HAZARDOUS INTERACTIONS WITH OTHER DRUGS

• Anticoagulants: effects of warfarin and acenocoumarol may be enhanced

Administration

RECONSTITUTION

–

ROUTE

• Oral

RATE OF ADMINISTRATION

–

COMMENTS

• Take with food
• Antacids and H_2-blockers should be taken 2–3 hours after administration of cefpodoxime

Other information

–

Cefprozil

Clinical use

Antibacterial agent

Dose in normal renal function

500 mg once or twice daily (depending on indication)

Pharmacokinetics

Molecular weight (daltons)	407.4
% Protein binding	35–45
% Excreted unchanged in urine	60–70
Volume of distribution (L/kg)	0.65
Half-life – normal/ESRF (hrs)	1.72/6

Dose in renal impairment GFR (mL/min)

30–50	Dose as in normal renal function
<30	500 mg loading dose followed by 50% of dose once daily

Dose in patients undergoing renal replacement therapies

CAPD	Unknown dialysability. Dose as in GFR < 30 mL/min
HD	Dialysed. Dose as in GFR < 30 mL/min
CAV/VVHD	Probably dialysed. Dose as in GFR < 30 mL/min

Important drug interactions

POTENTIALLY HAZARDOUS INTERACTIONS WITH OTHER DRUGS

• Anticoagulants: effect of warfarin and acenocoumarol enhanced

Administration

RECONSTITUTION

–

ROUTE

• Oral

RATE OF ADMINISTRATION

–

COMMENTS

–

Other information

• Haemodialysis removes 55% of dose during a 3-hour dialysis session

Cefradine

Clinical use

Antibacterial agent

Dose in normal renal function

Oral: 250–500 mg every 6 hours (or 500 mg–1 g every 12 hours)

Injection: 2–4 g daily (in four divided doses) (maximum 8 g/day)

Pharmacokinetics

Molecular weight (daltons)	349.4
% Protein binding	10
% Excreted unchanged in urine	100
Volume of distribution (L/kg)	0.25–0.46
Half-life – normal/ESRF (hrs)	0.7–1.3/6–15

Dose in renal impairment GFR (mL/min)

20–50	Dose as in normal renal function
10–20	Dose as in normal renal function
<10	250 mg every 6 hours

Dose in patients undergoing renal replacement therapies

CAPD	Dialysed. Dose as in GFR = <10 mL/min
HD	Dialysed. Dose as in GFR = <10 mL/min
CAV/VVHD	Unknown dialysability. Dose as in normal renal function

Important drug interactions

POTENTIALLY HAZARDOUS INTERACTIONS WITH OTHER DRUGS

• Anticoagulants: effects of warfarin and acenocoumarol may be enhanced

Administration

RECONSTITUTION

• IM: 2 mL of water for injection or sodium chloride 0.9% to each 500 mg
• IV bolus: 5 mL of water for injection, sodium chloride 0.9% or glucose 5% to each 500 mg
• IV infusions: 10 mL of suitable diluent to 1-g vial, then add to infusion solution

ROUTE

• Oral, IM, IV

RATE OF ADMINISTRATION

• IV bolus: over 3–5 minutes

COMMENTS

–

Other information

–

Ceftazidime

Clinical use

Antibacterial agent

Dose in normal renal function

1–2 g every 8–12 hours

Pharmacokinetics

Molecular weight (daltons)	637
% Protein binding	17
% Excreted unchanged in urine	60–85
Volume of distribution (L/kg)	0.28–0.4
Half-life – normal/ESRF (hrs)	1.2/13–25

Dose in renal impairment GFR (mL/min)

31–50	1 g every 12 hours
16–30	1 g every 24 hours
6–15	500 mg – 1 g every 24 hours
<5	500 mg – 1 g every 48 hours

Dose in patients undergoing renal replacement therapies

CAPD	Dialysed. 500 mg – 1 g every 24 hours
HD	Dialysed. 500 mg – 1 g every 24–48 hours
CAV/VVHD	Not dialysed. 500 mg – 1 g every 12 hours

Important drug interactions

POTENTIALLY HAZARDOUS INTERACTIONS WITH OTHER DRUGS

• Anticoagulants: effect of warfarin and acenocoumarol may be enhanced

Administration

RECONSTITUTION

Amount of water for injection to be added to vials:

• 1.5 mL to 500-mg vial for IM administration
• 5 mL to 500-mg vial for IV injection
• 3 mL to 1-g vial for IM administration
• 10 mL to 1-g vial for IV injection

ROUTE

• IV. IM rarely

RATE OF ADMINISTRATION

• 3–4 minutes bolus
• Infusion: over 30 minutes

COMMENTS

• May be given IP in CAPD fluid 125–250 mg/L fluid
• Reconstituted solutions vary in colour, but this is quite normal
• Compatible with most IV fluids, e.g. sodium chloride 0.9%, glucose saline, glucose 5%

Other information

• Vd increases with infection
• Ceftazidime levels can be monitored in patients requiring high doses with impaired renal function

Ceftriaxone

Clinical use

Antibacterial agent

Dose in normal renal function

1 g daily (severe infections: 2–4 g daily)
Gonorrhoea: single dose 250 mg IM

Pharmacokinetics

Molecular weight (daltons)	661.6
% Protein binding	90
% Excreted unchanged in urine	30–65
Volume of distribution (L/kg)	0.12–0.18
Half-life – normal/ESRF (hrs)	7–9/12–24

Dose in renal impairment GFR (mL/min)

20–50	Dose as in normal renal function
10–20	Dose as in normal renal function
<10	Dose as in normal renal function

Dose in patients undergoing renal replacement therapies

CAPD	Not dialysed. Dose as in normal renal function
HD	Not dialysed. Dose as in normal renal function
CAV/VVHD	Unknown dialysability. Dose as in normal renal function

Important drug interactions

POTENTIALLY HAZARDOUS INTERACTIONS WITH OTHER DRUGS

• Anticoagulants: effect of warfarin and acenocoumarol may be enhanced

Administration

RECONSTITUTION

• Bolus 250 mg: IV – 5 mL water for injection; IM – 1 mL 1% lidocaine hydrochloride
• Bolus 1 g: IV – 10 mL water for injection; IM – 3.5 mL 1% lidocaine hydrochloride
• Infusion: 2 g in 40 mL of calcium-free solution, e.g. sodium chloride 0.9%, glucose 5%
• Incompatible with calcium-containing solutions, e.g. Hartmann's, Ringer's

ROUTE

• IV, IM

RATE OF ADMINISTRATION

• Bolus: over 2–4 minutes
• Infusion: over at least 30 minutes

COMMENTS

• Doses of 50 mg/kg or over should be given by slow IV infusion
• For IM injection: doses greater than 1 g should be divided and injected at more than one site

Other information

• Calcium ceftriaxone has appeared as a precipitate in urine, or been mistaken as gallstones in patients receiving higher than recommended doses
• Monitor levels in dialysis patients
• For severe renal impairment maximum daily dose recommended = 2 g
• Contains 3.6 mmol sodium per gram of ceftriaxone
• In severe renal impairment accompanied by hepatic insufficiency, the plasma concentration of ceftriaxone should be determined at regular intervals and dosage adjusted

Cefuroxime (oral)

Clinical use

Antibacterial agent

Dose in normal renal function

125–500 mg every 12 hours
Gonorrhoea: single dose of 1 g

Pharmacokinetics

Molecular weight (daltons)	510.5
% Protein binding	35–50
% Excreted unchanged in urine	90
Volume of distribution (L/kg)	0.13–1.8
Half-life – normal/ESRF (hrs)	1.2/17

Dose in renal impairment GFR (mL/min)

20–50	Dose as in normal renal function
10–20	Dose as in normal renal function
<10	Dose as in normal renal function

Dose in patients undergoing renal replacement therapies

CAPD	Unknown dialysability. Dose as in normal renal function
HD	Dialysed. Dose as in normal renal function
CAV/VVHD	Unknown dialysability. Dose as in normal renal function

Important drug interactions

POTENTIALLY HAZARDOUS INTERACTIONS WITH OTHER DRUGS

• Anticoagulants: effects of warfarin and acenocoumarol may be enhanced

Administration

RECONSTITUTION

–

ROUTE

• Oral

RATE OF ADMINISTRATION

–

COMMENTS

• Take with or after food

Other information

–

Cefuroxime (parenteral)

Clinical use

Antibacterial agent

Dose in normal renal function

750 mg – 1.5 g every 6–8 hours (total dose 3–6 g daily)

Pharmacokinetics

Molecular weight (daltons)	446.4
% Protein binding	33
% Excreted unchanged in urine	90
Volume of distribution (L/kg)	0.13–1.8
Half-life – normal/ESRF (hrs)	1.2/17

Dose in renal impairment GFR (mL/min)

20–50	750 mg – 1.5 g every 8 hours
10–20	750 mg – 1.5 g every 8–12 hours
<10	750 mg – 1.5 g every 24 hours

Dose in patients undergoing renal replacement therapies

CAPD	Unknown dialysability. Dose as in GFR = <10 mL/min
HD	Dialysed. Dose as in GFR = <10 mL/min
CAV/VVHD	Unknown dialysability. Dose as in GFR = 10–20 mL/min

Important drug interactions

POTENTIALLY HAZARDOUS INTERACTIONS WITH OTHER DRUGS

• Anticoagulants: effects of warfarin and acenocoumarol may be enhanced

Administration

RECONSTITUTION

• IM: 1 mL of water for injection to each 250 mg
• IV bolus: 2 mL of water for injection to each 250 mg, but 15 mL of water for injection to 1.5 g
• IV infusion: 1.5 g in 50 mL of water for injection

ROUTE

• IM, IV

RATE OF ADMINISTRATION

• IV bolus: over 3–5 minutes
• IV infusion: over 30 minutes

COMMENTS

• Do not mix in syringe with aminoglycoside antibiotics
• Injection may also be reconstituted with: sodium chloride 0.9%, glucose 5%, glucose saline, Hartmann's solution
• Cefuroxime and metronidazole can be mixed (see manufacturer's guidelines)

Other information

• At high doses, care in patients receiving concurrent treatment with potent diuretics such as furosemide and aminoglycosides as combination can adversely affect renal function
• Each 750-mg vial ≡ 1.8 mmol sodium

Celecoxib

Clinical use

COX-2 inhibitor used for pain and inflammation of osteoarthritis or rheumatoid arthritis

Dose in normal renal function

200 mg once or twice daily

Pharmacokinetics

Molecular weight (daltons)	381.4
% Protein binding	97
% Excreted unchanged in urine	<3
Volume of distribution (L/kg)	400 litres
Half-life – normal/ESRF (hrs)	8–12/unchanged

Dose in renal impairment GFR (mL/min)

30–50	Dose as in normal renal function. Use with caution
10–30	Dose as in normal renal function, but avoid if possible
<10	Dose as in normal renal function, but only use if ESRD on dialysis

Dose in patients undergoing renal replacement therapies

CAPD	Unlikely dialysability. Start with low doses
HD	Unlikely dialysability. Start with low doses
CAV/VVHD	Unknown dialysability. Start with low doses

Important drug interactions

POTENTIALLY HAZARDOUS INTERACTIONS WITH OTHER DRUGS

- Ciclosporin: potential for increased risk of nephrotoxicity
- Cytotoxic agents: reduced excretion of methotrexate, possible increased risk of toxicity
- ACE inhibitors and AT-II antagonists: antagonism of hypotensive effect; increased risk of renal damage and hyperkalaemia

- Analgesics: avoid use of two or more NSAIDs, including aspirin (increased side-effects)
- Antibacterials: possible increased risk of convulsions with quinolones
- Antifungals: if used with fluconazole half the dose of celecoxib
- Antivirals: increased risk of haematological toxicity with zidovudine. NSAID plasma concentrations possibly increased by ritonavir
- Diuretics: risk of NSAID nephrotoxicity increased; possible antagonism of diuretic effect; increased risk of hyperkalaemia with potassium-sparing diuretics
- Lithium: reduced excretion of lithium, risk of toxicity
- Tacrolimus: increased risk of nephrotoxicity
- Warfarin: enhances anticoagulant effect

Administration

RECONSTITUTION

–

ROUTE

- Oral

RATE OF ADMINISTRATION

–

COMMENTS

–

Other information

- Clinical trials have shown renal effects similar to those observed with comparator NSAIDs. Monitor patient for deterioration in renal function and fluid retention
- Inhibition of renal prostaglandin synthesis by NSAIDs may interfere with renal function, especially in the presence of existing renal disease. Avoid if possible; if not, check serum creatinine 48–72 hours after starting NSAID. If raised, discontinue NSAID therapy
- Use normal doses in patients with ESRD on dialysis
- Use with caution in renal transplant recipients – can reduce intra-renal autocoid synthesis
- Celecoxib should be used with caution in uraemic patients predisposed to GI bleeding or uraemic coagulopathies

Celiprolol

Clinical use

Beta-adrenoceptor blocker: mild to moderate hypertension

Dose in normal renal function

200 mg daily (maximum 400 mg daily)

Pharmacokinetics

Molecular weight (daltons)	416
% Protein binding	25
% Excreted unchanged in urine	10
Volume of distribution (L/kg)	–
Half-life – normal/ESRF (hrs)	4–5/5

Dose in renal impairment GFR (mL/min)

20–50	Dose as in normal renal function
10–20	Dose as in normal renal function
<10	150–300 mg daily

Dose in patients undergoing renal replacement therapies

CAPD	Unknown dialysability. Dose as in GFR = <10 mL/min
HD	Unknown dialysability. Dose as in GFR = <10 mL/min
CAV/VVHD	Unknown dialysability. Dose as in normal renal function

Important drug interactions

POTENTIALLY HAZARDOUS INTERACTIONS WITH OTHER DRUGS

- Anaesthetics: enhanced hypotensive effect
- Anti-arrhythmics: increased risk of myocardial depression and bradycardia, with amiodarone increased risk of bradycardia and AV block
- Antidepressants: enhanced hypotensive effect with MAOIs and linezolid
- Calcium-channel blockers: increased risk of bradycardia and AV block with diltiazem; severe hypotension and heart failure occasionally with nifedipine; asystole, severe hypotension and heart failure with verapamil
- Moxisylyte: possible severe postural hypotension
- NSAIDs: antagonise hypotensive effect
- Sympathomimetics: risk of severe hypertension
- Antihypertensives: enhanced hypotensive effects. Increased risk of withdrawal hypertension with clonidine. Increased risk of first-dose hypotensive effect with post-synaptic alpha-blockers

Administration

RECONSTITUTION

–

ROUTE

- Oral

RATE OF ADMINISTRATION

–

COMMENTS

- Take half to one hour before food

Other information

- Manufacturers state – not recommended for patients with GFR < 15 mL/min

Certoparin (LMWH)

Clinical use

Prophylaxis of peri- and post-operative venous thromboembolism

Dose in normal renal function

3000 IU 1–2 hours before surgery then daily for 7–10 days

Pharmacokinetics

Molecular weight (daltons)	6000
% Protein binding	–
% Excreted unchanged in urine	Small amount
Volume of distribution (L/kg)	4–5.9 litres
Half-life – normal/ESRF (hrs)	4.3/–

Dose in renal impairment GFR (mL/min)

20–50	Dose as in normal renal function
10–20	Dose as in normal renal function
<10	Avoid

Dose in patients undergoing renal replacement therapies

CAPD	Unlikely dialysability. Avoid
HD	Unlikely dialysability. Avoid
CAV/VVHD	Unlikely dialysability. Dose as in normal renal function

Important drug interactions

POTENTIALLY HAZARDOUS INTERACTIONS WITH OTHER DRUGS

- Analgesics: aspirin enhances anticoagulant effect; increased risk of haemorrhage with intravenous diclofenac and with ketorolac (avoid concomitant use); possibly increased risk of bleeding with NSAIDs
- Nitrates: GTN infusion causes an increased excretion (reduced anticoagulant effect)

Administration

RECONSTITUTION

–

ROUTE

- SC

RATE OF ADMINISTRATION

–

COMMENTS

–

Other information

- The dose of protamine to neutralise the effect of certoparin is 1500 IU for each dose of certoparin
- Low molecular weight heparins are renally excreted and hence accumulate in severe renal impairment. While the doses recommended for prophylaxis against DVT and prevention of thrombus formation in extra-corporeal circuits are well tolerated in patients with ESRF, the doses recommended for treatment of DVT and PE have been associated with severe, sometimes fatal, bleeding episodes in such patients. Hence the use of unfractionated heparin would be preferable in these instances
- Heparin can suppress adrenal secretion of aldosterone leading to hypercalcaemia, particularly in patients with chronic renal impairment and diabetes mellitus

Cetirizine

Clinical use

Antihistamine: symptomatic relief of allergy such as hay fever, urticaria

Dose in normal renal function

10 mg daily

Pharmacokinetics

Molecular weight (daltons)	461.8
% Protein binding	93
% Excreted unchanged in urine	60–70
Volume of distribution (L/kg)	0.4–0.6
Half-life – normal/ESRF (hrs)	7–10/20

Dose in renal impairment GFR (mL/min)

20–50	Dose as in normal renal function
10–20	Dose as in normal renal function
<10	5 mg daily

Dose in patients undergoing renal replacement therapies

CAPD	Unlikely dialysability. Dose as in GFR = <10 mL/min
HD	Not dialysed. Dose as in GFR = <10 mL/min
CAV/VVHD	Unknown dialysability. Dose as in normal renal function

Important drug interactions

POTENTIALLY HAZARDOUS INTERACTIONS WITH OTHER DRUGS

• Concomitant use of terfenadine not recommended (risk of hazardous arrhythmias)

Administration

RECONSTITUTION

–

ROUTE

• Oral

RATE OF ADMINISTRATION

–

COMMENTS

• Available as tablets and solution

Other information

• Manufacturers recommend halving dose in renal impairment

Chloral hydrate

Clinical use

Insomnia (short-term use)

Dose in normal renal function

500 mg – 1 g at night (maximum 2 g/day)

Pharmacokinetics

Molecular weight (daltons)	165.4
% Protein binding	70–80
% Excreted unchanged in urine	<5
Volume of distribution (L/kg)	0.6
Half-life – normal/ESRF (hrs)	7–14/–

Dose in renal impairment GFR (mL/min)

20–50	Dose as in normal renal function
10–20	500 mg at night
<10	Avoid

Dose in patients undergoing renal replacement therapies

CAPD	Unknown dialysability. Avoid
HD	Dialysed. Avoid
CAV/VVHD	Unknown dialysability. Dose as in GFR = 10–20 mL/min

Important drug interactions

POTENTIALLY HAZARDOUS INTERACTIONS WITH OTHER DRUGS

• Anticoagulants: when chloral hydrate is added to or withdrawn from the drug regimen, or its dosage changed, careful monitoring of prothrombin time is required

Administration

RECONSTITUTION

–

ROUTE

• Oral – tablets/elixir

RATE OF ADMINISTRATION

–

COMMENTS

• Take with water (or milk) 15–30 minutes before bedtime

Other information

• Avoid in patients with marked hepatic or renal impairment, severe cardiac disease, marked gastritis and those susceptible to acute attacks of porphyria

• Chloral hydrate followed by intravenous furosemide may result in sweating, hot flushes, and variable blood pressure including hypertension

Chlorambucil

Clinical use

Antineoplastic agent. Hodgkin's disease, non-Hodgkin's lymphoma (NHL), chronic lymphocytic leukaemia (CLL), Waldenström's macroglobulinaemia (WM), ovarian carcinoma (OC), advanced breast cancer (ABC)

Dose in normal renal function

Hodgkin's disease = 0.2 mg/kg/day (4–8 wks)

NHL = 0.1–0.2 mg/kg/day (4–8 wks)

CLL = initially 0.15 mg/kg/day, then 4 weeks after 1st course ended 0.1 mg/kg/day

WM = initially 6–12 mg daily, 2–8 mg/day

OC = 0.2 mg/kg/day

ABC = 0.2 mg/kg/day – 6 wks (or 14–20 mg/day)

Pharmacokinetics

Molecular weight (daltons)	304.2
% Protein binding	99
% Excreted unchanged in urine	<1
Volume of distribution (L/kg)	0.86
Half-life – normal/ESRF (hrs)	1/–

Dose in renal impairment GFR (mL/min)

20–50	Dose as in normal renal function
10–20	Dose as in normal renal function
<10	Dose as in normal renal function

Dose in patients undergoing renal replacement therapies

CAPD	Not dialysed. Dose as in normal renal function
HD	Not dialysed. Dose as in normal renal function
CAV/VVHD	Not dialysed. Dose as in normal renal function

Important drug interactions

POTENTIALLY HAZARDOUS INTERACTIONS WITH OTHER DRUGS

• Patients who receive phenylbutazone may require reduced doses of chlorambucil

Administration

RECONSTITUTION

–

ROUTE

• Oral

RATE OF ADMINISTRATION

–

COMMENTS

–

Other information

• Chlorambucil is extensively metabolised in the liver, principally to phenylacetic acid mustard, which is pharmacologically active

• Chlorambucil is excreted in the urine, almost exclusively as metabolites

Chloramphenicol

Clinical use

Antibacterial agent

Dose in normal renal function

Oral/IV: 50 mg/kg/day in divided doses every 6 hours (maximum 100 mg/kg/day)

Eye drops: every 2 hours initially, continue for 48 hours after eye appears normal

Eye ointment: every 6–8 hours or at night (if using drops in the day)

Ear drops: 2–3 drops every 8–12 hours

Pharmacokinetics

Molecular weight (daltons)	323.1
% Protein binding	45–60
% Excreted unchanged in urine	10
Volume of distribution (L/kg)	0.5–1.0
Half-life – normal/ESRF (hrs)	1.6–3.3/3–7

Dose in renal impairment GFR (mL/min)

20–50	Dose as in normal renal function
10–20	Dose as in normal renal function
<10	Dose as in normal renal function

Dose in patients undergoing renal replacement therapies

CAPD	Not dialysed. Dose as in normal renal function
HD	Not dialysed. Dose as in normal renal function
CAV/VVHD	Not dialysed. Dose as in normal renal function

Important drug interactions

POTENTIALLY HAZARDOUS INTERACTIONS WITH OTHER DRUGS

• Anticoagulants: effects of warfarin and acenocoumarol enhanced

• Antidiabetics: effect of sulphonylureas enhanced

• Anti-epileptics: metabolism accelerated by phenobarbital (reduced plasma concentration of chloramphenicol). Increased plasma concentration of phenytoin (risk of toxicity)

• Ciclosporin: chloramphenicol possibly increases ciclosporin concentration

• Tacrolimus: chloramphenicol possibly increases tacrolimus concentration

Administration

RECONSTITUTION

• Chloromycetin: add 11.75 mL water for injection to 300-mg vial – gives 25 mg/mL; add 11 mL water for injection to 1.2-g vial – gives 100 mg/mL

• Kemicetin: 1-g vial – reconstitute with water for injection, sodium chloride 0.9% or glucose 5%:
  • 1.7 mL = 400 mg/mL solution
  • 3.2 mL = 250 mg/mL solution
  • 4.2 mL = 200 mg/mL solution
  • 9.2 mL = 100 mg/mL solution

ROUTE

• Oral, IV, IM (Kemicetine only), topically

RATE OF ADMINISTRATION

• IV: over at least 1 minute

COMMENTS

–

Other information

• Manufacturers recommend monitoring serum levels in patients with renal impairment – Micromedex therapeutic range 10–25 micrograms/mL

• Chloromycetin – 300-mg vial = 0.94 mmol sodium – 1.2-g vial = 3.75 mmol sodium

• Kemicetine – 1-g vial = 3.14 mmol sodium

Chlordiazepoxide

Clinical use

Anxiety (short-term use), alcohol withdrawal, muscle spasm

Dose in normal renal function

Anxiety: 30–100 mg daily in divided doses

Insomnia associated with anxiety, muscle spasm: 10–30 mg daily

Alcohol withdrawal: 25–100 mg repeated if necessary after 2–4 hours

Pharmacokinetics

Molecular weight (daltons)	299.8
% Protein binding	94–97
% Excreted unchanged in urine	<5
Volume of distribution (L/kg)	0.3–0.5
Half-life – normal/ESRF (hrs)	5–30/unchanged

Dose in renal impairment GFR (mL/min)

20–50	Dose as in normal renal function
10–20	Dose as in normal renal function
<10	50% of normal dose

Dose in patients undergoing renal replacement therapies

CAPD	Not dialysed. Dose as in GFR = <10 mL/min
HD	Not dialysed. Dose as in GFR = <10 mL/min
CAV/VVHD	Unknown dialysability. Dose as in normal renal function

Important drug interactions

POTENTIALLY HAZARDOUS INTERACTIONS WITH OTHER DRUGS

• Rifampicin may increase the metabolism of chlordiazepoxide
• Cimetidine inhibits metabolism of benzodiazepines

Administration

RECONSTITUTION

–

ROUTE

• Oral

RATE OF ADMINISTRATION

–

COMMENTS

• May be administered parenterally. By deep IM or slow IV – in doses similar to those stated for oral administration

Other information

• Active metabolite

Chloroquine

Clinical use

(1) Treatment of malaria.
(2) Prophylaxis and suppression of malaria.
(3) Treatment of amoebic hepatitis and abscess.
(4) Treatment of discoid and systemic lupus erythematosus.
(5) Treatment of rheumatoid arthritis.

Dose in normal renal function

Orally:
(1) 1 g chloroquine phosphate – in many cases followed by 500 mg 6–8 hours later then 500 mg/day for 2 days.
(2) 500 mg chloroquine phosphate once a week on the same day each week (start 1 week before exposure to risk and continue until 4 weeks after leaving the malarious area).
(3) 1 g chloroquine phosphate daily for 2 days followed by 250 mg every 12 hours for 2 or 3 weeks.
(4) 250 mg chloroquine phosphate every 12 hours for 1–2 weeks followed by a maintenance dose of 250 mg daily.
(5) 250 mg chloroquine phosphate daily.

Pharmacokinetics

Molecular weight (daltons)	319.9
% Protein binding	50–65
% Excreted unchanged in urine	40
Volume of distribution (L/kg)	Large
Half-life – normal/ESRF (hrs)	2–4/5–50 days

Dose in renal impairment GFR (mL/min)

20–50	Dose as in normal renal function
10–20	Dose as in normal renal function
<10	50% of normal dose

Dose in patients undergoing renal replacement therapies

CAPD	Not dialysed. Dose as in GFR = <10 mL/min
HD	Not dialysed. Dose as in GFR = <10 mL/min
CAV/VVHD	Not dialysed. Dose as in normal renal function

Important drug interactions

POTENTIALLY HAZARDOUS INTERACTIONS WITH OTHER DRUGS

• Anti-arrhythmics: increased risk of ventricular arrhythmias with amiodarone – avoid concomitant use
• Anti-epileptics: antagonism of anticonvulsant effect
• Other anti-malarials: increased risk of convulsions with mefloquine
• Digoxin: chloroquine possibly increases the plasma concentration of digoxin
• Ciclosporin: increases plasma ciclosporin concentration (increased risk of toxicity)

Administration

RECONSTITUTION

–

ROUTE

• Oral, IV, IM/SC in rare cases

RATE OF ADMINISTRATION

• IV infusion: administer dose 10 mg/kg of chloroquine base in sodium chloride 0.9% by slow IV infusion over 8 hours followed by three further 8-hour infusions containing 5 mg base/kg (total dose 25 mg base/kg over 32 hours)

COMMENTS

• Oral: do not take indigestion remedies at the same time of day as this medicine
• Chloroquine sulphate injection 5.45% w/v (equivalent to 40 mg chloroquine base per mL) is available

Other information

• Excretion is increased in alkaline urine
• Cautioned in patients with renal or hepatic disease
• Bone marrow suppression may occur with extended treatment

Chlorphenamine (chlorpheniramine)

Clinical use

Antihistamine: relief of allergy, pruritus and treatment or prophylaxis of anaphylaxis

Dose in normal renal function

Oral: 4 mg 4–6 times a day (maximum 24 mg/day)

IV/IM/SC: 10–20 mg (maximum 40 mg/day)

Pharmacokinetics

Molecular weight (daltons)	391 (chlorphenamine maleate)
% Protein binding	72
% Excreted unchanged in urine	20
Volume of distribution (L/kg)	6–12
Half-life – normal/ESRF (hrs)	14–24/–

Dose in renal impairment GFR (mL/min)

20–50	Dose as in normal renal function
10–20	4 mg four times a day
<10	4 mg 3–4 times a day

Dose in patients undergoing renal replacement therapies

CAPD	Unknown dialysability. Dose as in GFR = <10 mL/min
HD	Unknown dialysability. Dose as in GFR = <10 mL/min
CAV/VVHD	Unknown dialysability. Dose as in GFR = 10–20 mL/min

Important drug interactions

POTENTIALLY HAZARDOUS INTERACTIONS WITH OTHER DRUGS

• Inhibits phenytoin metabolism and can lead to phenytoin toxicity

Administration

RECONSTITUTION

–

ROUTE

• Oral, IV

RATE OF ADMINISTRATION

• Bolus over 1 minute

COMMENTS

• Injection reported to cause stinging or burning sensation at site of injection

Other information

• Tends to be more efficacious, but more sedating, than terfenadine in treatment of pruritus

• Increased cerebral sensitivity in patients with renal impairment

Chlorpromazine

Clinical use

Anti-emetic, anxiety and agitation, antipsychotic, hiccups

Dose in normal renal function

- Anti-emetic: Oral: 10–25 mg every 4–6 hours; IM: 25–50 mg every 3–4 hours
- Antipsychotic, anxiety and agitation: Oral: 25 mg every 8 hours initially, increase as necessary (up to 1 g daily); IM: 25–50 mg every 6–8 hours
- Hiccups: Oral: 25–50 mg every 6–8 hours; IM: 25–50 mg initially
- PR: 100 mg every 6–8 hours

Pharmacokinetics

Molecular weight (daltons)	319
% Protein binding	91–99
% Excreted unchanged in urine	<1
Volume of distribution (L/kg)	7.4
Half-life – normal/ESRF (hrs)	11–42/unchanged

Dose in renal impairment GFR (mL/min)

20–50	Dose as in normal renal function
10–20	Dose as in normal renal function
<10	Start with small dose

Dose in patients undergoing renal replacement therapies

CAPD	Not dialysed. Dose as in normal renal function. Start with small dose
HD	Not dialysed. Dose as in normal renal function. Start with small dose
CAV/VVHD	Unknown dialysability. Dose as in normal renal function

Important drug interactions

POTENTIALLY HAZARDOUS INTERACTIONS WITH OTHER DRUGS

- Anaesthetics: enhanced hypotensive effect
- Antidepressants: increased plasma level of tricyclics
- Anticonvulsant: antagonises effect, lowering anticonvulsant threshold
- ACE inhibitors and AT-II antagonists: severe postural hypotension
- Adrenergic neurone blockers: antagonism of hypotensive effect
- Sibutramine: increased risk of CNS toxicity – avoid concomitant use

Administration

RECONSTITUTION

–

ROUTE

- Oral, deep IM, PR (unlicensed)

RATE OF ADMINISTRATION

–

COMMENTS

–

Other information

- Start with small doses in severe renal impairment due to increased cerebral sensitivity

Chlorpropamide

Clinical use

Diabetes mellitus, diabetes insipidus

Dose in normal renal function

Diabetes mellitus: initially 250 mg daily (elderly 100–125 mg, but avoid). Maximum 500 mg daily

Diabetes insipidus: initially 100 mg daily

Pharmacokinetics

Molecular weight (daltons)	276.7
% Protein binding	88–96
% Excreted unchanged in urine	47
Volume of distribution (L/kg)	0.09–0.27
Half-life – normal/ESRF (hrs)	24–48/50–200

Dose in renal impairment GFR (mL/min)

20–50	50% of normal dose
10–20	Avoid
<10	Avoid

Dose in patients undergoing renal replacement therapies

CAPD	Unknown dialysability. Avoid
HD	Unknown dialysability. Avoid
CAV/VVHD	Unknown dialysability. Avoid

Important drug interactions

POTENTIALLY HAZARDOUS INTERACTIONS WITH OTHER DRUGS

• Analgesics: azapropazone, phenylbutazone and possibly other NSAIDs enhance the effects of the sulphonylureas

• Antibacterials: chloramphenicol, co-trimoxazole, 4-quinolones, sulphonamides, and trimethoprim enhance effect of sulphonylureas. Rifamycins reduce effect of sulphonylureas

• Antifungals: fluconazole and miconazole increase plasma concentrations of sulphonylureas

• Antihistamines: depressed thrombocyte count with concomitant use of oral antidiabetics and ketotifen

• Uricosurics: sulfinpyrazone enhances effect of sulphonylureas

Administration

RECONSTITUTION

–

ROUTE

• Oral

RATE OF ADMINISTRATION

–

COMMENTS

• Take with breakfast

Other information

• Chlorpropamide can enhance antidiuretic hormone and very rarely cause hyponatraemia

• Contra-indicated in patients with serious impairment of hepatic, renal or thyroid function – severe risk of metabolic acidosis

• Prolonged hypoglycaemia can occur in azotaemic patients

Chlortalidone (chlorthalidone)

Clinical use

Thiazide-like diuretic: hypertension, oedema, diabetes insipidus, mild to moderate heart failure

Dose in normal renal function

Hypertension: 25–50 mg daily

Oedema: 50 mg daily initially, or 100–200 mg alternate days

Diabetes insipidus: 100 mg every 12 hours initially, reducing to 50 mg daily where possible

Heart failure: 25–50 mg daily increasing to 100–200 mg daily

Pharmacokinetics

Molecular weight (daltons)	338.8
% Protein binding	76–90
% Excreted unchanged in urine	50
Volume of distribution (L/kg)	3.9
Half-life – normal/ESRF (hrs)	44–80/–

Dose in renal impairment GFR (mL/min)

20–50	Dose as in normal renal function
10–20	Dose as in normal renal function
<10	Avoid

Dose in patients undergoing renal replacement therapies

CAPD	Unknown dialysability. Avoid
HD	Not dialysed. Avoid
CAV/VVHD	Unknown dialysability. Dose as in normal renal function

Important drug interactions

POTENTIALLY HAZARDOUS INTERACTIONS WITH OTHER DRUGS

- ACE inhibitors and AT-II antagonists: enhanced hypotensive effect
- Anti-arrhythmics: toxicity of amiodarone, disopyramide, flecainide, and quinidine increased if hypokalaemia occurs. Action of lidocaine mexiletine and tocainide antagonised by hypokalaemia
- Antihistamines: hypokalaemia increases risk of ventricular arrhythmias with terfenadine
- Antihypertensives: enhanced hypotensive effect, increased risk of first-dose hypotensive effect of post-synaptic alpha-blockers such as prazosin
- Cardiac glycosides: increased risk of toxicity if hypokalaemia occurs
- Lithium: lithium excretion reduced by thiazides – increased plasma lithium concentration and risk of toxicity
- Antidiabetics: dosage of insulin or oral antidiabetic agents may need adjusting
- NSAIDs: increased risk of nephrotoxicity

Administration

RECONSTITUTION

–

ROUTE

- Oral

RATE OF ADMINISTRATION

–

COMMENTS

- A single dose at breakfast time is preferable

Other information

- Can precipitate diabetes mellitus and gout, and cause severe electrolyte disturbances and an increase in serum lipids

Ciclosporin

Clinical use

Immunosuppressant: prophylaxis of kidney transplant rejection, nephrotic syndrome, atopic dermatitis, psoriasis and rheumatoid arthritis

Dose in normal renal function

Kidney transplant prophylaxis: Oral: 2–15 mg/kg/day based on levels (see local protocol)

IV: one-third to one-half of oral dose (see local protocol)

Nephrotic syndrome: Oral: 2.5–5 mg/kg in two divided doses

Atopic dermatitis: Oral: 2.5–5 mg/kg in two divided doses

Rheumatoid arthritis: Oral: 2.5–4 mg/kg in two divided doses

Pharmacokinetics

Molecular weight (daltons)	1203
% Protein binding	96–99
% Excreted unchanged in urine	<1
Volume of distribution (L/kg)	3.5–7.4
Half-life – normal/ESRF (hrs)	3–16/(unchanged)

Dose in renal impairment
GFR (mL/min)

20–50	Dose as in normal renal function
10–20	Dose as in normal renal function
<10	Dose as in normal renal function

Dose in patients undergoing renal replacement therapies

CAPD	Not dialysed. Dose as in normal renal function, adjust according to levels
HD	Not dialysed. Dose as in normal renal function, adjust according to levels
CAV/VVHD	Not dialysed. Dose as in normal renal function, adjust according to levels

Important drug interactions

POTENTIALLY HAZARDOUS INTERACTIONS WITH OTHER DRUGS

• Increased risk of hyperkalaemia with ACE inhibitors, AT-II antagonists, potassium-sparing diuretics, potassium salts
• Increased risk of nephrotoxicity with NSAIDs, aminoglycosides, co-trimoxazole, trimethoprim, 4-quinolones, amphotericin, colchicine, melphalan
• Increased plasma ciclosporin levels with amiodarone, propafenone, chloramphenicol, doxycycline, erythromycin, clarithromycin, itraconazole, ketoconazole, miconazole, fluconazole, chloroquine, diltiazem, nicardipine, nifedipine, verapamil, high-dose methylprednisolone, danazol, progestogens, cimetidine, ritonavir, grapefruit juice
• Decreased plasma ciclosporin levels with rifampicin, IV trimethoprim, IV sulphadimidine, carbamazepine, phenobarbital, phenytoin, griseofulvin, octreotide, St John's Wort, ticlopidine
• Increased risk of neurotoxicity with doxorubicin
• Increased toxicity with methotrexate
• Increased risk of myopathy with HMG CoA reductase inhibitors
• Increased half-life with tacrolimus
• Mycophenolate mofetil: some studies show that ciclosporin decreases plasma MPA AUC levels – no dose change required
• Orlistat: absorption of ciclosporin possibly reduced

Administration

RECONSTITUTION

• Dilute 50 mg in 20–100 mL with sodium chloride 0.9% or glucose 5%

ROUTE

• Oral, IV peripherally or centrally

RATE OF ADMINISTRATION

• Over 2–6 hours peripherally or 1 hour centrally

COMMENTS

–

Other information

• To convert from IV to oral therapy multiply by 2–3 (usually 2.5)
• Dose and monitor blood levels in accordance with local protocol

Cidofovir

Clinical use

Treatment of CMV retinitis in patients with AIDS if other agents are unsuitable

Treatment of BK polyoma virus in transplant patients (unlicensed)

Dose in normal renal function

5 mg/kg weekly for 2 weeks then once every 2 weeks

(See 'Other information' for BK polyoma virus treatment)

Pharmacokinetics

Molecular weight (daltons)	279.2
% Protein binding	<6
% Excreted unchanged in urine	80–100
Volume of distribution (L/kg)	0.3–0.8
Half-life – normal/ESRF (hrs)	2.5 ± 0.5/30

Dose in renal impairment GFR (mL/min)

55–80	2.5–4 mg/kg/dose
<55	Avoid. See 'Other information'

Dose in patients undergoing renal replacement therapies

CAPD	Not dialysed. 0.5 mg/kg/dose
HD	Dialysed. 0.5 mg/kg/dose
CAV/VVHD	Unknown dialysability. 0.5 mg/kg/dose

Important drug interactions

POTENTIALLY HAZARDOUS INTERACTIONS WITH OTHER DRUGS

• None known

Administration

RECONSTITUTION

–

ROUTE

• IV infusion

RATE OF ADMINISTRATION

• Over 60 minutes

COMMENTS

• Dilute in 100 ml sodium chloride 0.9%

Other information

• Always administer with oral probenecid and intravenous sodium chloride 0.9%

• Administer 2 hours before dialysis session to benefit from peak concentration without having delayed clearance

• 52% of dose dialysed out with high-flux haemodialysis

• The manufacturer advises to avoid in renal failure but there is a paper which suggests theoretical doses (based on a 70-kg person): Brody et al. (1999) Pharmacokinetics of cidofovir in renal insufficiency and in continuous ambulatory peritoneal dialysis or high-flux haemodialysis. *Clinical Pharmacology and Therapeutics*. **65**(1)

CL_{CR} (mL/min/kg)	Dose (mg/kg)
1.3–1.8	5.0
1–1.2	4.0
0.8–0.9	3.0
0.7	2.5
0.5–0.6	2.0
0.4	1.5
0.2–0.3	1.0
0.1	0.5

• Information for the treatment of BK polyoma virus in transplant patients is from Pittsburgh. Starting dose was 0.25 mg/kg (if GFR<30 mL/min) in 100 mL sodium chloride 0.9% administered over 1 hour. Hydration pre and post dose with 1 litre of sodium chloride 0.9% if tolerated. If no change within 10–14 days, increase to 0.3–0.5 mg/kg; dose can be increased up to 1 mg/kg depending on response and side-effects. Most patients would need a cumulative dose of 1–1.5 mg/kg. Initially use *without* probenecid. Monitor blood and urine samples for PCR measurement of viral load

Cilazapril

Clinical use

ACE inhibitor: hypertension, congestive heart disease

Dose in normal renal function

• Essential hypertension: 1 mg – 2.5 mg daily (maximum 5 mg daily)
• Renovascular hypertension: 0.25–0.5 mg daily initially (adjust maintenance dose individually)
• Cardiac failure: 0.5 mg daily initially

Pharmacokinetics

Molecular weight (daltons)	435.5
% Protein binding	–
% Excreted unchanged in urine	91
Volume of distribution (L/kg)	20 litres
Half-life – normal/ESRF (hrs)	9/–

Dose in renal impairment GFR (mL/min)

40–50	Initially 1 mg once daily (maximum 5 mg daily)
10–40	Initially 0.5 mg once daily (maximum 2.5 mg daily)
<10	0.25–0.5 mg once daily and adjust according to response

Dose in patients undergoing renal replacement therapies

CAPD	Unknown dialysability. Dose as in GFR = <10 mL/min
HD	Dialysed. Dose as in GFR = <10 mL/min
CAV/VVHD	Unknown dialysability. Dose as in GFR = 10–40 mL/min

Important drug interactions

POTENTIALLY HAZARDOUS INTERACTIONS WITH OTHER DRUGS

• Anaesthetics: enhanced hypotensive effect
• Ciclosporin: decreased renal function and increased risk of hyperkalaemia
• NSAIDs: antagonism of hypotensive effect and increased risk of renal failure, hyperkalaemia
• Diuretics: enhanced hypotensive effect, hyperkalaemia with potassium-sparing diuretics
• Epoetin: increased risk of hyperkalaemia
• Lithium: ACE inhibitors reduce excretion of lithium (increased plasma lithium concentration)
• Potassium salts: hyperkalaemia
• Tacrolimus: decreased renal function and increased risk of hyperkalaemia

Administration

RECONSTITUTION
–

ROUTE

• Oral

RATE OF ADMINISTRATION
–

COMMENTS

• Take dose about the same time each day

Other information

• Data refer to active drug – cilazaprilat
• Symptomatic hypotension reported in patients with sodium or volume depletion, i.e. sickness, diarrhoea, on diuretics, low-sodium diet or post dialysis
• Renal failure has been reported in association with ACE inhibitors in patients with renal artery stenosis, post renal transplant, or those with congestive heart failure
• A high incidence of anaphylactoid reactions has been reported in patients dialysed with high-flux polyacrylonitrile membranes and treated concomitantly with an ACE inhibitor – this combination should therefore be avoided
• Hyperkalaemia and other side-effects are more common in patients with impaired renal function
• Close monitoring of renal function during therapy is necessary in those with renal insufficiency

Cimetidine

Clinical use

Gastric and duodenal ulcer treatment and prophylaxis, reflux oesophagitis, Zollinger-Ellison syndrome. (Unlicensed use: refractory uraemic pruritus)

Dose in normal renal function

- Oral: duodenal and gastric ulceration treatment: 800 mg at night, or 400 mg twice daily. Rarely, up to 2.4 g daily
- Prophylaxis: 400 mg at night or 400 mg twice daily
- Reflux oesophagitis: 400 mg every 6 hours
- IM: 200 mg every 4–6 hours, maximum 2.4 g daily
- IV bolus: 200 mg every 4–6 hours
- IV infusion: 400 mg every 4–6 hours intermittent or 50–100 mg/hour continuous, maximum 2.4 g daily
- Zollinger-Ellison syndrome: 400 mg every 6 hours

Pharmacokinetics

Molecular weight (daltons)	252
% Protein binding	20
% Excreted unchanged in urine	50–70
Volume of distribution (L/kg)	0.8–1.3
Half-life – normal/ESRF (hrs)	1.5–2/5

Dose in renal impairment GFR (mL/min)

20–50	Dose as in normal renal function
10–20	50% of normal dose
<10	25–50% of normal dose

Dose in patients undergoing renal replacement therapies

CAPD	Not dialysed. Dose as in GFR = <10 mL/min
HD	Dialysed. Dose as in GFR = <10 mL/min
CAV/VVHD	Unknown dialysability. Dose as in GFR = 10–20 mL/min

Important drug interactions

POTENTIALLY HAZARDOUS INTERACTIONS WITH OTHER DRUGS

- Anti-arrhythmics: increased plasma concentration of many anti-arrhythmics
- Anticoagulants: enhanced effect of acenocoumarol and warfarin
- Anti-epileptics: inhibits metabolism of carbamazepine, phenytoin and valproate. Plasma levels increased
- Ciclosporin: possibly increases ciclosporin levels
- Theophylline: inhibits metabolism. Plasma levels increased

Administration

RECONSTITUTION

–

ROUTE

- Oral, IM, IV

RATE OF ADMINISTRATION

- IV infusion: 400 mg in 100 mL sodium chloride 0.9% or glucose 5% over 30–60 minutes
- IV bolus: 200 mg over at least 5 minutes. Dilute larger doses to 10 mL and give over at least 10 minutes
- Continuous IV infusion: 50–100 mg/hour

COMMENTS

- Avoid bolus if possible

Other information

- Inhibits tubular secretion of creatinine
- Uraemic patients susceptible to mental confusion

Cinnarizine

Clinical use

Treatment of vestibular disorders, motion sickness, vascular disease

Dose in normal renal function

30 mg three times a day

Motion sickness: 30 mg 2 hours before travel then 15 mg every 8 hours when required

Vascular disease: 75 mg 2–3 times daily

Pharmacokinetics

Molecular weight (daltons)	368.5
% Protein binding	80
% Excreted unchanged in urine	<20
Volume of distribution (L/kg)	No data
Half-life – normal/ESRF (hrs)	3–6/–

Dose in renal impairment GFR (mL/min)

20–50	Dose as in normal renal function
10–20	Dose as in normal renal function
<10	Dose as in normal renal function

Dose in patients undergoing renal replacement therapies

CAPD	Unlikely to be dialysed. Dose as in normal renal function
HD	Unlikely to be dialysed. Dose as in normal renal function
CAV/VVHD	Unlikely to be dialysed. Dose as in normal renal function

Important drug interactions

POTENTIALLY HAZARDOUS INTERACTIONS WITH OTHER DRUGS

• None known

Administration

RECONSTITUTION

–

ROUTE

• Oral

RATE OF ADMINISTRATION

–

COMMENTS

–

Other information

–

Ciprofloxacin

Clinical use

Antibacterial agent

Dose in normal renal function

Oral: 250–750 mg every 12 hours
IV: 100–400 mg every 12 hours

Pharmacokinetics

Molecular weight (daltons)	331
% Protein binding	20–40
% Excreted unchanged in urine	50–70
Volume of distribution (L/kg)	2.5
Half-life – normal/ESRF (hrs)	3–6/6–9

Dose in renal impairment GFR (mL/min)

20–50	Dose as in normal renal function
10–20	50% of normal dose
<10	50% of normal dose

Dose in patients undergoing renal replacement therapies

CAPD	Not dialysed. Oral: 250 mg every 8–12 hours. IV: 100 mg every 12 hours
HD	Not dialysed. Oral: 250–500 mg every 12 hours. IV: 100–200 mg every 12 hours
CAV/VVHD	Dialysed. Oral: 500–750 mg every 12 hours. IV: 200–400 mg every 12 hours

Important drug interactions

POTENTIALLY HAZARDOUS INTERACTIONS WITH OTHER DRUGS

- Tacrolimus: increased levels – anecdotally
- Analgesics: increased risk of convulsions with NSAIDs
- Anticoagulants: anticoagulant effect enhanced
- Ciclosporin: variable response. No interaction seen locally. Some reports of increased nephrotoxicity
- Theophylline: possibly increased risk of convulsions. Increased plasma levels of theophylline

Administration

RECONSTITUTION

–

ROUTE

- Oral, IV

RATE OF ADMINISTRATION

- Infusion: over 30–60 minutes

COMMENTS

- Swallow tablets whole, do not chew
- Do not take milk, iron preparations, indigestion remedies or phosphate binders at the same time as ciprofloxacin orally

Other information

- IP ciprofloxacin in CAPD, dose range 25 mg/L to 100 mg/L
- In CAPD peritonitis *oral* ciprofloxacin up to 500 mg two times daily may be administered
- The bioavailability of the oral and IV forms are approximately equivalent
- Only very small amounts dialysed

Cisapride (unlicensed product)

Clinical use

Dyspepsia, gastro-oesophageal reflux and other symptoms of impaired gastric motility

Dose in normal renal function

10 mg 3–4 times a day (once daily for maintenance therapy)

Pharmacokinetics

Molecular weight (daltons)	484
% Protein binding	98
% Excreted unchanged in urine	<1
Volume of distribution (L/kg)	2.4
Half-life – normal/ESRF (hrs)	7–10/–

Dose in renal impairment GFR (mL/min)

20–50	5 mg 3–4 times a day and titrate as necessary
10–20	5 mg 3–4 times a day and titrate as necessary
<10	5 mg 3–4 times a day and titrate as necessary

Dose in patients undergoing renal replacement therapies

CAPD	Unknown dialysability. Dose as in GFR = <10 mL/min
HD	Unknown dialysability. Dose as in GFR = <10 mL/min
CAV/VVHD	Unknown dialysability. Dose as in GFR = 10–20 mL/min

Important drug interactions

POTENTIALLY HAZARDOUS INTERACTIONS WITH OTHER DRUGS

• Ciclosporin: higher and earlier peak ciclosporin level in blood/plasma

• Antibacterials: macrolides can possibly inhibit metabolism (risk of ventricular arrhythmias)
• Antifungals: azoles inhibit metabolism (ventricular arrhythmias reported)
• Anticoagulants: effects enhanced
• Any CYP 450 inhibitors, e.g. antivirals: risk of prolongation of QT interval and ventricular arrhythmias – avoid concomitant use
• Drugs that prolong QT interval, e.g. some anti-arrhythmics, antihistamines: avoid concomitant use
• Cimetidine: increases bioavailability of cisapride
• Grapefruit juice: increases bioavailability of cisapride
• Drugs that affect electrolyte balance, e.g. diuretics: avoid concomitant use

Administration

RECONSTITUTION

–

ROUTE

• Oral

RATE OF ADMINISTRATION

–

COMMENTS

• Preferably take 15–30 minutes before a meal

Other information

• Start with low dose and increase according to response providing patient can tolerate it
• Predominantly metabolised hepatically to inactive renally excreted metabolites

Cisplatin

Clinical use

Antineoplastic agent: testicular and metastatic ovarian tumours, also cervical tumours, lung carcinoma, and bladder cancer

Dose in normal renal function

- Single agent therapy: 50–120 mg/m² as a single IV dose every 3–4 weeks or 15–20 mg/m² IV daily for 5 days every 3–4 weeks
- Combination therapy: 20 mg/m² and upward, IV every 3–4 weeks

Pharmacokinetics

Molecular weight (daltons)	300
% Protein binding	90
% Excreted unchanged in urine	27–45
Volume of distribution (L/kg)	0.5
Half-life – normal/ESRF (hrs)	0.3–0.5/–

Dose in renal impairment GFR (mL/min)

20–50	See 'Other information'
10–20	See 'Other information'
<10	See 'Other information'

Dose in patients undergoing renal replacement therapies

CAPD	Unknown dialysability. Dose as in GFR = <10 mL/min
HD	Dialysed. Dose as in GFR = <10 mL/min
CAV/VVHD	Unknown dialysability. Dose as in GFR = 10–20 mL/min

Important drug interactions

POTENTIALLY HAZARDOUS INTERACTIONS WITH OTHER DRUGS

- Antibacterials: aminoglycosides, vancomycin and capreomycin increase risk of nephrotoxicity and possibility of ototoxicity

Administration

RECONSTITUTION

- BMS cisplatin: no reconstitution necessary
- FAULDING/PHARMACIA cisplatin: dissolve in water for injection to form a 1 mg/mL solution (use within 20 hours, protect from light, store at room temperature)

ROUTE

- IV infusion

RATE OF ADMINISTRATION

- Over 6–8 hours

COMMENTS

- Pretreatment hydration with 1–2 L of fluid infused for 8–12 hours prior to cisplatin dose is recommended in order to initiate diuresis. The drug is then well-diluted in sodium chloride 0.9% or glucose saline solutions to ensure hydration and maintain urine output. Adequate hydration *must* be maintained during the following 24 hours, with potassium and magnesium supplementation given as necessary
- Cisplatin solutions react with aluminium – do not use equipment containing aluminium

Other information

- Dose modification depends not only on the degree of renal dysfunction, but also on the intended dose and the therapeutic end-point. In general, any patient with a GFR < 70 mL/min should be highlighted as 'at risk' from cisplatin renal toxicity. Furthermore, dose modification will depend on the risk/benefit ratio for that patient. Consequently, the clinical decision may range from complete omission of cisplatin if palliation is intended, to treatment at full dose if cure is possible, with the damage to renal function being justified on the balance of the benefit to the patient of the chemotherapy. An alternative approach is consideration of a change to carboplatin, which can be dosed specifically according to GFR
- Ototoxicity, nephrotoxicity and myelo-suppression reported. Check hearing, renal function and haematology before treatment and before each subsequent course (also during treatment)
- Hypomagnesaemia, hypocalcaemia and hyperuricaemia observed
- The addition of mannitol to the infusion may aid diuresis and protect the kidneys

Citalopram

Clinical use

SSRI antidepressant, used for depressive illness, panic disorder

Dose in normal renal function

10–60 mg daily
Oral drops: 8–48 mg (4 drops = 10 mg tablet)

Pharmacokinetics

Molecular weight (daltons)	405.3 (hydrobromide)
% Protein binding	<80
% Excreted unchanged in urine	12–23
Volume of distribution (L/kg)	12.3
Half-life – normal/ESRF (hrs)	35/prolonged by 35%

Dose in renal impairment GFR (mL/min)

20–50	Dose as in normal renal function
10–20	Dose as in normal renal function
<10	Dose as in normal renal function. Use with caution

Dose in patients undergoing renal replacement therapies

CAPD	Unlikely to be dialysed. Dose as in GFR = <10 mL/min
HD	Not dialysed. Dose as in GFR = <10 mL/min
CAV/VVHD	Unlikely to be dialysed. Dose as in GFR = 10–20 mL/min

Important drug interactions

POTENTIALLY HAZARDOUS INTERACTIONS WITH OTHER DRUGS

• Analgesics: risk of CNS toxicity increased with tramadol

• Anticoagulants: effect of acenocoumarol and warfarin possibly enhanced
• Antidepressants: enhanced CNS effects with MAOI and moclobemide – avoid concomitant use; plasma concentration of some tricyclics increased; increased serotonergic effect with St John's Wort – avoid concomitant use
• Anti-epileptics: convulsive threshold lowered
• Terfenadine: increased risk of arrythmias
• Antivirals: plasma concentration possibly increased by ritonavir
• Lithium: increased risk of CNS effects
• Sibutramine: increased risk of CNS toxicity (avoid concomitant use)
• Linezolid: use with care, possibly increased risk of side-effects
• Anti-malarials: artemether with lumefantrine – manufacturer advises avoid concomitant use

Administration

RECONSTITUTION

–

ROUTE

• Oral

RATE OF ADMINISTRATION

–

COMMENTS

–

Other information

• Only 1% of drug is removed by haemodialysis
• There is reduced clearance of citalopram in severe renal failure
• The company does not advise citalopram once the GFR < 20 mL/min

Cladribine

Clinical use

Treatment of hairy-cell leukaemia (HCL), chronic lymphocytic leukaemia (CLL) in patients who have failed to respond to standard regimens

Dose in normal renal function

HCL: 0.09 mg/kg (3.6 mg/m^2) daily for 7 days

CLL: 0.12 mg/kg (4.8 mg/m^2) daily for 2 hours on days 1 to 5 of a 28-day cycle or according to local protocol

Pharmacokinetics

Molecular weight (daltons)	285.7
% Protein binding	20
% Excreted unchanged in urine	18
Volume of distribution (L/kg)	9
Half-life – normal/ESRF (hrs)	3–22/no data

Dose in renal impairment GFR (mL/min)

20–50	Use with caution. See 'Other information'
10–20	Use with caution. See 'Other information'
<10	Use with caution. See 'Other information'

Dose in patients undergoing renal replacement therapies

CAPD	Unknown dialysability. Dose as in GFR = <10 mL/min
HD	Unknown dialysability. Dose as in GFR = <10 mL/min
CAV/VVHD	Unknown dialysability. Dose as in GFR = 10–20 mL/min

Important drug interactions

POTENTIALLY HAZARDOUS INTERACTIONS WITH OTHER DRUGS

• Caution when administering with any other immunosuppressive or myelosuppressive therapy

Administration

RECONSTITUTION

–

ROUTE

• IV infusion

RATE OF ADMINISTRATION

• 24 hours or 2 hours depending on condition being treated

COMMENTS

• Add to 100–500 mL of sodium chloride 0.9%

Other information

• Regular monitoring is recommended in renal failure

• Acute renal insufficiency has developed in some patients receiving high-dose cladribine

• There is inadequate data on dosing of patients with renal insufficiency therefore use according to clinical need

• Study showed that <10% of dose is excreted in urine as metabolites and <20% as parent drug

Clarithromycin

Clinical use

Antibacterial agent; adjunct in treatment of duodenal ulcers by eradication of *H. pylori*

Dose in normal renal function

Oral: 250–500 mg every 12 hours
IV: 500 mg every 12 hours

Pharmacokinetics

Molecular weight (daltons)	748
% Protein binding	70
% Excreted unchanged in urine	15
Volume of distribution (L/kg)	2–4
Half-life – normal/ESRF (hrs)	2.3–6/prolonged

Dose in renal impairment GFR (mL/min)

20–50	Dose as in normal renal function
10–20	Oral: 250–500 mg every 12–24 hours
IV: 250–500 mg every 12 hours
<10	Oral: 250 mg every 12–24 hours
IV: 250 mg every 12 hours

Dose in patients undergoing renal replacement therapies

CAPD	Unknown dialysability. Dose as in GFR = <10 mL/min
HD	Dialysed. Dose as in GFR = <10 mL/min
CAV/VVHD	Unknown dialysability. Dose as in GFR = 10–20 mL/min

Important drug interactions

POTENTIALLY HAZARDOUS INTERACTIONS WITH OTHER DRUGS

- Antibacterials: increased plasma concentration of rifabutin
- Anticoagulants: effect of acenocoumarol and warfarin is potentially enhanced
- Anticonvulsants: increased plasma carbamazepine concentration
- Antidepressants: avoid concomitant use with reboxetine
- Antihistamines: inhibits the metabolism of terfenadine (risk of hazardous arrhythmias)
- Antimuscarinics: avoid concomitant use with tolterodine
- Antipsychotics: increased risk of arrhythmias with pimozide – avoid concomitant use
- Antivirals: oral clarithromycin reduces absorption of ritonavir and zidovudine. Ritonavir increases clarithromycin concentration. Increased risk of rash with efavirenz
- Anxiolytics: inhibits metabolism of midazolam
- Ciclosporin: increases plasma ciclosporin concentration (although may take ~ 5 days after starting clarithromycin before increase in ciclosporin levels is seen)
- Tacrolimus: increased plasma tacrolimus levels
- Theophylline: increased plasma theophylline concentration

Administration

RECONSTITUTION

- Add 10 mL water for injection to vial (500 mg)

ROUTE

- IV infusion into one of the larger proximal veins
- Not to be administered by bolus or IM injection

RATE OF ADMINISTRATION

- Over 60 minutes

COMMENTS

- Add reconstituted product to 250 mL glucose 5% or sodium chloride 0.9%. (Stable in 100 mL, but more likely to cause phlebitis, pain and inflammation at the injection site.)

Other information

- Use with caution in renal or hepatic failure

Clindamycin

Clinical use

Antibacterial agent

Dose in normal renal function

- Oral: 150–450 mg every 6 hours. Endocarditis prophylaxis – 600 mg 1 hour before procedure
- IV/IM: 0.6–4.8 g daily in 2–4 divided doses. Prophylaxis – 300 mg 15 minutes before procedure then 150 mg 6 hours later

Pharmacokinetics

Molecular weight (daltons)	479.5 (as hydrochloride, in capsules)
	505 (as phosphate, in injection)
% Protein binding	60–95
% Excreted unchanged in urine	10–13
Volume of distribution (L/kg)	0.6–1.2
Half-life – normal/ESRF (hrs)	2–4/3–5

Dose in renal impairment GFR (mL/min)

20–50	Dose as in normal renal function
10–20	Dose as in normal renal function
<10	Dose as in normal renal function

Dose in patients undergoing renal replacement therapies

CAPD	Not dialysed. Dose as in normal renal function
HD	Not dialysed. Dose as in normal renal function
CAV/VVHD	Not dialysed. Dose as in normal renal function

Important drug interactions

POTENTIALLY HAZARDOUS INTERACTIONS WITH OTHER DRUGS

- Muscle relaxants: enhanced neuromuscular blockade
- Erythromycin: antagonism demonstrated in vitro, manufacturers recommend that the two drugs should not be administered concurrently

Administration

RECONSTITUTION

–

ROUTE

- Oral, IV infusion, IM

RATE OF ADMINISTRATION

- 10–60 minutes

COMMENTS

- Dilute prior to IV administration. Up to 900 mg in at least 50 mL of diluent. Over 900 mg in 100 mL of diluent. Compatible diluents: sodium chloride 0.9% or glucose 5%
- Administration of more than 1200 mg in a single 1-hour infusion is not recommended
- Single IM injections of greater than 600 mg are not recommended

Other information

- Capsules should be swallowed whole with a glass of water
- Pseudomembranous colitis may occur
- Periodic kidney and LFTs should be carried out during prolonged therapy
- Dosage may require reduction in patients with severe renal impairment due to prolonged half-life

Clodronate sodium

Clinical use

Bisphosphonate for: (1) management of osteolytic lesions, hypercalcaemia and bone pain associated with skeletal metastases in patients with breast cancer or multiple myeloma; (2) maintenance of acceptable serum Ca^{2+} levels in patients with hypercalcaemia of malignancy

Dose in normal renal function

(1) Loron/Bonefos: 1600–3200 mg daily
Loron 520: 1040–2080 mg daily

(2) 300 mg daily for 7–10 days or a single-dose infusion of 1.5 g

Pharmacokinetics

Molecular weight (daltons)	360.9
% Protein binding	36
% Excreted unchanged in urine	70–90
Volume of distribution (L/kg)	0.25
Half-life – normal/ESRF (hrs)	13/increased

Dose in renal impairment GFR (mL/min)

20–50	Dose as in normal renal function
10–20	50% of normal dose
<10	25% of normal dose

Dose in patients undergoing renal replacement therapies

CAPD	Not dialysed. Dose as in GFR = <10 mL/min
HD	Dialysed. Dose as in GFR = <10 mL/min
CAV/VVHD	Unknown dialysability. Dose as in GFR = 10–20 mL/min

Important drug interactions

POTENTIALLY HAZARDOUS INTERACTIONS WITH OTHER DRUGS

• None known

Administration

RECONSTITUTION

–

ROUTE

• Oral, IV infusion

RATE OF ADMINISTRATION

1 Single infusion: 1500 mg over 4 hours.

2 Multiple infusions: 300 mg over at least 2 hours.

COMMENTS

1 Single infusion: 1500 mg sodium clodronate to 500 mL sodium chloride 0.9% or glucose 5%.

2 Multiple infusions: 300 mg sodium clodronate to 500 mL sodium chloride 0.9% or glucose 5%.

• Multiple infusions should be repeated on successive days until normocalcaemia is achieved or to a maximum of 7–10 days

• Whichever method of infusion is employed, most patients will achieve normocalcaemia within 5 days

Other information

• Renal failure has been associated with IV use of biphosphonates. Smaller doses (up to 300 mg daily) over 2–3 hours are less likely to be associated with renal impairment than high doses by short IV infusion

• Reversible elevations of creatinine have been reported. Renal function should be monitored during treatment

• Orally: avoid food for one hour before and after treatment, particularly calcium-containing products; also avoid iron, mineral supplements and antacids

Clomethiazole (chlormethiazole)

Clinical use

Alcohol withdrawal; sedation; restlessness and agitation

Dose in normal renal function

• Alcohol withdrawal: 2–4 capsules stat then:

day 1: 3 capsules three or four times daily

day 2: 2 capsules three or four times daily

day 3: 1 capsule four times daily

Reduce over a further 4–6 days, give a total treatment of not more than 9 days

• Insomnia: 1–2 capsules at night

• Restlessness and agitation: 1 capsule three times daily

Pharmacokinetics

Molecular weight (daltons)	162
% Protein binding	65
% Excreted unchanged in urine	0.1–5
Volume of distribution (L/kg)	4–16
Half-life – normal/ESRF (hrs)	4–6/unchanged

Dose in renal impairment GFR (mL/min)

20–50	Dose as in normal renal function
10–20	Dose as in normal renal function
<10	Dose as in normal renal function

Dose in patients undergoing renal replacement therapies

CAPD	Unknown dialysability. Dose as in normal renal function
HD	Dialysed. Dose as in normal renal function
CAV/VVHD	Unknown dialysability. Dose as in normal renal function

Important drug interactions

POTENTIALLY HAZARDOUS INTERACTIONS WITH OTHER DRUGS

• Cimetidine: inhibits metabolism of clomethiazole

Administration

RECONSTITUTION

–

ROUTE

• Oral

RATE OF ADMINISTRATION

–

COMMENTS

• Syrup should be stored in a fridge

Other information

• Clomethiazole has a high hepatic extraction ratio

• Increased cerebral sensitivity in renal impairment

• Manufacturers recommend caution should be observed in patients with chronic renal disease

Clomipramine

Clinical use

Depressive illness, phobic and obsessional states;
adjunctive treatment of cataplexy associated with
narcolepsy

Dose in normal renal function

10–250 mg daily

Pharmacokinetics

Molecular weight (daltons)	351.3
% Protein binding	97
% Excreted unchanged in urine	–
Volume of distribution (L/kg)	12
Half-life – normal/ESRF (hrs)	19–37/–

Dose in renal impairment GFR (mL/min)

20–50	Dose as in normal renal function
10–20	Start at lower doses and monitor effect
<10	Start at lower doses and monitor effect

Dose in patients undergoing renal replacement therapies

CAPD	Not dialysed. Dose as in GFR = < 10 mL/min
HD	Not dialysed. Dose as in GFR = < 10 mL/min
CAV/VVHD	Not dialysed. Dose as in GFR = 10–20 mL/min

Important drug interactions

POTENTIALLY HAZARDOUS INTERACTIONS WITH
OTHER DRUGS

• Alcohol: enhanced sedative effect
• Anti-arrhythmics: increased risk of ventricular
arrhythmias with drugs which prolong QT
interval
• Anthypertensives: hypotensive effect enhanced,
antagonism of adrenergic neurone blockers and
clonidine
• Antipsychotics: increased risk of ventricular
arrhythmias
• Beta-blockers: increased risk of ventricular
arrhythmias with sotalol
• MAOIs: CNS excitation and hypertension –
tricyclics should not be started until 2 weeks
after stopping MAOI; MAOI should not be
started until at least 1 week after tricyclic has
stopped
• Anti-epileptics: convulsive threshold can be
lowered
• Antihistamines: increased risk of ventricular
arrhythmias with terfenadine
• Sibutramine: increased risk of CNS toxicity
• Sympathomimetics: hypertension and arrhythmias
reported

Administration

RECONSTITUTION

–

ROUTE

• Oral, IV, IM

RATE OF ADMINISTRATION

• Initially: infuse over 1.5–3 hours
• If satisfactory response: infusion duration may be
decreased to a minimum of 45 minutes

COMMENTS

• IV infusion: initially 25–50 mg in 200–500 mL
of sodium chloride 0.9% or glusose 5%. If
satisfactory response, increase dose, but volume
of infusion fluid may be reduced to a minimum of
125 mL
• IM injection: 25 mg increasing to maximum
150 mg daily
• Monitor blood pressure during the infusion as
hypotension may occur

Other information

• Normal doses have been used in dialysis patients
long-term, but caution as parent drug and active
metabolites may accumulate

Clonazepam

Clinical use

Benzodiazepine: anticonvulsant, anxiolytic

Dose in normal renal function

1–8 mg/day

Pharmacokinetics

Molecular weight (daltons)	315.7
% Protein binding	47–86
% Excreted unchanged in urine	<1
Volume of distribution (L/kg)	1.5–4.5
Half-life – normal/ESRF (hrs)	18–45/–

Dose in renal impairment GFR (mL/min)

20–50	Dose as in normal renal function
10–20	Dose as in normal renal function
<10	Dose as in normal renal function

Dose in patients undergoing renal replacement therapies

CAPD	Unknown dialysability. Dose as in normal renal function
HD	Not dialysed. Dose as in normal renal function
CAV/VVHD	Unknown dialysability. Dose as in normal renal function

Important drug interactions

POTENTIALLY HAZARDOUS INTERACTIONS WITH OTHER DRUGS

• None known

Administration

RECONSTITUTION

• IV bolus: add the contents of the diluent ampoule (1 mL water for injection) to the contents of the clonazepam ampoule (1 mg in 1 mL solvent)
• IV infusion: up to 3 mg (3 ampoules) added to 250 mL sodium chloride 0.9%, glucose 5%, glucose/sodium chloride 0.9%

ROUTE

• Oral, IV bolus or infusion

RATE OF ADMINISTRATION

• IV bolus: 1 mg over approximately 30 seconds

COMMENTS

• IV infusion of clonazepam is potentially hazardous (especially if prolonged), calling for close and constant observation and best carried out in specialist centres with ICU facilities. Risks include apnoea, hypotension and deep unconsciousness

Other information

• In long-term administration, active metabolites may accumulate and lower doses should be used
• Clonazepam is one of several agents which are used in restless leg syndrome and has also been tried in the management of intractable hiccup where chlorpromazine has failed

Clonidine

Clinical use

All grades of essential and secondary hypertension
Treatment of migraine

Dose in normal renal function

0.05–0.1 mg three times a day, increasing gradually
to 1.8 mg or more

Slow IV: 150–300 micrograms (maximum
750 micrograms in 24 hours)

Migraine: 50–75 micrograms twice daily

Pharmacokinetics

Molecular weight (daltons)	266
% Protein binding	20–40
% Excreted unchanged in urine	45
Volume of distribution (L/kg)	3–6
Half-life – normal/ESRF (hrs)	6–23/39–42

Dose in renal impairment
GFR (mL/min)

20–50	Dose as in normal renal function
10–20	Dose as in normal renal function
<10	Dose as in normal renal function

Dose in patients undergoing renal replacement therapies

CAPD	Not dialysed. Dose as in normal renal function
HD	Not dialysed. Dose as in normal renal function
CAV/VVHD	Unknown dialysability. Dose as in normal renal function

Important drug interactions

POTENTIALLY HAZARDOUS INTERACTIONS WITH
OTHER DRUGS

- Antidepressants: tricyclics antagonise hypotensive effect and also increase risk of hypertension on clonidine withdrawal
- Beta-adrenoreceptor antagonists: increased risk of hypertension on withdrawal

Administration

RECONSTITUTION

–

ROUTE

- Oral, IV

RATE OF ADMINISTRATION

–

COMMENTS

–

Other information

- Use in renal impairment: clonidine plasma concentrations for a given dose are 2–3 times higher in patients with severe renal impairment. However, blood pressure control appears satisfactory and adverse effects are not increased
- Clearance of clonidine by haemodialysis is not sufficient to require an additional post-dialysis dose
- Clonidine withdrawal: rebound hypertension if drug is abruptly withdrawn
- Tricyclic antidepressants may decrease efficacy

Clopidogrel

Clinical use

Antiplatelet, used for reduction of atherosclerotic events, and in non-ST segment elevation acute coronary syndrome (unstable angina or non-Q-wave myocardial infarction)

Dose in normal renal function

75 mg daily

Acute coronary syndrome: 300 mg loading dose then 75 mg daily (with aspirin 75–325 mg daily)

Pharmacokinetics

Molecular weight (daltons)	419.9
% Protein binding	98
% Excreted unchanged in urine	50
Volume of distribution (L/kg)	–
Half-life – normal/ESRF (hrs)	8/–

Dose in renal impairment GFR (mL/min)

20–50	Dose as in normal renal function
10–20	Dose as in normal renal function
<10	Dose as in normal renal function

Dose in patients undergoing renal replacement therapies

CAPD	Unlikely dialysability. Dose as in normal renal function
HD	Unlikely dialysability. Dose as in normal renal function
CAV/VVHD	Unlikely dialysability. Dose as in normal renal function

Important drug interactions

POTENTIALLY HAZARDOUS INTERACTIONS WITH OTHER DRUGS

• Warfarin: enhanced anticoagulant effect, manufacturer advises to avoid concomitant use

Administration

RECONSTITUTION

–

ROUTE

• Oral

RATE OF ADMINISTRATION

–

COMMENTS

–

Other information

• Due to limited therapeutic experience the manufacturer advises caution when using clopidogrel in patients with renal impairment

Co-amoxiclav (amoxicillin/clavulanic acid)

Clinical use

Antibacterial agent

Dose in normal renal function

For treatment of infections: IV – 1.2 g every
8 hours (increasing to every 6 hours in severe
infection); Oral – 375–625 mg three times daily

Pharmacokinetics

Molecular weight (daltons)	Amoxicillin: 365.4; clavulanic acid: 199.2
% Protein binding	Amoxicillin: 15–25; clavulanic acid: 22
% Excreted unchanged in urine	Amoxicillin: 50–70; clavulanic acid: 60
Volume of distribution (L/kg)	Amoxicillin: 0.26; clavulanic acid: 0.3
Half-life – normal/ESRF (hrs)	Amoxicillin: 0.9–2.3/5–20; clavulanic acid: 0.8–1.0

Dose in renal impairment
GFR (mL/min)

30–50	Dose as in normal renal function
10–30	IV: 1.2 g every 12 hours Oral: dose as in normal renal function
<10	IV: 1.2 g stat followed by 600 mg–1.2 g IV every 12 hours Oral: 375 mg three times daily

Dose in patients undergoing renal replacement therapies

CAPD	Dialysed. Dose as in GFR = <10 mL/min
HD	Dialysed. Dose as in GFR = <10 mL/min
CAV/VVHD	Dialysed. Dose as in GFR = 10–20 mL/min

Important drug interactions

POTENTIALLY HAZARDOUS INTERACTIONS WITH OTHER DRUGS

- Anticoagulants: effects of acenocoumarol and warfarin are potentially enhanced
- Oral contraceptives: potentially reduced efficacy
- Methotrexate: reduced excretion thereby increasing risk of toxicity

Administration

RECONSTITUTION

- IV: 600 mg with 10 mL water for injection; 1.2 g with 20 mL water for injection

ROUTE

- Oral, IV

RATE OF ADMINISTRATION

- IV bolus: over 3–4 minutes
- Infusion: infuse over 30–40 minutes in 100 mL sodium chloride 0.9%

COMMENTS

- IV preparation is less stable in infusion solutions containing glucose, dextran or bicarbonate. May be injected into drip tubing over period of 3–4 minutes
- Do not mix with aminoglycosides

Other information

- CSM has advised that cholestatic jaundice may occur if treatment exceeds a period of 14 days or up to 6 weeks after treatment has been stopped. The incidence of cholestatic jaundice occurring with co-amoxiclav is higher in males than in females and prevalent particularly in men over the age of 65 years
- The probability of co-amoxiclav-associated cholestatic jaundice is six times more common than with amoxicillin
- Each 1.2-g vial contains: sodium 3.1 mmol, potassium 1 mmol

Co-beneldopa (Madopar)

Clinical use

Treatment of parkinsonism

Dose in normal renal function

150–800 mg daily in divided doses after meals
(expressed as levodopa)

Pharmacokinetics

Molecular weight (daltons)	293.7 (benserazide), 197.2 (levodopa)
% Protein binding	None (benserazide), 5–8 (levodopa)
% Excreted unchanged in urine	None (benserazide), 11 (levodopa)
Volume of distribution (L/kg)	No data (benserazide), 0.9–1.6 (levodopa)
Half-life – normal/ESRF (hrs)	1.5 (benserazide), 1–3 (levodopa)

Dose in renal impairment GFR (mL/min)

20–50	Dose as in normal renal function
10–20	Dose as in normal renal function
<10	Dose as in normal renal function

Dose in patients undergoing renal replacement therapies

CAPD	Unknown dialysability. Dose as in normal renal function
HD	Unknown dialysability. Dose as in normal renal function
CAV/VVHD	Unknown dialysability. Dose as in normal renal function

Important drug interactions

POTENTIALLY HAZARDOUS INTERACTIONS WITH OTHER DRUGS

• Bupropion: increased risk of side-effects of levodopa
• Anaesthetics: risk of arrhythmias with volatile liquid anaesthetics such as halothane
• Antidepressants: hypertensive crisis with MAOIs and linezolid (including moclobemide) – avoid for at least 2 weeks after stopping MAOI
• Ferrous sulphate: reduces AUC of levodopa by 30–50%, clinically significant in some but not all patients

Administration

RECONSTITUTION

–

ROUTE

• Oral

RATE OF ADMINISTRATION

–

COMMENTS

–

Other information

• Can be used to treat restless legs syndrome
• Urine may be red-tinged and turn dark on standing, due to metabolites
• Serum uric acid and blood urea nitrogen levels are occasionally elevated

Co-careldopa (Sinemet)

Clinical use

Treatment of parkinsonism

Dose in normal renal function

75–200 mg carbidopa daily in divided doses after meals with 0.75–2 g levodopa (up to 800 mg with carbidopa)

Pharmacokinetics

Molecular weight (daltons)	244.2 (carbidopa), 197.2 (levodopa)
% Protein binding	36 (carbidopa), 5–8 (levodopa)
% Excreted unchanged in urine	30 (carbidopa), 11 (levodopa)
Volume of distribution (L/kg)	No data (carbidopa), 0.9–1.6 (levodopa)
Half-life – normal/ESRF (hrs)	2 (carbidopa), 1–3/unknown (levodopa)

Dose in renal impairment GFR (mL/min)

20–50	Dose as in normal renal function
10–20	Dose as in normal renal function
<10	Dose as in normal renal function

Dose in patients undergoing renal replacement therapies

CAPD	Unknown dialysability. Dose as in normal renal function
HD	Unknown dialysability. Dose as in normal renal function
CAV/VVHD	Unknown dialysability. Dose as in normal renal function

Important drug interactions

POTENTIALLY HAZARDOUS INTERACTIONS WITH OTHER DRUGS

- Bupropion: increased risk of side-effects of levodopa
- Anaesthetics: risk of arrhythmias with volatile liquid anaesthetics such as halothane
- Antidepressants: hypertensive crisis with MAOIs and linezolid (including moclobemide) – avoid for at least 2 weeks after stopping MAOI
- Ferrous sulphate: reduces AUC of levodopa by 30–50%, clinically significant in some but not all patients

Administration

RECONSTITUTION

–

ROUTE

- Oral

RATE OF ADMINISTRATION

–

COMMENTS

–

Other information

- Can be used to treat restless legs syndrome
- May cause dark urine

Co-codamol (paracetamol & codeine phosphate)

Clinical use

Analgesia

Dose in normal renal function

1–2 tablets up to four times a day

Pharmacokinetics

Molecular weight (daltons)	Paracetamol: 151; codeine: 299 (codeine phosphate mw = 406)
% Protein binding	Paracetamol: 20–30; codeine: 7
% Excreted unchanged in urine	Paracetamol: 1–4; codeine: <5
Volume of distribution (L/kg)	Paracetamol: 0.9–1.0; codeine: 3–4
Half-life – normal/ESRF (hrs)	Paracetamol: 2/unchanged; codeine: 2.5–3.5/–

Dose in renal impairment GFR (mL/min)

20–50	Dose as in normal renal function
10–20	75–100% of normal dose
<10	50–100% of normal dose

Dose in patients undergoing renal replacement therapies

CAPD	Unknown dialysability. Dose as in GFR = <10 mL/min
HD	Unknown dialysability. Dose as in GFR = <10 mL/min
CAV/VVHD	Unknown dialysability. Dose as in GFR = 10–20 mL/min

Important drug interactions

POTENTIALLY HAZARDOUS INTERACTIONS WITH OTHER DRUGS

• None known

Administration

RECONSTITUTION

–

ROUTE

• Oral

RATE OF ADMINISTRATION

–

COMMENTS

• Available in two strengths: (1) 8/500: 8 mg codeine phosphate/500 mg paracetamol; (2) 30/500: 30 mg codeine phosphate/ 500 mg paracetamol

• 30/500 formulation: may cause drowsiness, due to increased cerebral sensitivity in patients with renal failure

Other information

• Effervescent formulations of Solpadol and Tylex (30/500) should be avoided in renal impairment. They contain 18.6 mmol and 13.6 mmol sodium per tablet respectively

• Caution is recommended when giving paracetamol to patients with renal impairment. Plasma concentrations of the glucuronide and sulphate conjugates of paracetamol are increased in patients with moderate renal impairment and in patients on dialysis. Paracetamol itself may be regenerated from these metabolites

• In renal impairment, opioid analgesics may produce a prolonged effect with increased cerebral sensitivity

• Increased risk of constipation in ESRF especially with 30/500 preparation

Codeine

Clinical use

Analgesic, anti-diarrhoeal, cough suppressant

Dose in normal renal function

30–60 mg up to four times a day

Pharmacokinetics

Molecular weight (daltons)	Codeine: 299; codeine phosphate: 406
% Protein binding	7
% Excreted unchanged in urine	<5
Volume of distribution (L/kg)	3–4
Half-life – normal/ESRF (hrs)	2.5–3.5/–

Dose in renal impairment GFR (mL/min)

20–50	Dose as in normal renal function
10–20	75% of normal dose
<10	50% of normal dose

Dose in patients undergoing renal replacement therapies

CAPD	Unknown dialysability. Dose as in GFR = <10 mL/min
HD	Unknown dialysability. Dose as in GFR = <10 mL/min
CAV/VVHD	Unknown dialysability. Dose as in GFR = 10–20 mL/min

Important drug interactions

POTENTIALLY HAZARDOUS INTERACTIONS WITH OTHER DRUGS

• None known

Administration

RECONSTITUTION

–

ROUTE

• Oral, IV, IM, SC

RATE OF ADMINISTRATION

• IV bolus

COMMENTS

–

Other information

• Increased risk of drowsiness due to increased cerebral sensitivity in patients with renal failure
• Increased risk of constipation – care in patients on CAPD

Co-dydramol (paracetamol & dihydrocodeine)

Clinical use

Analgesia

Dose in normal renal function

1–2 tablets up to four times a day

Pharmacokinetics

Molecular weight (daltons)	Paracetamol: 151; dihydrocodeine: 452
% Protein binding	Paracetamol: 20–30; dihydrocodeine: –
% Excreted unchanged in urine	Paracetamol: 1–4; dihydrocodeine: 13–22
Volume of distribution (L/kg)	Paracetamol: 0.9–1.0; dihydrocodeine: 1.1
Half-life – normal/ESRF (hrs)	Paracetamol: 2/unchanged; dihydrocodeine: 3.4–4.5/6 +

Dose in renal impairment GFR (mL/min)

20–50	1–2 tablets every 6 hours
10–20	75–100% of dose every 6 hours
<10	50–100% of dose every 6–8 hours

Dose in patients undergoing renal replacement therapies

CAPD	Not dialysed. Dose as in GFR = <10 mL/min
HD	Not dialysed. Dose as in GFR = <10 mL/min
CAV/VVHD	Unknown dialysability. Dose as in GFR = 10–20 mL/min

Important drug interactions

POTENTIALLY HAZARDOUS INTERACTIONS WITH OTHER DRUGS

• None known

Administration

RECONSTITUTION

–

ROUTE

• Oral

RATE OF ADMINISTRATION

–

COMMENTS

–

Other information

• Active metabolites of dihydrocodeine accumulate in renal impairment (drowsiness/lightheadedness/constipation). Increased cerebral sensitivity in patients with renal failure

Colchicine

Clinical use

Acute gout. Short-term prophylaxis during initial therapy with allopurinol and uricosuric drugs

Dose in normal renal function

Acute: 1 mg then 0.5 mg every 2–3 hours until pain relieved or vomiting/diarrhoea occurs. Maximum of 6 mg per course. Do not repeat course within 3 days

Short-term prophylaxis: 500 micrograms 2–3 times per day

Pharmacokinetics

Molecular weight (daltons)	399
% Protein binding	30–50
% Excreted unchanged in urine	5–20
Volume of distribution (L/kg)	1–2
Half-life – normal/ESRF (hrs)	19/40

Dose in renal impairment GFR (mL/min)

20–50	Dose as in normal renal function
10–20	Dose as in normal renal function
<10	50% of normal dose

Dose in patients undergoing renal replacement therapies

CAPD	Unknown dialysability. Dose as in GFR = <10 mL/min
HD	Not dialysed. Dose as in GFR = <10 mL/min
CAV/VVHD	Unknown dialysability. Dose as in GFR = 10–20 mL/min

Important drug interactions

POTENTIALLY HAZARDOUS INTERACTIONS WITH OTHER DRUGS

• Ciclosporin: risk of myopathy or rhabdomyolysis, also increased blood-ciclosporin concentrations and nephrotoxicity

Administration

RECONSTITUTION

–

ROUTE

• Oral

RATE OF ADMINISTRATION

–

COMMENTS

–

Other information

• If nausea, vomiting or diarrhoea occur, stop therapy
• In ESRD colchicine can be administered concurrently with allopurinol, but seek specialist advice

Colestipol

Clinical use

Hyperlipidaemias, particularly type IIa

Dose in normal renal function

5 g once or twice daily, increased if necessary at intervals of 1–2 months, to a maximum of 30 g daily

Pharmacokinetics

Molecular weight (daltons)	–
% Protein binding	0
% Excreted unchanged in urine	0
Volume of distribution (L/kg)	Not absorbed
Half-life – normal/ESRF (hrs)	Not absorbed

Dose in renal impairment GFR (mL/min)

20–50	Dose as in normal renal function
10–20	Dose as in normal renal function
<10	Dose as in normal renal function

Dose in patients undergoing renal replacement therapies

CAPD	Not dialysed. Dose as in normal renal function
HD	Not dialysed. Dose as in normal renal function
CAV/VVHD	Not dialysed. Dose as in normal renal function

Important drug interactions

POTENTIALLY HAZARDOUS INTERACTIONS WITH OTHER DRUGS

• Anticoagulants: may enhance *or* reduce effects of acenocoumarol, phenindione, warfarin

• Ciclosporin: no reports of an interaction. However, ciclosporin levels should be carefully monitored if colestipol and ciclosporin are prescribed concurrently, as colestipol may interfere with ciclosporin absorption

Administration

RECONSTITUTION

–

ROUTE

• Oral

RATE OF ADMINISTRATION

–

COMMENTS

• Other drugs should be taken at least 1 hour before or 4–6 hours after colestipol to reduce possible interference with absorption

• Colestipol granules may be administered as a suspension in water or a flavoured vehicle

• Colestipol orange contains 32.5 mg aspartame (18.2 mg phenylalanine) per sachet

Other information

• Colestipol may interfere with the absorption of fat soluble vitamins

Colestyramine (cholestyramine)

Clinical use

Hyperlipidaemias, pruritis associated with partial biliary obstruction and primary biliary cirrhosis, diarrhoeal disorders

Dose in normal renal function

• Lipid reduction: 12–24 g daily (in single or up to four divided doses). Maximum 36 g daily
• Pruritis: 4–8 g daily
• Diarrhoeal disorders: 12–24 g daily. Maximum 36 g daily

Pharmacokinetics

Molecular weight (daltons)	–
% Protein binding	0
% Excreted unchanged in urine	0
Volume of distribution (L/kg)	Not absorbed
Half-life – normal/ESRF (hrs)	Not absorbed

Dose in renal impairment GFR (mL/min)

20–50	Dose as in normal renal function
10–20	Dose as in normal renal function
<10	Dose as in normal renal function

Dose in patients undergoing renal replacement therapies

CAPD	Not dialysed. Dose as in normal renal function
HD	Not dialysed. Dose as in normal renal function
CAV/VVHD	Not dialysed. Dose as in normal renal function

Important drug interactions

POTENTIALLY HAZARDOUS INTERACTIONS WITH OTHER DRUGS

• Anticoagulants: effect of acenocoumarol, phenindione and warfarin may be enhanced or reduced
• Valproate, cardiac glycosides, MMF: absorption reduced

Administration

RECONSTITUTION

• Mix with water, or a suitable liquid such as fruit juice, and stir to a uniform consistency
• May also be mixed with skimmed milk, thin soups, apple sauce, etc

ROUTE

• Oral

RATE OF ADMINISTRATION

–

COMMENTS

• Do not take in dry form
• Administer other drugs at least 1 hour before or 4–6 hours after colestyramine
• Prepare powder immediately prior to administration

Other information

• Hyperchloraemic acidosis occasionally reported on prolonged use of colestyramine
• On chronic use, an increased bleeding tendency may occur associated with vitamin K deficiency

Co-proxamol (paracetamol & dextropropoxyphene)

Clinical use

Analgesia

Dose in normal renal function

1–2 tablets, three or four times daily. Maximum 8 tablets daily

Pharmacokinetics

Molecular weight (daltons)	Paracetamol: 151 Dextropropoxyphene HCl: 376
% Protein binding	Paracetamol: 20–30 Dextropropoxyphene HCl: 80
% Excreted unchanged in urine	Paracetamol: 1–4 Dextropropoxyphene HCl: 1
Volume of distribution (L/kg)	Paracetamol: 0.9–1 Dextropropoxyphene HCl: ~16
Half-life – normal/ESRF (hrs)	Paracetamol: 2/unchanged Dextropropoxyphene HCl: 6–12/–

Dose in renal impairment GFR (mL/min)

20–50	Dose as in normal renal function
10–20	75–100% of normal dose
<10	50–100% of normal dose

Dose in patients undergoing renal replacement therapies

CAPD	Unknown dialysability. Dose as in GFR = <10 mL/min
HD	Unknown dialysability. Dose as in GFR = <10 mL/min
CAV/VVHD	Unknown dialysability. Dose as in GFR = 10–20 mL/min

Important drug interactions

POTENTIALLY HAZARDOUS INTERACTIONS WITH OTHER DRUGS

• None known

Administration

RECONSTITUTION

–

ROUTE

• Oral

RATE OF ADMINISTRATION

–

COMMENTS

• May cause drowsiness – increased cerebral sensitivity in patients with renal failure

Other information

• Caution is recommended when giving paracetamol to patients with renal impairment. Plasma concentrations of the glucuronide and sulphate conjugates of paracetamol are increased in patients with moderate renal impairment and in patients on dialysis

• In renal impairment, opioid analgesics may produce a prolonged effect with increased cerebral sensitivity

• The elimination of the drug is prolonged and plasma concentrations are increased so that adjustment of the dose may be necessary

Cortisone acetate

Clinical use

Glucocorticoid replacement in adrenocortical insufficiency

Dose in normal renal function

25–37.5 mg daily in divided doses

Pharmacokinetics

Molecular weight (daltons)	402.5
% Protein binding	90–95
% Excreted unchanged in urine	0
Volume of distribution (L/kg)	0.3
Half-life – normal/ESRF (hrs)	0.5–2/3.5

Dose in renal impairment GFR (mL/min)

20–50	Dose as in normal renal function
10–20	Dose as in normal renal function
<10	Dose as in normal renal function

Dose in patients undergoing renal replacement therapies

CAPD	Not dialysed. Dose as in normal renal function
HD	Not dialysed. Dose as in normal renal function
CAV/VVHD	Unknown dialysability. Dose as in normal renal function

Important drug interactions

POTENTIALLY HAZARDOUS INTERACTIONS WITH OTHER DRUGS

• Anticoagulants: anticoagulant effect of acenocoumarol and warfarin possibly altered
• Rifamycins accelerate metabolism of corticosteroids
• Anti-epileptics: carbamazepine, phenobarbital, phenytoin and primidone accelerate metabolism of corticosteroids
• Increased risk of hypokalaemia with amphotericin

Administration

RECONSTITUTION
–

ROUTE
• Oral

RATE OF ADMINISTRATION
–

COMMENTS
–

Other information

• Treatment of adrenocortical insufficiency with hydrocortisone is now generally preferred since cortisone itself is inactive and must be converted by the liver to hydrocortisone, its active metabolite, and hence, in some liver disorders, its bioavailability is less reliable
• Mineralocorticoid activity is usually supplemented by fludrocortisone acetate by mouth
• Cortisone acetate has been used in the treatment of many allergic and inflammatory disorders, but prednisolone or other synthetic glucocorticoids are generally preferred because of their reduced sodium-retaining properties

Co-trimoxazole (trimethoprim & sulfamethoxazole)

Clinical use

Antibacterial agent for treatment and prophylaxis of *Pneumocystis carinii* pneumonitis (PCP); acute exacerbations of chronic bronchitis and urinary tract infections (UTIs) on microbiological advice

Dose in normal renal function

PCP: 120 mg/kg in 2–4 divided doses

Oral prophylaxis: 480–960 mg daily or 960 mg on alternate days

Acute exacerbations of chronic bronchitis and UTIs on microbiological advice:

IV: 960 mg – 1.44 g of co-trimoxazole twice a day

Oral: 960 mg of co-trimoxazole twice a day

Pharmacokinetics

Molecular weight (daltons)	Sulfamethoxazole: 253 Trimethoprim: 290
% Protein binding	Sulfamethoxazole: 50 Trimethoprim: 30–70
% Excreted unchanged in urine	Sulfamethoxazole: 70 Trimethoprim: 40–70
Volume of distribution (L/kg)	Sulfamethoxazole 0.28–0.38 (altered in uraemia) Trimethoprim: 1–2.2
Half-life – normal/ESRF (hrs)	Sulfamethoxazole: 10/20–50 Trimethoprim: 9–13/20–49

Dose in renal impairment GFR (mL/min)

30–50	Dose as in normal renal function
15–30	60 mg/kg twice daily for 3 days then 30 mg/kg twice daily (PCP); or 50% of dose
<15	30 mg/kg twice daily (PCP); or 50% of dose (This should only be given if haemodialysis facilities are available)

Dose in patients undergoing renal replacement therapies

CAPD	Not dialysed. Dose as in GFR = <15 mL/min
HD	Dialysed. Dose as in GFR = <15 mL/min
CAV/VVHD	Dialysed. Dose as in GFR = 15–30 mL/min

Important drug interactions

POTENTIALLY HAZARDOUS INTERACTIONS WITH OTHER DRUGS

- Anticoagulants: effect of warfarin enhanced
- Antidiabetics: effect of sulphonylureas enhanced
- Anti-epileptics: antifolate effect and plasma concentration of phenytoin increased
- Anti-malarials: increased risk of antifolate effect with pyrimethamine
- Ciclosporin: increased risk of nephrotoxicity. No significant changes in ciclosporin levels
- Cytotoxics: increased risk of haematological toxicity with azathioprine and mercaptopurine. Antifolate effect of methotrexate increased

Administration

RECONSTITUTION

–

ROUTE

- IV, oral

RATE OF ADMINISTRATION

- Over 30 minutes – 1½ hours centrally (or 2–3 hours for high doses) (unlicensed)

COMMENTS

- For an IV infusion dilute 5 mL co-trimoxazole strong solution with 125 mL sodium chloride 0.9% or glucose 5% and infuse over 1½ hours
- Alternatively, dilute 5 mL to 75 mL glucose 5% and administer over 1 hour
- Can infuse undiluted solution via central line (unlicensed)

Other information

- Alternative dosing for acute exacerbations of chronic bronchitis and UTIs on microbiological advice only not PCP
- After 2–3 days plasma samples collected 12 hours post dose should have levels of sulfamethoxazole not higher than 150 micrograms/mL. If higher, stop treatment until levels fall below 120 micrograms/mL
- Plasma levels of trimethoprim should be 5 micrograms/mL or higher for optimum efficacy for PCP
- Folic acid supplementation may be necessary during chronic therapy
- Monthly blood counts advisable

Cyclizine

Clinical use

Nausea, vomiting, vertigo, motion sickness, labyrinthine disorders

Dose in normal renal function

50 mg up to three times daily

Pharmacokinetics

Molecular weight (daltons)	266
% Protein binding	–
% Excreted unchanged in urine	<1
Volume of distribution (L/kg)	–
Half-life – normal/ESRF (hrs)	20/–

Dose in renal impairment GFR (mL/min)

20–50	Dose as in normal renal function
10–20	Dose as in normal renal function
<10	Dose as in normal renal function

Dose in patients undergoing renal replacement therapies

CAPD	Unknown dialysability. Dose as in normal renal function
HD	Unknown dialysability. Dose as in normal renal function
CAV/VVHD	Unknown dialysability. Dose as in normal renal function

Important drug interactions

POTENTIALLY HAZARDOUS INTERACTIONS WITH OTHER DRUGS

• Other antihistamines: concomitant use of terfenadine and mizolastine not recommended – increased risk of hazardous arrhythmias

Administration

RECONSTITUTION

–

ROUTE

• IV, IM, oral

RATE OF ADMINISTRATION

• Slow IV

COMMENTS

• Increased cerebral sensitivity in patients with renal failure

Other information

–

Cyclophosphamide

Clinical use

Antineoplastic agent. (1) Immunosuppression of autoimmune diseases. (2) Treatment of malignant disease

Dose in normal renal function

1 Oral (for autoimmune disease): 1–5 mg/kg/day
IV: usually 0.5–1 g/m² repeated at intervals, e.g. monthly (pulse therapy)
2 50–250 mg/m² daily

Pharmacokinetics

Molecular weight (daltons)	279
% Protein binding	Parent drug 13: alkylating metabolites 50–60
% Excreted unchanged in urine	10–15
Volume of distribution (L/kg)	0.62
Half-life – normal/ESRF (hrs)	4–7.5/10

Dose in renal impairment GFR (mL/min)

20–50	Dose as in normal renal function
10–20	75–100% of normal dose
<10	50–75% of normal dose

Dose in patients undergoing renal replacement therapies

CAPD	Dialysed. Dose as in GFR = <10 mL/min. Following dose do not perform CAPD exchange for 12 hours
HD	Dialysed. Dose as in GFR = <10 mL/min. Dose at minimum of 12 hours before HD session
CAV/VVHD	Dialysed. Dose as in GFR = 10–20 mL/min

Important drug interactions

POTENTIALLY HAZARDOUS INTERACTIONS WITH OTHER DRUGS

• Other cytotoxics: increased toxicity with high-dose cyclophosphamide and pentostatin – avoid concomitant use

Administration

RECONSTITUTION

• Add 5 mL water for injection to each 100 mg
• (sodium chloride 0.9% for Endoxana)

ROUTE

• Oral, IV

RATE OF ADMINISTRATION

• Directly into vein over 2–3 minutes, or directly into tubing of fast-running IV infusion with patient supine

COMMENTS

• IV route occasionally used for pulse therapy. Can be administered as an IV infusion

Other information

• Patients receiving chronic indefinite therapy may be at increased risk of developing urothelial carcinoma
• If patient is anuric and on dialysis, neither the cyclophosphamide nor its metabolites nor mesna should appear in the urinary tract. The use of mesna may therefore be unnecessary, although this would be a clinical decision
• If the patient is still passing urine, mesna should be given to prevent urothelial toxicity

Cycloserine

Clinical use

Antibacterial agent: treatment of active pulmonary or extra-pulmonary tuberculosis

Dose in normal renal function

Initially 250 mg every 12 hours for 2 weeks, increased according to blood concentration and response to maximum 500 mg every 12 hours

Pharmacokinetics

Molecular weight (daltons)	102
% Protein binding	<20
% Excreted unchanged in urine	60–70
Volume of distribution (L/kg)	0.11–0.26
Half-life – normal/ESRF (hrs)	10/–

Dose in renal impairment GFR (mL/min)

20–50	250–500 mg every 12–24 hours. Monitor blood levels weekly
10–20	250–500 mg every 12–24 hours. Monitor blood levels weekly
<10	250 mg every 24 hours. Monitor blood levels weekly

Dose in patients undergoing renal replacement therapies

CAPD	Unknown dialysability. Dose as in GFR = <10 mL/min
HD	Dialysed. Dose as in GFR = <10 mL/min
CAV/VVHD	Likely to be dialysed. Dose as in GFR = 10–20 mL/min

Important drug interactions

POTENTIALLY HAZARDOUS INTERACTIONS WITH OTHER DRUGS

• Increased plasma concentration of phenytoin – risk of toxicity
• Alcohol: increased risk of seizures

Administration

RECONSTITUTION

–

ROUTE

• Oral

RATE OF ADMINISTRATION

–

COMMENTS

• May cause drowsiness – increased cerebral sensitivity in patients with renal impairment
• Blood concentration monitoring is required especially in renal impairment, if dose exceeds 500 mg daily, or if signs of toxicity. Blood concentration should not exceed 30 mg/L
• Contra-indicated in severe renal insufficiency

Other information

• Can cause CNS toxicity
• Pyridoxine has been used in an attempt to treat or prevent neurological reactions, but its value is unproven

Cyproterone acetate

Clinical use

(1) Control of libido in severe hypersexuality and sexual deviation in adult male. (2) Management of patients with prostatic cancer (LHRH 'flare', palliative treatment, hot flushes)

Dose in normal renal function

(1) Control of hypersexuality: 50 mg twice daily
(2) Prostatic cancer: 200–300 mg/day

Pharmacokinetics

Molecular weight (daltons)	417
% Protein binding	–
% Excreted unchanged in urine	<1
Volume of distribution (L/kg)	10–30
Half-life – normal/ESRF (hrs)	38/–

Dose in renal impairment GFR (mL/min)

20–50	Dose as in normal renal function
10–20	Dose as in normal renal function
<10	Dose as in normal renal function

Dose in patients undergoing renal replacement therapies

CAPD	Unknown dialysability. Dose as in normal renal function
HD	Unknown dialysability. Dose as in normal renal function
CAV/VVHD	Unknown dialysability. Dose as in normal renal function

Important drug interactions

POTENTIALLY HAZARDOUS INTERACTIONS WITH OTHER DRUGS

• None known

Administration

RECONSTITUTION

–

ROUTE

• Oral

RATE OF ADMINISTRATION

–

COMMENTS

• May cause drowsiness – increased CNS sensitivity in patients with renal impairment

Other information

• The CSM has advised that in view of the hepatotoxicity associated with long-term doses of 300 mg daily, the use of cyproterone acetate in prostatic cancer should be restricted to short courses to cover testosterone flare associated with gonadorelin analogues, treatment of hot flushes after orchidectomy or gonadorelin analogues and for patients who have not responded to (or are intolerant of) other treatments

• Direct hepatic toxicity including jaundice, hepatitis and hepatic failure have been reported. LFTs should be performed before treatment and whenever symptoms suggestive of hepatotoxicity occur

Cytarabine

Clinical use

Antineoplastic agent: acute leukaemias

Dose in normal renal function

'High-dose infusional therapy': 1–3 g/m²
every 12 hours for up to 6 days
'Low-dose (conventional) therapy': 100 mg/m²

Pharmacokinetics

Molecular weight (daltons)	243
% Protein binding	13
% Excreted unchanged in urine	6
Volume of distribution (L/kg)	2.6
Half-life – normal/ESRF (hrs)	0.5–3/unchanged

Dose in renal impairment GFR (mL/min)

20–50   100% of conventional low-dose regimen. For high dose, see 'Other information'

10–20   100% of conventional low-dose regimen. For high dose, see 'Other information'

<10   100% of conventional low-dose regimen. for high dose, see 'Other information'

Dose in patients undergoing renal replacement therapies

CAPD   Not dialysed. Dose as in GFR = <10 mL/min

HD   Not dialysed. Dose as in GFR = <10 mL/min

CAV/VVHD   Unknown dialysability. Dose as in GFR = <10 mL/min

Important drug interactions

POTENTIALLY HAZARDOUS INTERACTIONS WITH OTHER DRUGS

• None known

Administration

RECONSTITUTION

• Reconstitute/dilute with water for injection BP, glucose 5%, sodium chloride 0.9%

ROUTE

• Cytarabine injection (Faulding) only: IV infusion, IV injection, IM, SC, (20 mg/mL available for intrathecal use)
• Cytosar: IV infusion, IV injection, SC

RATE OF ADMINISTRATION

• IV injection: rapid
• IV infusion: infuse over 1–24 hours (1 hour is adequate for high dose)

COMMENTS

• Cytarabine injection (Faulding): administered intrathecally for leukaemic meningitis in doses up to 10–30 mg/m² three times a week
• As a rule, patients have been seen to tolerate higher doses when given by rapid IV injection as compared with slow infusion. This difference is due to the rapid metabolism of cytarabine and the consequent short duration of action of the high dose

Other information

Elevated baseline serum creatinine (>1.2 mg/dl) was an independent risk factor for the development of neurotoxicity during treatment with high-dose cytarabine. Furthermore, retrospective analysis implicates impaired renal function as an independent risk factor for high-dose cytarabine-induced cerebral and cerebellar toxicity. The incidence of neurotoxicity was 86–100% following administration of high-dose cytarabine to patients with CL_{CR} <40 mL/min and 60–76% following administration to patients with CL_{CR} <60 mL/min. In contrast, when patients with CL_{CR} >60 mL/min received high-dose cytarabine, the incidence of neurotoxicity was found to be 8%, which correlates with the overall incidence of this adverse effect. Accordingly, it has been suggested that high-dose cytarabine should be used with caution in patients with impaired renal function. For CL_{CR} of 30–45 mL/min, 50% of normal cytarabine dose should be prescribed and for CL_{CR} of 45–60 mL/min, 60% of normal cytarabine dose (high-dose regimen) should be prescribed. High-dose cytarabine should be avoided for CL_{CR} = 30 mL/min or less

Cytomegalovirus (CMV) human immunoglobulin (unlicensed product)

Clinical use

Prophylaxis for renal transplant recipients at risk of primary cytomegalovirus (CMV) disease. Treatment of CMV disease (usually with ganciclovir)

Dose in normal renal function

See local protocols

Pharmacokinetics

Molecular weight (daltons)	150
% Protein binding	N/A
% Excreted unchanged in urine	0
Volume of distribution (L/kg)	1
Half-life – normal/ESRF (hrs)	50

Dose in renal impairment GFR (mL/min)

20–50	Dose as in normal renal function
10–20	Dose as in normal renal function
<10	Dose as in normal renal function

Dose in patients undergoing renal replacement therapies

CAPD	Not dialysed. Dose as in normal renal function
HD	Not dialysed. Dose as in normal renal function
CAV/VVHD	Not dialysed. Dose as in normal renal function

Important drug interactions

POTENTIALLY HAZARDOUS INTERACTIONS WITH OTHER DRUGS

• Ciclosporin: no effect on efficacy of CMV immunoglobulin

Administration

RECONSTITUTION

–

ROUTE

• IV peripherally or centrally

RATE OF ADMINISTRATION

–

COMMENTS

• Follow guidelines supplied by company

Other information

• Can give 10 mg IV chlorphenamine 1 hour before administration

• Monitor for anaphylaxis, have adrenaline available

• Do not mix with any other drugs or infusion fluids

Daclizumab

Clinical use

Humanised murine/human monoclonal anti-CD25
antibody for prophylaxis of acute allograft
rejection, in combination with maintenance
immunosuppressants

Dose in normal renal function

1 mg/kg within 24 hours of transplantation, then
1 mg/kg every 14 days for five doses

Pharmacokinetics

Molecular weight (daltons)	Large
% Protein binding	–
% Excreted unchanged in urine	–
Volume of distribution (L/kg)	5.3 litres
Half-life – normal/ESRF (hrs)	270–919

Dose in renal impairment
GFR (mL/min)

20–50	Dose as in normal renal function
10–20	Dose as in normal renal function
<10	Dose as in normal renal function

Dose in patients undergoing renal replacement therapies

CAPD	Not dialysed. Dose as in normal renal function
HD	Not dialysed. Dose as in normal renal function
CAV/VVHD	Unlikely dialysability. Dose as in normal renal function

Important drug interactions

POTENTIALLY HAZARDOUS INTERACTIONS WITH
OTHER DRUGS

• None known

Administration

RECONSTITUTION

–

ROUTE

• IV infusion

RATE OF ADMINISTRATION

• Over 15 minutes

COMMENTS

• Add required dose to 50 mL of sodium chloride
0.9%

• Stable for 24 hours at 2–8 °C if prepared
aseptically

Other information

–

Dalteparin sodium (LMWH)

Clinical use

1 Peri and post-operative surgical thromboprophylaxis

2 Prevention of thrombus formation in extra-corporeal circulation during HD

3 Treatment of DVT

4 Unstable coronary artery disease

Dose in normal renal function

Dose according to risk of thrombosis:

Moderate risk: 2500 IU (antifactor Xa) SC 1–2 hours prior to surgery, thereafter 2500 IU SC daily for 5 days

High risk: 2500 IU (antifactor Xa) SC 1–2 hours prior surgery, 2500 IU 12 hours later, thereafter 5000 IU SC daily for 5 days

Treatment of DVT: 200 units/kg (maximum 18,000 units as a single dose) or 100 units/kg twice daily

Unstable coronary artery disease: 120 units/kg every 12 hours (maximum 10,000 units twice daily) for 5–8 days

Pharmacokinetics

Molecular weight (daltons)	Average mw = 4000–6000
% Protein binding	–
% Excreted unchanged in urine	–
Volume of distribution (L/kg)	0.06–0.13
Half-life – normal/ESRF (hrs)	3.8/prolonged

Dose in renal impairment GFR (mL/min)

20–50	Dose as in normal renal function
10–20	Dose as in normal renal function only for prophylaxis doses – see 'Other information'
<10	Dose as in normal renal function only for prophylaxis doses – see 'Other information'

Dose in patients undergoing renal replacement therapies

CAPD	Not dialysed. Dose as in GFR < 10 mL/min
HD	Not dialysed. Dose as in GFR < 10 mL/min
CAV/VVHD	Not dialysed. Dose as in GFR = 10–20 mL/min

Important drug interactions

POTENTIALLY HAZARDOUS INTERACTIONS WITH OTHER DRUGS

• Anticoagulant/antiplatelet agents, e.g. aspirin, dextran, warfarin, may enhance effects of dalteparin

• Increased risk of haemorrhage with ketorolac

• Nitrates: GTN infusion increases excretion

Administration

RECONSTITUTION

–

ROUTE

• SC injection into abdominal wall (pre-filled syringes)

• IV bolus/infusion (ampoules)

RATE OF ADMINISTRATION

–

COMMENTS

• Dalteparin solution for injection (ampoules) is compatible with sodium chloride 0.9% and glucose 5%

Other information

• Dalteparin is also indicated for prevention of clotting in the extra-corporeal circulation during haemodialysis or haemofiltration

• Dose for >4-hour session: IV bolus of 30–40 IU (antifactor Xa) per kg body-weight, followed by infusion of 10–15 IU/kg/hour. Dose for <4-hour session: as above or single IV bolus injection of 5000 IU

• Antifactor Xa levels should be regularly monitored in new patients on haemodialysis during the first weeks, later less frequent monitoring is generally required. Consult manufacturer's literature

- Low molecular weight heparins are renally excreted and hence accumulate in severe renal impairment. While the doses recommended for prophylaxis against DVT and prevention of thrombus formation in extra-corporeal circuits are well tolerated in patients with ESRF, the doses recommended for treatment of DVT and PE have been associated with severe, sometimes fatal, bleeding episodes in such patients. Hence the use of unfractionated heparin would be preferable in these instances

- Bleeding may be provoked especially at high doses corresponding with antifactor Xa levels greater than 1.5 IU/mL

- The prolongation of the APTT induced by dalteparin is fully neutralised by protamine, but the anti-Xa activity is only neutralised to about 25–50%

- 1 mg of protamine inhibits the effect of 100 IU (antifactor Xa) of dalteparin

- Heparin can suppress adrenal secretion of aldosterone leading to hypercalcaemia, particularly in patients with chronic renal impairment and diabetes mellitis

Danaparoid (unlicensed preparation)

Clinical use

Prophylaxis of DVT and PE, thromboembolic disease requiring parenteral anticoagulation in patients with heparin-induced thrombocytopenia (HIT). Anticoagulation for haemodialysis

Dose in normal renal function

DVT and PE: 750 units twice daily for 7–10 days (SC)

HIT: 2500 units IV bolus (BWt <55 kg: 1250 units, >90 kg: 3750 units) then an infusion of 400 units/hour for 2 hours, 300 units/hour for 2 hours then 200 units/hour for 5 days

Monitor anti-Xa activity in patients >90 kg and with renal impairment

Pharmacokinetics

Molecular weight (daltons)	Approx 5500
% Protein binding	–
% Excreted unchanged in urine	40–50
Volume of distribution (L/kg)	8–9
Half-life – normal/ESRF (hrs)	18–28/>31

Dose in renal impairment GFR (mL/min)

20–50	Dose as in normal renal function
10–20	Use with caution
<10	Use with caution – reduce second and subsequent doses

Dose in patients undergoing renal replacement therapies

CAPD	Not dialysed. Dose as in GFR = <10 ml/min
HD	Not dialysed. Dose as in GFR = <10 ml/min
CAV/VVHD	Not dialysed. Dose as in GFR = 10–20 ml/min

Important drug interactions

POTENTIALLY HAZARDOUS INTERACTIONS WITH OTHER DRUGS

• Enhances effects of oral anticoagulants
• Interferes with laboratory monitoring of prothrombin time – monitor anticoagulation closely

Administration

RECONSTITUTION

• Glucose 5% or sodium chloride 0.9%

ROUTE

• SC, IV

RATE OF ADMINISTRATION

• See dose

COMMENTS

–

Other information

Can also be used for haemodialysis anticoagulation:

• 2/3 times a week dialysis:

First and second dialysis: 3750 units IV bolus prior to dialysis. (If patient weighs <55 kg then give 2500 unit IV bolus.)

Subsequent dialysis: 3000 units by IV bolus prior to dialysis, provided there are no fibrin threads in the bubble chamber. (If patient weighs <55 kg then give 2000 unit IV bolus.)

• Daily dialysis:

1st dialysis: 3750 units IV bolus prior to dialysis (if patient <55 kg give 2500 units).

2nd dialysis: 2500 units IV bolus prior to dialysis (if patient <55 kg give 2000 units).

Prior to the second and subsequent dialysis a specimen should be drawn for plasma anti-Xa levels (to be used for dosing a third and subsequent dialysis).

Expected pre-dialysis ranges of anti-Xa levels:

1 If plasma anti-Xa levels are <0.3 U/mL then third or subsequent dialysis dose should be 3000 units. For patients weighing <55 kg use 2000 units.

2 If plasma anti-Xa levels are 0.3–0.35 U/mL then third or subsequent dialysis dose should be 2500 units. For patients weighing <55 kg use 1500 units.

3 If plasma anti-Xa levels are 0.35–0.4 U/mL then third or subsequent dialysis dose should be 2000 units. For patients weighing <55 kg use 1500 units.

4 If plasma anti-Xa levels are >0.4 U/mL then do not give any danaparoid before dialysis. However, if fibrin threads form in the bubble chamber, then

the patient may be given 1500 units by IV bolus (irrespective of the patient's weight).

- During dialysis the plasma anti-Xa level should be between 0.5–0.8 U/mL

- If needed take a blood sample prior to every dialysis and during dialysis (at 30 minutes and at 4 hours)

- Available from BS Durban

- Information from Organon: protamine is no use as an antidote for bleeding complications.

If no anti-Xa monitoring is available then the first four dialysis sessions should have pre-dialysis IV bolus of 3750, 3750, 3000 and 2500 units respectively, then 2500 units thereafter. Take blood sample prior to 4th and 7th dialysis to ensure there is no accumulation

- Oozing from puncture sites has been noted 24–36 hours post dose

Dapsone

Clinical use

Treatment and prophylaxis of leprosy, dermatitis herpetiformis, PCP, malaria prophylaxis

Dose in normal renal function

Leprosy: 1–2 mg/kg or 100 mg daily

PCP: 100 mg daily in one or two divided doses

Dermatitis herpetiformis: 50–300 mg daily

Malaria prophylaxis: 100 mg weekly in combination with pyrimethamine 12.5 mg weekly

Pharmacokinetics

Molecular weight (daltons)	248.3
% Protein binding	50–80
% Excreted unchanged in urine	20
Volume of distribution (L/kg)	No data
Half-life – normal/ESRF (hrs)	10–50

Dose in renal impairment GFR (mL/min)

20–50	Dose as in normal renal function
10–20	Dose as in normal renal function, use with caution
<10	50–100 mg daily, use with caution. No dose reduction is required for malaria prophylaxis. See 'Other information'

Dose in patients undergoing renal replacement therapies

CAPD	Likely to be dialysed. Dose as in GFR < 10 mL/min
HD	Dialysed. Dose as in GFR < 10 mL/m
CAV/VVHD	Likely to be dialysed. Dose as in GFR = 10–20 mL/min

Important drug interactions

POTENTIALLY HAZARDOUS INTERACTIONS WITH OTHER DRUGS

• None known

Administration

RECONSTITUTION

–

ROUTE

• Oral

RATE OF ADMINISTRATION

–

COMMENTS

–

Other information

• Greater risk of haemolytic side-effects in patients with G-6-PD deficiency

• Regular blood counts are recommended in patients with severe anaemia or renal impairment, weekly for the first month then monthly for 6 months and then semi-annually

• Almost all patients lose 1–2 g of haemoglobin

• The dose for herpetiformis can be reduced if the patient is on a gluten-free diet

• One study used dapsone in a haemodialysis patient for bullous dermatosis, they initiated therapy at 100 mg but had to reduce the dose to 50 mg due to haemolytic effects. (*Int J Dermatol.* (2002) **41**(11): 778–80)

Darbepoetin alfa

Clinical use

Treatment of anaemia associated with chronic renal failure, and adult cancer patients with non-haematological malignancies receiving chemotherapy

Dose in normal renal function

Renal failure: 0.45 micrograms/kg once a week, dose is adjusted by 25% every 4 weeks according to response

May sometimes be given fortnightly once patients have been stabilised

Cancer: 2.25 micrograms/kg once a week, adjust doses by 50% every 4 weeks according to response

Pharmacokinetics

Molecular weight (daltons)	38,000
% Protein binding	–
% Excreted unchanged in urine	–
Volume of distribution (L/kg)	0.05
Half-life – normal/ESRF (hrs)	21 (IV), 49 (SC)/unchanged

Dose in renal impairment
GFR (mL/min)

20–50	Dose as in normal renal function
10–20	Dose as in normal renal function
<10	Dose as in normal renal function

Dose in patients undergoing renal replacement therapies

CAPD	Not dialysed. Dose as in normal renal function
HD	Not dialysed. Dose as in normal renal function
CAV/VVHD	Not dialysed. Dose as in normal renal function

Important drug interactions

POTENTIALLY HAZARDOUS INTERACTIONS WITH OTHER DRUGS

• Ciclosporin and tacrolimus: monitor ciclosporin and tacrolimus levels, since these drugs are bound to red blood cells there is a potential risk of a drug interaction as haemoglobin concentration increases

• ACE inhibitors and AT-II antagonists: increased risk of hyperkalaemia

Administration

RECONSTITUTION

–

ROUTE

• SC, IV

RATE OF ADMINISTRATION

–

COMMENTS

–

Other information

• To convert to darbepoetin from epoetin, divide weekly epoetin dose by 200

• Same dose may be given either SC or IV – monitor response

• Pretreatment checks and appropriate correction/treatment needed for iron, folate and B_{12} deficiency, infection, inflammation or aluminium toxicity to produce optimum response to therapy

• Concomitant iron therapy (200–300 mg elemental oral iron) needed daily. IV iron may be needed for patients with very low serum ferritin (<100 nanograms/mL)

• May increase heparin requirement during HD

• There are reports of pure red cell aplasia (PRCA) associated with epoetin therapy. This is a very rare condition and results in failure of the production of erythroid elements (i.e. red blood cell precursors) in the bone marrow, which in turn results in profound anaemia. This is possibly due to an immune response to the protein backbone of R-HuEPO. The antibodies formed as a result of this immune response render the patient unresponsive to the therapeutic effects of epoetin alfa, epoetin beta and darbepoetin

Daunorubicin

Clinical use

Antineoplastic agent: acute leukaemias

Dose in normal renal function

30–45 mg/m^2, or as for local protocol

Pharmacokinetics

Molecular weight (daltons)	564
% Protein binding	50–90
% Excreted unchanged in urine	25–30
	(over 7 days)
Volume of distribution (L/kg)	23
Half-life – normal/ESRF (hrs)	18–27/–

Dose in renal impairment GFR (mL/min)

20–50	Dose as in normal renal function – see 'Other information'
10–20	Dose as in normal renal function – see 'Other information'
<10	Dose as in normal renal function – see 'Other information'

Dose in patients undergoing renal replacement therapies

CAPD	Unlikely dialysability. Dose as in GFR = <10 mL/min
HD	Unlikely dialysability. Dose as in GFR = <10 mL/min
CAV/VVHD	Unknown dialysability. Dose as in GFR = 10–20 mL/min

Important drug interactions

POTENTIALLY HAZARDOUS INTERACTIONS WITH OTHER DRUGS

• None known

Administration

RECONSTITUTION

• Reconstitute 20 mg vial with 4 mL water for injection giving a concentration of 5 mg/mL. Dilute calculated dose of daunorubicin further in sodium chloride 0.9% to give a final concentration of 1 mg/mL

ROUTE

• IV

RATE OF ADMINISTRATION

• 1 mg/mL solution should be infused over 20 minutes into the tubing or a side arm of a rapidly flowing IV infusion of sodium chloride 0.9%

COMMENTS

• Do not administer IM or SC: extremely irritating to tissues

Other information

• Daunorubicin is potentially cardiotoxic
• Monitor blood uric acid and urea levels
• Daunorubicin is extensively metabolised. The liver clears 40–50% of drug largely into bile
• Manufacturer's literature suggests that in patients with a serum creatinine of 105–265 micromol/L, the dose should be reduced to 75% of normal, and if the creatinine is >265 micromol/L, the dose should be 50% of normal
• A liposomal formulation of daunorubicin is now available (DaunoXome). Dilute to 0.2–1 mg/mL with glucose 5% and administer over 30–60 minutes

Deferiprone

Clinical use

Orally administered chelator used in the treatment of transfusional iron overload, or aluminium toxicity in haemodialysis patients

Dose in normal renal function

75 mg/kg/day in 2–4 divided doses

Pharmacokinetics

Molecular weight (daltons)	139.2
% Protein binding	No information
% Excreted unchanged in urine	15 – see 'Other information'
Volume of distribution (L/kg)	1.55–1.73
Half-life – normal/ESRF (hrs)	1.0–2.5/unknown

Dose in renal impairment GFR (mL/min)

20–50	Dose as in normal renal function
10–20	Give 50% dose and monitor
<10	Give 50% dose and monitor

Dose in patients undergoing renal replacement therapies

CAPD	Unknown dialysability. Dose as in GFR < 10 ml/min
HD	Dialysed. Dose as in GFR < 10 ml/min
CAV/VVHD	Dialysed. Dose as in GFR = 10–20 ml/min

Important drug interactions

POTENTIALLY HAZARDOUS INTERACTIONS WITH OTHER DRUGS

• None known

Administration

RECONSTITUTION

–

ROUTE

• Oral

RATE OF ADMINISTRATION

–

COMMENTS

–

Other information

• Deferiprone is hepatically metabolised (>85%) to predominantly glucuronide conjugates (no chelating activity). Deferiprone, the glucuronide conjugates, and deferiprone-complexed iron are cleared principally by the kidney with 80% of the dose recovered in the urine

• Side-effects include reversible neutropenia, agranulocytosis, musculoskeletal and joint pain, subclinical ototoxicity, plus case reports of systemic vasculitis and fatal SLE

• Can cause subnormal serum zinc levels

• Reddish-brown discolouration of the urine reported in 40% of thalassaemia patients undergoing deferiprone therapy

• Deferiprone removed aluminium in vitro from blood samples of 46 patients undergoing chronic haemodialysis. Only patients with serum aluminium concentrations >80 micrograms/mL were included. Deferiprone removed the aluminium faster and more effectively from higher molecular weight proteins than desferrioxamine. (Canteros-Piccotto MA et al. (1996) Nephrol Dial Transplant. 11(7): 1488–9)

Defibrotide

Clinical use

Treatment of severe veno-occlusive disease, or peripheral obliterative arterial disease

Dose in normal renal function

400–1200 mg daily in 1–3 divided doses,
or
10–40 mg/kg (up to a maximum of 60 mg/kg) daily in four divided doses

Pharmacokinetics

Molecular weight (daltons)	45,000–55,000
% Protein binding	Unknown
% Excreted unchanged in urine	IV – 85
	Oral – 3.6–6.5
Volume of distribution (L/kg)	0.04–0.05
Half-life – normal/ESRF (hrs)	9.8–27.1 minutes

Dose in renal impairment GFR (mL/min)

20–50	Dose as in normal renal function
10–20	Dose as in normal renal function
<10	Dose as in normal renal function

Dose in patients undergoing renal replacement therapies

CAPD	Unknown dialysability – Dose as in GFR < 10 ml/min
HD	Unknown dialysability – Dose as in GFR < 10 ml/min
CAV/VVHD	Unknown dialysability – Dose as in GFR = 10–20 ml/min

Important drug interactions

POTENTIALLY HAZARDOUS INTERACTIONS WITH OTHER DRUGS

• Increased risk of haemorrhage with other antithrombotic agents

Administration

RECONSTITUTION

–

ROUTE

• Oral, IV

RATE OF ADMINISTRATION

• In 100 mL sodium chloride 0.9% over 2 hours

COMMENTS

–

Other information

• Defibrotide is eliminated via both the urine and faeces due to non-saturable renal and saturable hepatic processes

• Preliminary data suggest defibrotide may be useful in preventing fibrin deposition in the circuitry of dialysis machines. The dose is given as a bolus of 100–400 mg, repeated at 60-minute intervals

• IV injection results in a dose-dependent increase in the plasma concentration of 6-deoxyribose. Despite the short elimination half-life, fibrinolytic effects have been described in the absence of any detectable concentrations of 6-deoxyribose

• Hypotension has been reported following IV administration to patients undergoing haemodialysis

• Ankle oedema and palpitations have been reported with defibrotide therapy

Deflazacort

Clinical use

Glucocorticoid, used for suppression of inflammatory and allergic disorders

Dose in normal renal function

3–18 mg daily
(Acute disorders up to 120 mg daily initially)

Pharmacokinetics

Molecular weight (daltons)	441.5
% Protein binding	40
% Excreted unchanged in urine	18
Volume of distribution (L/kg)	1.2
Half-life – normal/ESRF (hrs)	1.1–1.9/ unchanged

Dose in renal impairment GFR (mL/min)

20–50	Dose as in normal renal function
10–20	Dose as in normal renal function
<10	Dose as in normal renal function

Dose in patients undergoing renal replacement therapies

CAPD	Unlikely dialysability. Dose as in normal renal function
HD	Not dialysed. Dose as in normal renal function
CAV/VVHD	Unlikely dialysability. Dose as in normal renal function

Important drug interactions

POTENTIALLY HAZARDOUS INTERACTIONS WITH OTHER DRUGS

- Antibacterials: rifamycins accelerate metabolism of corticosteroids (reduced effect)
- Anticoagulants: anticoagulant effect of acenocoumarol and warfarin possibly altered
- Anti-epileptics: carbamazepine, phenobarbital, phenytoin and primidone accelerate metabolism of corticosteroids (reduced effect)
- Antifungals: increased risk of hypokalaemia with amphotericin (avoid concomitant use unless required to control reactions)
- Ciclosporin: increases half-life of deflazacort

Administration

RECONSTITUTION

–

ROUTE

- Oral

RATE OF ADMINISTRATION

–

COMMENTS

–

Other information

- 6 mg of deflazacort is equivalent to 5 mg prednisolone

Desferrioxamine

Clinical use

Chelating agent used in the treatment of acute iron poisoning and chronic iron or aluminium overload

Dose in normal renal function

20–60 mg/kg/day. Exact dosages should be determined for each individual

Pharmacokinetics

Molecular weight (daltons)	657
% Protein binding	<10
% Excreted unchanged in urine	30–35
Volume of distribution (L/kg)	2–2.5
Half-life – normal/ESRF (hrs)	6/–

Dose in renal impairment GFR (mL/min)

20–50	Dose as in normal renal function
10–20	Dose as in normal renal function
<10	50% of normal dose

Dose in patients undergoing renal replacement therapies

CAPD	Treatment of aluminium overload: 1 g once or twice each week prior to final exchange of the day by slow IV infusion, IM, SC or IP
HD	Treatment of aluminium overload: 1 g once each week administered during the last hour of dialysis as a slow IV infusion
CAV/VVHD	Dose schedule unknown. Metal chelates will be removed by dialysis

Important drug interactions

POTENTIALLY HAZARDOUS INTERACTIONS WITH OTHER DRUGS

• Avoid prochlorperazine, methotrimeprazine (prolonged unconsciousness)

Administration

RECONSTITUTION

• Dissolve contents of one vial (500 mg) in 5 mL of water for injection = 10% solution. If for IV administration, the 10% solution can be diluted with sodium chloride 0.9%, glucose 5% or glucose/sodium chloride

ROUTE

• IV, SC (bolus or continuous infusion)
• IM, IP (CAPD, CCPD), oral (acute iron poisoning)

RATE OF ADMINISTRATION

• IV (acute overdose): max 15 mg/kg/hour. Reduce after 4–6 hours so that total dose does not exceed 80 mg/kg/24 hours
• SC: infuse over 8–12 hours. Local irritation may occur

COMMENTS

• The urine in patients treated with desferrioxamine for severe iron intoxication may appear orange/red
• SC infusion is about 90% as effective as IV administration which is now the route of choice in transfusion-related iron overload
• For oral administration, 5–10 g should be dissolved in 50–100 mL water
• IM injection is less effective than SC

Other information

• Studies suggest that during HD only a small amount of plasma desferrioxamine transfers across dialysis membrane
• Contra-indicated in patients with severe renal disease except those on dialysis
• Desferrioxamine may predispose to development of infection with Yersinia species
• In haemodialysis patients treated with desferrioxamine post dialysis, the half-life has been found to be extended to 19 hours between dialysis sessions
• In treatment of acute iron poisoning, effectiveness of treatment is dependent on an adequate urine output. If oliguria or anuria develop, PD or HD may be necessary

Desirudin (unlicensed product)

Clinical use

Prophylaxis of DVT in patients undergoing hip and knee replacement surgery

Dose in normal renal function

15 mg 5–15 minutes before surgery then 15 mg twice daily for 9–12 days or until mobile

Pharmacokinetics

Molecular weight (daltons)	6963.4
% Protein binding	No data
% Excreted unchanged in urine	40–50
Volume of distribution (L/kg)	0.25
Half-life – normal/ESRF (hrs)	2–3/–

Dose in renal impairment GFR (mL/min)

30–61   Dose as in normal renal function. Aim for APTT <0.85 seconds

<30   Avoid

Dose in patients undergoing renal replacement therapies

CAPD	Not dialysed. Avoid
HD	Not dialysed. Avoid
CAV/VVHD	Not dialysed. Avoid

Important drug interactions

POTENTIALLY HAZARDOUS INTERACTIONS WITH OTHER DRUGS

• Anticoagulants, antiplatelets, NSAIDs, heparin and dextran – increased risk of bleeding

Administration

RECONSTITUTION

• With diluent supplied

ROUTE

• SC

RATE OF ADMINISTRATION

–

COMMENTS

• 7% of dose is metabolised by the kidneys

Other information

• The effect is poorly reversible
• APTT levels can be reduced by IV DDAVP
• Available on a 'named patient' basis from Aventis Pharma

Desloratadine

Clinical use

Antihistamine, used for symptomatic relief of allergy such as hay fever, urticaria

Dose in normal renal function

5 mg daily

Pharmacokinetics

Molecular weight (daltons)	310.8
% Protein binding	83–87
% Excreted unchanged in urine	40.6 (as active metabolites)
Volume of distribution (L/kg)	–
Half-life – normal/ESRF (hrs)	19–40 (average: 27)

Dose in renal impairment GFR (mL/min)

20–50	Dose as in normal renal function
10–20	Dose as in normal renal function
<10	5 mg every 48 hours

Dose in patients undergoing renal replacement therapies

CAPD	Unlikely to be dialysed. Dose as in GFR = <10 mL/min
HD	Not dialysed. Dose as in GFR = <10 mL/min
CAV/VVHD	Unlikely to be dialysed. Dose as in normal renal function

Important drug interactions

POTENTIALLY HAZARDOUS INTERACTIONS WITH OTHER DRUGS

• None known

Administration

RECONSTITUTION

–

ROUTE

• Oral

RATE OF ADMINISTRATION

–

COMMENTS

–

Other information

• Desloratadine is a metabolite of loratadine

Desmopressin (DDAVP)

Clinical use

Diabetes insipidus, nocturnal enuresis

Post-biopsy bleeding (unlicensed indication)

Pre-biopsy prophylaxis (unlicensed indication)

Dose in normal renal function

Diabetes insipidus: Oral: 0.2–1.2 mg daily in three divided doses, IV: 1–4 micrograms daily, Inhaled: 10–40 micrograms in one or two divided doses

Nocturnal enuresis: Oral: 200–400 micrograms at bedtime, Inhaled: 20–40 micrograms at bedtime

Biopsy: Males: 16 micrograms, Females: 12 micrograms or 300–400 nanograms/kg

Pharmacokinetics

Molecular weight (daltons)	1070
% Protein binding	0
% Excreted unchanged in urine	N/A
Volume of distribution (L/kg)	–
Half-life – normal/ESRF (hrs)	6–24/–

Dose in renal impairment GFR (mL/min)

20–50	Dose as in normal renal function
10–20	Dose as in normal renal function
<10	Dose as in normal renal function

Dose in patients undergoing renal replacement therapies

CAPD	Unlikely dialysability. Dose as in normal renal function
HD	Unlikely dialysability. Dose as in normal renal function
CAV/VVHD	Unlikely dialysability. Dose as in normal renal function

Important drug interactions

POTENTIALLY HAZARDOUS INTERACTIONS WITH OTHER DRUGS

• None known

Administration

RECONSTITUTION

• Dilute dose to 50 mL with sodium chloride 0.9%

ROUTE

• IV peripherally, intranasally, oral, SC, IM

RATE OF ADMINISTRATION

• Over 20 minutes

COMMENTS

• Do not inject at a faster rate – greater risk of tachyphylaxis

• In patients with ischaemic heart disease, infuse more slowly – increased risk of acute ischaemic event

Other information

• Emergency treatment of more generalised bleeding unresponsive to normal treatments: 0.1–0.5 micrograms/kg four times a day + IV oestrogens conjugated (Premarin) (unlicensed) 0.6 mg/kg/day for up to 5 days

• DDAVP works as a haemostatic by stimulating factor VIII production

• Onset of action less than 1 hour. Duration of effect 4–8 hours

Dexamethasone

Clinical use

Corticosteroid: cerebral oedema, suppression of inflammatory and allergic disorders, rheumatic disease, shock

Anti-emetic (unlicensed indication)

Dose in normal renal function

Cerebral oedema: 20 mg IV followed by 4 mg IV or IM every 6 hours

Oral: 0.5–10 mg daily, IV: 0.5–20 mg

Shock: 2–6 mg/kg IV repeated if required after 2–6 hours

Pharmacokinetics

Molecular weight (daltons)	393
% Protein binding	70
% Excreted unchanged in urine	8
Volume of distribution (L/kg)	0.6–1
Half-life – normal/ESRF (hrs)	3/–

Dose in renal impairment GFR (mL/min)

20–50	Dose as in normal renal function
10–20	Dose as in normal renal function
<10	Dose as in normal renal function

Dose in patients undergoing renal replacement therapies

CAPD	Not dialysed. Dose as in normal renal function
HD	Not dialysed. Dose as in normal renal function
CAV/VVHD	Removal unlikely. Dose as in normal renal function

Important drug interactions

POTENTIALLY HAZARDOUS INTERACTIONS WITH OTHER DRUGS

- Amphotericin: increased risk of hypokalaemia
- Anticoagulants: anticoagulant effect of acenocoumarol and warfarin possibly altered
- Rifampicin: accelerates dexamethasone metabolism
- Anti-epileptics: accelerate dexamethasone metabolism

Administration

RECONSTITUTION

–

ROUTE

- Oral, IV or IM

RATE OF ADMINISTRATION

- IV slowly over not less than 5 minutes. If underlying cardiac pathology, infusion over 20–30 minutes advised

COMMENTS

–

Other information

- Dexamethasone sodium phosphate 5 mg = dexamethasone 4 mg
- Injection solution can be administered orally or via naso-gastric tube
- Tablets will disperse in water

Dexketoprofen

Clinical use

NSAID, used for musculoskeletal pain, dysmenorrhoea, dental pain

Dose in normal renal function

12.5 mg every 4–6 hours
or 25 mg every 8 hours

Pharmacokinetics

Molecular weight (daltons)	254
% Protein binding	99
% Excreted unchanged in urine	<10
Volume of distribution (L/kg)	0.24
Half-life – normal/ESRF (hrs)	1.65/–

Dose in renal impairment GFR (mL/min)

20–50	Dose as in normal renal function but use with caution
10–20	Dose as in normal renal function but avoid if posssible
<10	Dose as in normal renal function but only if ESRD on dialysis

Dose in patients undergoing renal replacement therapies

CAPD	Dialysed. Dose as for GFR < 10 mL/min
HD	Dialysed. Dose as for GFR < 10 mL/min
CAV/VVHD	Dialysed. Dose as for GFR = 10–20 mL/min

Important drug interactions

POTENTIALLY HAZARDOUS INTERACTIONS WITH OTHER DRUGS

- Ciclosporin: increased risk of nephrotoxicity
- Lithium: excretion decreased
- Cytotoxic agents: reduced excretion of methotrexate
- Anticoagulants: effects of acenocoumarol and warfarin enhanced
- Antidiabetic agents: effects of sulphonylureas enhanced
- Anti-epileptic agents: effects of phenytoin enhanced
- ACE inhibitors and AT-II antagonists: antagonism of hypotensive effect; increased risk of renal damage and hyperkalaemia
- Antibacterials: increased risk of convulsions with quinolones
- Antivirals: increased haematological toxicity with zidovudine; plasma concentration possibly increased by ritonavir
- Other analgesics: avoid concomitant administration of two or more NSAIDs, including aspirin (increased side-effects)
- Diuretics: risk of nephrotoxicity increased; risk of hyperkalaemia with potassium-sparing diuretics
- Tacrolimus: increased risk of nephrotoxicity

Administration

RECONSTITUTION

–

ROUTE

- Oral

RATE OF ADMINISTRATION

–

COMMENTS

–

Other information

- Inhibition of renal prostaglandin synthesis by NSAIDs may interfere with renal function, especially in the presence of existing renal disease. Avoid if possible; if not, check serum creatinine 48–72 hours after starting NSAID. If raised, discontinue NSAID therapy
- Use normal doses in patients with ESRD on dialysis
- Use with caution in renal transplant recipients – can reduce intra-renal autocoid synthesis
- Dexketoprofen should be used with caution in uraemic patients predisposed to GI bleeding or uraemic coagulopathies

Diamorphine

Clinical use

Opiate analgesic. Control of severe pain, pain relief in myocardial infarction

Dose in normal renal function

SC/IM: 5–10 mg 4-hourly increasing dose as necessary

IV: 2.5–5 mg. Elderly patients – reduce dose by half

Pharmacokinetics

Molecular weight (daltons)	424
% Protein binding	30–40
% Excreted unchanged in urine	<10
Volume of distribution (L/kg)	40–50 litres
Half-life – normal/ESRF (hrs)	1.7–3.5 minutes/–

Dose in renal impairment GFR (mL/min)

20–50	Dose as in normal renal function
10–20	Use small doses, e.g. 2.5 mg SC/IM approx 6-hourly and titrate to response
<10	Use small doses, e.g. 2.5 mg SC/IM approx 8-hourly and titrate to response

Dose in patients undergoing renal replacement therapies

CAPD	Not dialysed. Dose as in GFR = <10 mL/min
HD	Dialysed. Dose as in GFR = <10 mL/min
CAV/VVHD	Unknown dialysability. Dose as in GFR = 10–20 mL/min

Important drug interactions

POTENTIALLY HAZARDOUS INTERACTIONS WITH OTHER DRUGS

- Anti-arrhythmics: delayed absorption of mexiletine
- Antipsychotics: enhanced sedative and hypotensive effect

Administration

RECONSTITUTION

- 1 mL water for injection or sodium chloride 0.9% (less may be used, e.g. for SC injection use 0.1 mL for 10 mg)

ROUTE

- IV, IM, SC

RATE OF ADMINISTRATION

- IV: 1 mg/minute

COMMENTS

- Monitor BP and respiratory rates

Other information

- Increased cerebral sensitivity in renal impairment which can result in excessive sedation and serious respiratory depression necessitating ventilation
- More potent than morphine
- *Extreme caution* with regular dosing – accumulation of active metabolites may occur
- Naloxone for effect-reversal must be readily available if required

Diazepam

Clinical use

Benzodiazepine: peri-operative sedation (IV), anxiolytic, muscle relaxant, status epilepticus

Dose in normal renal function

Pre-med: 0.1–0.2 mg/kg IV

PR: 10–30 mg

Anxiety: 2 mg three times a day, increasing if necessary to 15–30 mg daily in divided doses

Insomnia: 5–15 mg at night

Status epilepticus: IV: 10–20 mg repeat if required, infusion 3 mg/kg over 24 hours, PR: 500 micrograms/kg

Pharmacokinetics

Molecular weight (daltons)	285
% Protein binding	94–99
% Excreted unchanged in urine	<1
Volume of distribution (L/kg)	1.1–1.8
Half-life – normal/ESRF (hrs)	20–90/unchanged

Dose in renal impairment GFR (mL/min)

20–50	Dose as in normal renal function
10–20	Use small doses and titrate to response
<10	Use small doses and titrate to response

Dose in patients undergoing renal replacement therapies

CAPD	Not dialysed. Dose as in GFR = <10 mL/min
HD	Not dialysed. Dose as in GFR = <10 mL/min
CAV/VVHD	Unknown dialysability. Dose as in GFR = 10–20 mL/min

Important drug interactions

POTENTIALLY HAZARDOUS INTERACTIONS WITH OTHER DRUGS

- Antivirals: ritonavir and amprenavir increases the plasma concentration of diazepam
- Isoniazid inhibits metabolism of diazepam
- Rifampicin enhances metabolism of diazepam

Administration

RECONSTITUTION

–

ROUTE

- IV injection, infusion, oral, PR

RATE OF ADMINISTRATION

- 5 mg (1 mL)/minute

COMMENTS

- Injection can be mixed with sodium chloride 0.9% or glucose 5% to 40 mg in 500 mL

Other information

- Active metabolites renally excreted therefore accumulate in renal impairment
- Increased cerebral sensitivity in renal impairment which may result in excessive sedation and encephalopathy
- Always have flumazenil available to reverse effect
- Protein binding decreased in ESRD
- Vd increased in ESRD
- IV emulsion formulation (Diazemuls) less likely to cause thrombophlebitis

Diclofenac

Clinical use

NSAID and analgesic

Dose in normal renal function

75–150 mg daily in divided doses

Pharmacokinetics

Molecular weight (daltons)	318
% Protein binding	99
% Excreted unchanged in urine	<1
Volume of distribution (L/kg)	0.12–0.17
Half-life – normal/ESRF (hrs)	1–2/unchanged

Dose in renal impairment GFR (mL/min)

20–50	Dose as in normal renal function
10–20	Dose as in normal renal function, but avoid if possible
<10	Dose as in normal renal function, but only use if ESRD on dialysis

Dose in patients undergoing renal replacement therapies

CAPD	Not dialysed. Dose as in normal renal function
HD	Not dialysed. Dose as in normal renal function
CAV/VVHD	Not dialysed. Dose as in normal renal function

Important drug interactions

POTENTIALLY HAZARDOUS INTERACTIONS WITH OTHER DRUGS

- Ciclosporin: increased risk of nephrotoxicity
- Lithium: excretion decreased
- Cytotoxic agents: reduced excretion of methotrexate
- Anticoagulants: effects of acenocoumarol and warfarin enhanced
- Antidiabetic agents: effects of sulphonylureas enhanced
- Anti-epileptic agents: effects of phenytoin enhanced

- ACE inhibitors and AT-II antagonists: antagonism of hypotensive effect; increased risk of renal damage and hyperkalaemia
- Antibacterials: increased risk of convulsions with quinolones
- Antivirals: increased haematological toxicity with zidovudine; plasma concentration possibly increased by ritonavir
- Other analgesics: avoid concomitant administration of two or more NSAIDs, including aspirin (increased side-effects)
- Diuretics: risk of nephrotoxicity increased; risk of hyperkalaemia with potassium-sparing diuretics
- Tacrolimus: increased risk of nephrotoxicity

Administration

RECONSTITUTION

–

ROUTE

- Oral, IV, IM, PR

RATE OF ADMINISTRATION

- 25–50 mg over 15–60 minutes, 75 mg over 30–120 minutes
- Continuous infusion of 5 mg/hour

COMMENTS

- Dilute 75 mg in 100–500 mL of sodium chloride 0.9% or glucose 5% buffered with 0.5 mL sodium bicarbonate 8.4%

Other information

- Diclofenac should be used with caution in uraemic patients predisposed to GI bleeding or uraemic coagulopathies
- Inhibition of renal prostaglandin synthesis by NSAIDs may interfere with renal function, especially in the presence of existing renal disease. Avoid if possible; if not, check serum creatinine 48–72 hours after starting NSAID. If raised, discontinue NSAID therapy
- Use normal doses in patients with ESRD on dialysis
- Use with great caution in renal transplant recipients – can reduce intra-renal autocoid synthesis

Didanosine

Clinical use

Nucleoside reverse transcriptase inhibitor for treatment of HIV in combination with other antiretroviral drugs

Dose in normal renal function

Greater than 60 kg: 400 mg daily in 1–2 divided doses

Less than 60 kg: 250 mg daily in 1–2 divided doses

Pharmacokinetics

Molecular weight (daltons)	236.2
% Protein binding	<5
% Excreted unchanged in urine	20
Volume of distribution (L/kg)	54 litres
Half-life – normal/ESRF (hrs)	1.4/4.1

Dose in renal impairment GFR (mL/min)

>60	<60kg: 250 mg daily in one or two divided doses >60kg: 400 mg daily in one or two divided doses
30–59	<60kg: 150 mg daily in one or two divided doses >60kg: 200 mg daily in one or two divided doses
10–29	<60kg: 100 mg daily >60kg: 150 mg daily
<10	<60kg: 75 mg daily >60kg: 100 mg daily

Dose in patients undergoing renal replacement therapies

CAPD	Not dialysed. Dose as in GFR = <10 mL/min
HD	Partially dialysed. Dose as in GFR = <10 mL/min
CAV/VVHD	Partially dialysed. Dose as in GFR = 10–29 mL/min

Important drug interactions

POTENTIALLY HAZARDOUS INTERACTIONS WITH OTHER DRUGS

• Antivirals: ganciclovir and tenofovir can increase plasma didanosine concentration
• Antimicrobials: ciprofloxacin, tetracyclines and other antibiotics affected by indigestion remedies – do not administer within 2 hours of didanosine

Administration

RECONSTITUTION
–

ROUTE
• Oral

RATE OF ADMINISTRATION
–

COMMENTS
• Give dose after dialysis on dialysis days, and at the same time on non-dialysis days

Other information

• Haemodialysis removes 20–35% of the dose
• Administer 30 minutes before meals
• Magnesium content of tablets 8.6 mEq
• Chew, crush or disperse tablet in at least 30 mL of water
• Can be diluted in apple juice
• Ingestion with food decreases absorption by 50%

Diflunisal

Clinical use

NSAID and analgesic

Dose in normal renal function

250–500 mg twice daily

Pharmacokinetics

Molecular weight (daltons)	250
% Protein binding	99
% Excreted unchanged in urine	<3
Volume of distribution (L/kg)	0.1
Half-life – normal/ESRF (hrs)	5–20/62

Dose in renal impairment GFR (mL/min)

20–50	Dose as in normal renal function
10–20	50% of normal dose, but avoid if possible
<10	50% of normal dose, but only use if ESRD on dialysis

Dose in patients undergoing renal replacement therapies

CAPD	Not dialysed. Dose as in normal renal function
HD	Not dialysed. Dose as in normal renal function
CAV/VVHD	Not dialysed. Dose as in normal renal function

Important drug interactions

POTENTIALLY HAZARDOUS INTERACTIONS WITH OTHER DRUGS

- Ciclosporin: increased risk of nephrotoxicity
- Antibacterials: increased risk of convulsions with quinolones
- Lithium: decreased excretion

- Cytotoxic agents: decreased excretion of methotrexate
- Anticoagulants: effects of acenocoumarol and warfarin enhanced
- Antidiabetic agents: effects of sulphonylureas enhanced
- Anti-epileptic agents: effects of phenytoin enhanced
- ACE inhibitors and AT-II antagonists: antagonism of hypotensive effect; increased risk of renal damage and hyperkalaemia
- Tacrolimus: increased risk of nephrotoxicity

Administration

RECONSTITUTION

–

ROUTE

- Oral

RATE OF ADMINISTRATION

–

COMMENTS

–

Other information

- Diflunisal should be used with caution in uraemic patients predisposed to GI bleeding or uraemic coagulopathies
- Inhibition of renal prostaglandin synthesis by NSAIDs may interfere with renal function, especially in the presence of existing renal disease. Avoid use of NSAIDs if possible; if not, check serum creatinine 48–72 hours after starting NSAID. If raised, discontinue NSAID therapy
- Use normal doses in patients with ESRD on dialysis
- Use with great caution in renal transplant recipients – can reduce intra-renal autocoid synthesis

Digitoxin

Clinical use

Heart failure, supraventricular arrhythmias

Dose in normal renal function

Maintenance dose: 100 micrograms daily or on alternate days; may be increased to 200 micrograms daily if necessary

Pharmacokinetics

Molecular weight (daltons)	765
% Protein binding	>90
% Excreted unchanged in urine	20–25
Volume of distribution (L/kg)	0.6
Half-life – normal/ESRF (hrs)	144–200/210

Dose in renal impairment
GFR (mL/min)

20–50	Dose as in normal renal function
10–20	Dose as in normal renal function
<10	Give 50–75% of normal dose

Dose in patients undergoing renal replacement therapies

CAPD	Not dialysed. Dose as in GFR = <10 mL/min
HD	Not dialysed. Dose as in GFR = <10 mL/min
CAV/VVHD	Unknown dialysability. Dose as in GFR = 10–20 mL/min

Important drug interactions

POTENTIALLY HAZARDOUS INTERACTIONS WITH OTHER DRUGS

- Anti-arrhythmics: amiodarone increases digitoxin levels
- Antifungals: increased toxicity if hypokalaemia occurs with amphotericin; plasma levels of digitoxin increased by itraconazole
- Calcium-channel blockers: increased digitoxin levels
- Diuretics: increased digitoxin toxicity if hypokalaemia occurs
- Anti-malarials: quinine, hydroxychloroquine and chloroquine increase plasma levels of digitoxin

Administration

RECONSTITUTION

–

ROUTE

- Oral

RATE OF ADMINISTRATION

–

COMMENTS

–

Other information

- Vd decreased by uraemia
- Digitoxin is largely metabolised in the liver where 8–10% is converted to digoxin. More digitoxin is converted to digoxin in severe renal impairment

Digoxin

Clinical use

Atrial fibrillation, cardiac failure

Dose in normal renal function

Digitalisation: 1–1.5 mg in divided doses over 24 hours followed by 62.5–500 micrograms daily adjusted according to response

Pharmacokinetics

Molecular weight (daltons)	781
% Protein binding	20–30
% Excreted unchanged in urine	76–85, IV: 50–70
Volume of distribution (L/kg)	5–8
Half-life – normal/ESRF (hrs)	30–40/84–104

Dose in renal impairment GFR (mL/min)

Digitalisation using 750 micrograms – 1 mg
Interval between normal or reduced doses may need to be lengthened

20–50	125–250 micrograms per day
10–20	125–250 micrograms per day. Monitor levels
<10	Dose commonly 62.5 micrograms three times a week after HD, or 62.5 micrograms daily. Monitor levels

Dose in patients undergoing renal replacement therapies

CAPD	Not dialysed. Dose as in GFR = <10 mL/min
HD	Not dialysed. Dose as in GFR = <10 mL/min
CAV/VVHD	Unknown dialysability. Dose as in GFR = 10–20 mL/min

Important drug interactions

POTENTIALLY HAZARDOUS INTERACTIONS WITH OTHER DRUGS

- Anti-arrhythmics: amiodarone, propafenone and quinidine increase digoxin plasma level (halve maintenance dose of digoxin)
- Quinine: increases plasma concentration of digoxin (halve maintenance dose)
- Calcium-channel blockers: increase digoxin plasma levels
- Diuretics: increase toxicity if hypokalaemia occurs; effects enhanced by spironolactone
- Concurrent erythromycin or omeprazole administration decreases digoxin clearance
- Antifungals: increased toxicity if hypokalaemia occurs with amphotericin; plasma concentration of digoxin increased by itraconazole
- Anti-malarials: quinine, hydroxychloroquine and chloroquine raise plasma concentrations of digoxin; increased risk of bradycardia with mefloquine
- Ciclosporin: raised digoxin serum/blood levels
- ACE inhibitors and AT-II antagonists: increases digoxin plasma concentrations
- Antidepressants: digoxin levels reduced by St John's Wort

Administration

RECONSTITUTION

–

ROUTE

- Oral, IV

RATE OF ADMINISTRATION

- IV: infuse over 30 minutes – 2 hours

COMMENTS

- IV administration, dilute dose to 50 mL with sodium chloride 0.9%
- IV dosing may be used for very rapid control (infused over 1–2 hours)

Other information

- If possible take blood sample prior to commencing therapy for determination of Digoxin Immunoreactive Like Substance
- Complex kinetics in renal impairment. Vd and total body clearance reduced in ESRD
- Steady-state plasma monitoring advisable. Normal range 0.8–2 nanograms/mL
- Hypokalaemia, hypomagnesaemia, marked hypercalcaemia and hypothyroidism increase toxicity
- Increases uraemic GI symptoms
- Concomitant administration of phosphate binders reduce GI absorption by up to 25%

Dihydrocodeine

Clinical use

Analgesia

Dose in normal renal function

Oral: 30 mg every 4–6 hrs
SC/IM: up to 50 mg every 4–6 hrs

Pharmacokinetics

Molecular weight (daltons)	452
% Protein binding	–
% Excreted unchanged in urine	13–22
Volume of distribution (L/kg)	1.1
Half-life – normal/ESRF (hrs)	3.4–4.5/>6

Dose in renal impairment GFR (mL/min)

20–50	Dose as in normal renal function
10–20	Avoid or use small doses and titrate to response
<10	Avoid or use small doses and titrate to response

Dose in patients undergoing renal replacement therapies

CAPD	Unknown dialysability. Dose as in GFR = <10 mL/min
HD	Unknown dialysability. Dose as in GFR = <10 mL/min
CAV/VVHD	Unknown dialysability. Dose as in GFR = 10–20 mL/min

Important drug interactions

POTENTIALLY HAZARDOUS INTERACTIONS WITH OTHER DRUGS

• None known

Administration

RECONSTITUTION
–

ROUTE
• Oral, IM, SC

RATE OF ADMINISTRATION
–

COMMENTS
–

Other information

• Increased and prolonged effect in renal impairment, enhancing respiratory depression and constipation
• Increased CNS sensitivity in renal impairment
• Accumulation of active metabolites can occur – caution
• Effects can be reversed by naloxone
• Oral liquid formulation contains ethanol – caution if patient on metronidazole

Diltiazem

Clinical use

Calcium-channel blocker: prophylaxis and
treatment of angina, hypertension

Dose in normal renal function

Angina: 60–120 mg three times daily
Hypertension: 180–480 mg daily

Pharmacokinetics

Molecular weight (daltons)	451
% Protein binding	98
% Excreted unchanged in urine	<10
Volume of distribution (L/kg)	3–5
Half-life – normal/ESRF (hrs)	2/3.5

Dose in renal impairment GFR (mL/min)

20–50	Dose as in normal renal function
10–20	Dose as in normal renal function
<10	Dose as in normal renal function

Dose in patients undergoing renal replacement therapies

CAPD	Not dialysed. Dose as in normal renal function
HD	Not dialysed. Dose as in normal renal function
CAV/VVHD	Unknown dialysability. Dose as in normal renal function

Important drug interactions

POTENTIALLY HAZARDOUS INTERACTIONS WITH
OTHER DRUGS

• Ciclosporin: increases ciclosporin plasma
  concentrations
• Tacrolimus: increases tacrolimus plasma
  concentration
• Antivirals: ritonavir and amprenavir increase
  diltiazem concentrations
• Increased risk of bradycardia and AV block and
  myocardial depression if prescribed with
  amiodarone
• Metabolism increased by rifampicin
• Enhances effect of carbamazepine and increases
  plasma levels of phenytoin
• Risk of bradycardia and AV block if co-prescribed
  with beta-blockers
• Increased plasma concentration of digoxin
• Enhances effect of theophylline

Administration

RECONSTITUTION

–

ROUTE

• Oral

RATE OF ADMINISTRATION

–

COMMENTS

–

Other information

• Active metabolites
• Monitor heart rate early on in therapy. If falls
  below 50 beats/minute, do not increase dose
• Maintain patient on same brand

Dipyridamole

Clinical use

Antiplatelet agent

Dose in normal renal function

100–200 mg three times daily
Modified release: 200 mg twice daily

Pharmacokinetics

Molecular weight (daltons)	505
% Protein binding	99
% Excreted unchanged in urine	–
Volume of distribution (L/kg)	2.4
Half-life – normal/ESRF (hrs)	12/–

Dose in renal impairment GFR (mL/min)

20–50	Dose as in normal renal function
10–20	Dose as in normal renal function
<10	Dose as in normal renal function

Dose in patients undergoing renal replacement therapies

CAPD	Not dialysed. Dose as in normal renal function
HD	Not dialysed. Dose as in normal renal function
CAV/VVHD	Not dialysed. Dose as in normal renal function

Important drug interactions

POTENTIALLY HAZARDOUS INTERACTIONS WITH OTHER DRUGS

• Effects of adenosine enhanced and extended
• Anticoagulants: enhanced effect

Administration

RECONSTITUTION

–

ROUTE

• Oral, slow IV

RATE OF ADMINISTRATION

–

COMMENTS

–

Other information

–

Disopyramide

Clinical use

Ventricular and supraventricular arrhythmias

Dose in normal renal function

100–200 mg four times daily

IV: 2 mg/kg over 5 minutes to a maximum of 150 mg

Infusion: 400 micrograms/kg/hour

Pharmacokinetics

Molecular weight (daltons)	340
% Protein binding	40–80
% Excreted unchanged in urine	35–65
Volume of distribution (L/kg)	0.8–2.6
Half-life – normal/ESRF (hrs)	5–8/10–18

Dose in renal impairment GFR (mL/min)

20–50	100 mg every 8 hours or 150 mg every 12 hours
10–20	100 mg every 12 hours
<10	150 mg every 24 hours (monitor levels)

Dose in patients undergoing renal replacement therapies

CAPD	Not dialysed. Dose as in GFR = <10 mL/min
HD	Not dialysed. Dose as in GFR = <10 mL/min
CAV/VVHD	Unknown dialysability. Dose as in GFR = 10–20 mL/min

Important drug interactions

POTENTIALLY HAZARDOUS INTERACTIONS WITH OTHER DRUGS

• Amiodarone increases risk of ventricular arrhythmias

• Increased myocardial depression with any anti-arrhythmic, beta-blockers or verapamil

• Plasma levels: reduced by rifampicin and phenytoin, increased by erythromycin

• Increased risk of ventricular arrhythmias with mizolastine, tricyclic antidepressants, antipsychotics or ritonavir

Administration

RECONSTITUTION

–

ROUTE

• Oral, IV

RATE OF ADMINISTRATION

• Not >3 mL/minute

COMMENTS

• May be given by IV infusion peripherally at rate of 0.4 mg/kg/hour in glucose 5%, sodium chloride 0.9% or compound sodium lactate

Other information

• Use with caution in patients with impaired renal function

• Do not give renally impaired patients sustained-release preparations

• Optimum therapeutic plasma level 2–5 mg/L

• Haemoperfusion can be used in cases of severe poisoning

Dobutamine

Clinical use

Inotropic agent

Dose in normal renal function

2.5–10 micrograms/kg/minute up to
40 micrograms/kg/minute according to response

Pharmacokinetics

Molecular weight (daltons)	301.4
% Protein binding	–
% Excreted unchanged in urine	<10
Volume of distribution (L/kg)	0.25
Half-life – normal/ESRF (hrs)	2 minutes/–

Dose in renal impairment GFR (mL/min)

20–50	Dose as in normal renal function
10–20	Dose as in normal renal function
<10	Dose as in normal renal function

Dose in patients undergoing renal replacement therapies

CAPD	Not dialysed. Dose as in normal renal function
HD	Not dialysed. Dose as in normal renal function
CAV/VVHD	Not dialysed. Dose as in normal renal function

Important drug interactions

POTENTIALLY HAZARDOUS INTERACTIONS WITH OTHER DRUGS

• Antagonised by beta-blockers

Administration

RECONSTITUTION

–

ROUTE

• Continuous IV infusion centrally via CRIP (or peripherally via a large vein)

RATE OF ADMINISTRATION

• Varies with dose

COMMENTS

• Dilute to at least 50 mL with sodium chloride 0.9% or glucose 5% (less than 5 mg/ml)
• 250 mg may be diluted in as little as 50 mL diluent

Other information

• Cardiac and BP monitoring advised
• Sodium bicarbonate rapidly inactivates dobutamine
• Solution may turn pink, but potency is unaffected by this
• Can cause hypokalaemia

Docetaxel

Clinical use

Treatment of breast cancer and non-small-cell lung cancer unresponsive to alternative therapies

Dose in normal renal function

Breast cancer: 100 mg/m^2 every 3 weeks

In combination with doxorubicin (50 mg/m^2), dose of 75 mg/m^2

Non-small-cell lung cancer: 75 mg/m^2 every 3 weeks

Pharmacokinetics

Molecular weight (daltons)	807.9
% Protein binding	>95
% Excreted unchanged in urine	6
Volume of distribution (L/kg)	113 litres
Half-life – normal/ESRF (hrs)	4 min(α)/ 36 min(β)/ 11.1 hr(γ)

Dose in renal impairment GFR (mL/min)

20–50	Dose as in normal renal function
10–20	Dose as in normal renal function
<10	Dose as in normal renal function

Dose in patients undergoing renal replacement therapies

CAPD	Unlikely dialysability. Dose as in normal renal function
HD	Unlikely dialysability. Dose as in normal renal function
CAV/VVHD	Unlikely dialysability. Dose as in normal renal function

Important drug interactions

POTENTIALLY HAZARDOUS INTERACTIONS WITH OTHER DRUGS

- Ciclosporin: possibly inhibits metabolism of ciclosporin
- Doxorubicin: increased clearance of docetaxel

Administration

RECONSTITUTION

- With diluent provided

ROUTE

- IV

RATE OF ADMINISTRATION

- Over 1 hour

COMMENTS

- Allow vials to come to room temperature for 5 minutes
- Doses of up to 200 mg can be added to 250-mL infusion bags of glucose 5% or sodium chloride 0.9%
- Doses greater than 200 mg should be diluted to a concentration of 0.74 mg/mL
- Administer within 4 hours of dilution

Other information

- Give premedication with oral dexamethasone 16 mg daily for 3 days, starting 1 day before commencing chemotherapy

Domperidone

Clinical use

Acute nausea and vomiting (including that caused by levodopa and bromocriptine); functional dyspepsia

Dose in normal renal function

Nausea and vomiting: adults 10–20 mg orally at 4–8-hourly intervals

PR: 30–60 mg every 4–8 hours

Pharmacokinetics

Molecular weight (daltons)	426
% Protein binding	>90
% Excreted unchanged in urine	<1
Volume of distribution (L/kg)	5.7
Half-life – normal/ESRF (hrs)	7.5/–

Dose in renal impairment GFR (mL/min)

20–50	Dose as in normal renal function
10–20	Dose as in normal renal function
<10	Dose as in normal renal function

Dose in patients undergoing renal replacement therapies

CAPD	Unknown dialysability. Dose as in normal renal function
HD	Unknown dialysability. Dose as in normal renal function
CAV/VVHD	Unknown dialysability. Dose as in normal renal function

Important drug interactions

POTENTIALLY HAZARDOUS INTERACTIONS WITH OTHER DRUGS

• None known

Administration

RECONSTITUTION

–

ROUTE

• Oral, PR

RATE OF ADMINISTRATION

–

COMMENTS

• Treatment of acute nausea and vomiting: maximum period of treatment is 12 weeks
• Treatment of functional dyspepsia: administer before food; maximum period of treatment is 12 weeks

Other information

• Domperidone has the advantage over metoclopramide and the phenothiazines of being less likely to cause central effects, such as sedation and dystonic reactions, as it does not readily cross the blood–brain barrier

Donepezil hydrochloride

Clinical use

Treatment of dementia in mild to moderate Alzheimer's disease

Dose in normal renal function

5 mg daily increasing to 10 mg daily

Pharmacokinetics

Molecular weight (daltons)	416
% Protein binding	95
% Excreted unchanged in urine	17
Volume of distribution (L/kg)	12
Half-life – normal/ESRF (hrs)	70/unchanged

Dose in renal impairment GFR (mL/min)

20–50	Dose as in normal renal function
10–20	Dose as in normal renal function
<10	Dose as in normal renal function

Dose in patients undergoing renal replacement therapies

CAPD	Unlikely to be dialysed. Dose as in normal renal function
HD	Unlikely to be dialysed. Dose as in normal renal function
CAV/VVHD	Unlikely to be dialysed. Dose as in normal renal function

Important drug interactions

POTENTIALLY HAZARDOUS INTERACTIONS WITH OTHER DRUGS

- Ketoconazole: increases donepezil concentration by 30%
- Erythromycin, fluoxetine, itraconazole and other CYP 3A4 and CYP 2D6 inhibitors: inhibit donepezil metabolism, will increase donepezil levels
- Rifampicin, carbamazepine, phenytoin, alcohol: may reduce donepezil levels

Administration

RECONSTITUTION

–

ROUTE

- Oral

RATE OF ADMINISTRATION

–

COMMENTS

–

Other information

- Metabolised via CYP 450 3A4 and 2D6 so may interact with other drugs metabolised by these pathways

Dopamine

Clinical use

Increase renal blood perfusion at low 'renal' dose. At higher dose, has inotropic effect and eventually is vasoconstricting

Dose in normal renal function

Renal dose: 2–5 micrograms/kg/min

Inotropic dose: 5–10 micrograms/kg/min

Vasoconstricting dose: >10 micrograms/kg/min

NB: individual patient sensitivity may affect these ranges

Pharmacokinetics

Molecular weight (daltons)	190
% Protein binding	–
% Excreted unchanged in urine	–
Volume of distribution (L/kg)	–
Half-life – normal/ESRF (hrs)	2 min/–

Dose in renal impairment GFR (mL/min)

20–50	Dose as in normal renal function
10–20	Dose as in normal renal function
<10	Dose as in normal renal function

Dose in patients undergoing renal replacement therapies

CAPD	Not dialysed. Dose as in normal renal function
HD	Not dialysed. Dose as in normal renal function
CAV/VVHD	Not dialysed. Dose as in normal renal function

Important drug interactions

POTENTIALLY HAZARDOUS INTERACTIONS WITH OTHER DRUGS

• Ciclosporin: may reduce risk of ciclosporin nephrotoxicity
• Antidepressants: hypertensive crisis with MAOIs

Administration

RECONSTITUTION

–

ROUTE

• IV peripherally into *large* vein (centrally for inotropic dose). Central route always preferable

RATE OF ADMINISTRATION

• Via CRIP as indicated below

COMMENTS

• Add 200 mg to 250 mL sodium chloride 0.9% or glucose 5%, then Renal Dose (mL/hour) = 0.1875 x patient's weight in kg, i.e. for 60 kg patients, dose is 11.25 mL/hour of this solution
• Minimum dilution 200 mg in 50 mL
• Not compatible with sodium bicarbonate – rapid deactivation of dopamine

Other information

• Causes renal vasoconstriction at inotropic dose
• Cardiac and BP monitoring advised
• Very severe tissue damage caused by extravasation
• 'Renal effects' consist of a mixture of renal/splanchnic vasodilation, a direct tubular (diuretic) effect, and improved perfusion secondary to an increase in cardiac output

Dopexamine

Clinical use

Inotropic support in heart failure associated with cardiac surgery

Dose in normal renal function

IV infusion: 0.5 micrograms/kg/minute and may be increased to 1 microgram/kg/minute and then in increments (0.5–1 micrograms/kg/minute) up to 6 micrograms/kg/minute at not less than 15-minute intervals

Pharmacokinetics

Molecular weight (daltons)	429
% Protein binding	–
% Excreted unchanged in urine	10
Volume of distribution (L/kg)	0.45
Half-life – normal/ESRF (hrs)	Mean 7 minutes/–

Dose in renal impairment GFR (mL/min)

20–50	Dose as in normal renal function and adjust to response
10–20	Dose as in normal renal function and adjust to response
<10	Dose as in normal renal function and adjust to response

Dose in patients undergoing renal replacement therapies

CAPD	Unknown dialysability. Dose as in normal renal function
HD	Unknown dialysability. Dose as in normal renal function
CAV/VVHD	Unknown dialysability. Dose as in normal renal function

Important drug interactions

POTENTIALLY HAZARDOUS INTERACTIONS WITH OTHER DRUGS

- Antidepressants: risk of hypertensive crisis with MAOIs
- Beta-blockers: risk of severe hypertension
- Other sympathomimetics: risk of severe hypertension

Administration

RECONSTITUTION

–

ROUTE

- By intravenous infusion into a central or large peripheral vein

RATE OF ADMINISTRATION

- See dosage instructions

COMMENTS

- IV infusion of 400 or 800 micrograms/mL in glucose 5% or sodium chloride 0.9%
- Peripheral administration: concentration of infusion solution must not exceed 1 mg/mL
- Central administration: concentration not >4 mg/mL
- During the administration of dopexamine the rate of administration and duration of therapy should be adjusted according to the patient's response as determined by heart rate and rhythm, blood pressure, urine flow and measurement of cardiac output

Other information

- The duration of therapy is dependent upon the patient's overall response to treatment
- Avoid abrupt withdrawal

Dornase alfa

Clinical use

To improve pulmonary function in cystic fibrosis

Dose in normal renal function

2.5 mg (2500 units) daily via nebuliser can be increased to twice daily if over 21 years of age

Pharmacokinetics

Molecular weight (daltons)	29,250
% Protein binding	–
% Excreted unchanged in urine	No data
Volume of distribution (L/kg)	–
Half-life – normal/ESRF (hrs)	11 (from lungs in rats)

Dose in renal impairment GFR (mL/min)

20–50	Dose as in normal renal function
10–20	Dose as in normal renal function
<10	Dose as in normal renal function

Dose in patients undergoing renal replacement therapies

CAPD	Unlikely dialysability. Dose as in normal renal function
HD	Unlikely dialysability. Dose as in normal renal function
CAV/VVHD	Unlikely dialysability. Dose as in normal renal function

Important drug interactions

POTENTIALLY HAZARDOUS INTERACTIONS WITH OTHER DRUGS

• None known

Administration

RECONSTITUTION

–

ROUTE

• Nebulised

RATE OF ADMINISTRATION

–

COMMENTS

• <15% of dose is systemically absorbed

Other information

• No pharmacokinetic data available, little systemic absorption therefore little accumulation expected
• Use undiluted using recommended jet nebuliser/compressor system. Refer to data sheet

Dothiepin (Dosulepin)

Clinical use

Tricyclic antidepressant

Dose in normal renal function

50–225 mg daily

Pharmacokinetics

Molecular weight (daltons)	332
% Protein binding	80–90
% Excreted unchanged in urine	56 (mainly as metabolites)
Volume of distribution (L/kg)	11–78
Half-life – normal/ESRF (hrs)	14–24/–

Dose in renal impairment GFR (mL/min)

20–50	Dose as in normal renal function
10–20	Start with small dose, i.e. 25 mg at night
<10	Start with small dose, i.e. 25 mg at night

Dose in patients undergoing renal replacement therapies

CAPD	Not dialysed. Dose as in GFR = <10 mL/min
HD	Not dialysed. Dose as in GFR = <10 mL/min
CAV/VVHD	Unknown dialysability. Dose as in GFR = 10–20 mL/min

Important drug interactions

POTENTIALLY HAZARDOUS INTERACTIONS WITH OTHER DRUGS

• MAOIs: CNS excitation and hypertension
• SSRIs: may increase dothiepin blood levels
• Anti-epileptics: antagonism – reduced convulsive threshold
• Antihistamines: increased antimuscarinic and sedative effects; increased risk of arrhythmias with terfenadine and mizolastine
• Adrenaline/noradrenaline: hypertension and arrhythmias
• Alcohol: enhanced effect
• Anti-arrhythmics: increased risk of ventricular arrhythmias with drugs which prolong the QT interval, e.g. amiodarone, disopyramide, procainamide, quinidine
• Antihypertensives: enhanced hypotensive effect. Increased risk of ventricular arrhythmias with sotalol
• Antivirals: increased plasma concentration by ritonavir
• Sibutramine: increased risk of CNS toxicity – avoid concomitant use

Administration

RECONSTITUTION

–

ROUTE

• Oral

RATE OF ADMINISTRATION

–

COMMENTS

–

Other information

• Metabolites are active and partly renally excreted. Metabolites accumulate and cause excessive sedation
• 25–50 mg usually effective without too much sedation

Doxapram

Clinical use

Post-operative respiratory depression; acute respiratory failure

Dose in normal renal function

Post-operative respiratory depression: IV injection 0.5–1.5 mg/kg repeated at hourly intervals or IV infusion 2–5 mg/minute, adjust according to response

Pharmacokinetics

Molecular weight (daltons)	433
% Protein binding	–
% Excreted unchanged in urine	<5
Volume of distribution (L/kg)	0.58–2.74
Half-life – normal/ESRF (hrs)	2.4–4.1/–

Dose in renal impairment GFR (mL/min)

20–50	Dose as in normal renal function
10–20	Dose as in normal renal function
<10	Dose as in normal renal function

Dose in patients undergoing renal replacement therapies

CAPD	Unknown dialysability. Dose as in normal renal function
HD	Unknown dialysability. Dose as in normal renal function
CAV/VVHD	Unknown dialysability. Dose as in normal renal function

Important drug interactions

POTENTIALLY HAZARDOUS INTERACTIONS WITH OTHER DRUGS

• None known

Administration

RECONSTITUTION

–

ROUTE

• IV bolus, IV infusion

RATE OF ADMINISTRATION

• IV injection: over at least 30 seconds
• IV infusion post-operative: 2–3 mg/minute, adjust according to response
• IV infusion acute respiratory failure: 1.5–4 mg/minute, adjust according to response

COMMENTS

• Doxapram has a narrow margin of safety, the minimum effective dosage should be used and maximum recommended dosages should not be exceeded

Other information

• Unlike naloxone, doxapram does not reverse the other effects of opioid analgesics (i.e. analgesia)

Doxazosin

Clinical use

Alpha-adrenoceptor blocker: hypertension; benign prostatic hyperplasia

Dose in normal renal function

Hypertension: 1 mg daily, increased after 1–2 weeks to 2 mg daily, and thereafter to 4 mg daily, if necessary; maximum 16 mg daily

Doxazosin XL: 4–8 mg once daily

Pharmacokinetics

Molecular weight (daltons)	548
% Protein binding	98
% Excreted unchanged in urine	<5
Volume of distribution (L/kg)	1–1.7
Half-life – normal/ESRF (hrs)	9.5–12.5/13

Dose in renal impairment GFR (mL/min)

20–50	Dose as in normal renal function
10–20	Dose as in normal renal function
<10	Dose as in normal renal function

Dose in patients undergoing renal replacement therapies

CAPD	Not dialysed. Dose as in normal renal function
HD	Not dialysed. Dose as in normal renal function
CAV/VVHD	Not dialysed. Dose as in normal renal function

Important drug interactions

POTENTIALLY HAZARDOUS INTERACTIONS WITH OTHER DRUGS

- Anaesthetics: enhanced hypotensive effect
- Antidepressants: enhanced hypotensive effect
- Beta-blockers: increased first-dose hypotensive effect
- Calcium-channel blockers: enhanced hypotensive effect
- Diuretics: increased first-dose hypotensive effect
- Moxisylyte: possible severe postural hypotension

Administration

RECONSTITUTION

–

ROUTE

- Oral

RATE OF ADMINISTRATION

–

COMMENTS

–

Other information

- At steady state, the half-life is calculated at 22 hours (elimination $t_{1/2}$) providing action of 24 hours duration

Doxepin

Clinical use

Tricyclic antidepressant

Dose in normal renal function

Initially 75 mg daily, increased as necessary to maximum 300 mg daily in three divided doses

Pharmacokinetics

Molecular weight (daltons)	316
% Protein binding	95
% Excreted unchanged in urine	<1
Volume of distribution (L/kg)	20
Half-life – normal/ESRF (hrs)	8–25/10–30

Dose in renal impairment GFR (mL/min)

20–50	Dose as in normal renal function
10–20	Dose as in normal renal function
<10	Dose as in normal renal function

Dose in patients undergoing renal replacement therapies

CAPD	Not dialysed. Dose as in normal renal function
HD	Not dialysed. Dose as in normal renal function
CAV/VVHD	Not dialysed. Dose as in normal renal function

Important drug interactions

POTENTIALLY HAZARDOUS INTERACTIONS WITH OTHER DRUGS

- Alcohol: enhanced effect
- Altretamine: risk of severe postural hypotension
- Other antidepressants: risk of enhanced CNS effects and excitation with MAOIs
- Antihistamines: enhanced antimuscarinic and sedative effects. Increased risk of ventricular arrhythmias with terfenadine and mizolastine
- Sympathomimetics: increased risk of hypertension and ventricular arrhythmias
- Anti-arrhythmics: increased risk of ventricular arrhythmias with drugs which prolong the QT interval, e.g. amiodarone, disopyramide, procainamide, quinidine
- Anti-epileptics: effects antagonised (convulsive threshold lowered)
- Antihypertensives: enhanced hypotensive effect
- Beta-blockers: risk of ventricular arrhythmias with sotalol
- Sibutramine: increased risk of CNS toxicity – avoid concomitant use
- Antivirals: increased plasma concentrations by ritonavir
- Anti-malarials: avoid concomitant use with artemether with lumefantrine

Administration

RECONSTITUTION

–

ROUTE

- Oral

RATE OF ADMINISTRATION

–

COMMENTS

–

Other information

–

Doxorubicin

Clinical use

Antineoplastic agent: acute leukaemias, lymphomas, sarcomas, and malignant neoplasms of bladder, breast, lung, ovary, stomach and thyroid

Dose in normal renal function

60–75 mg/m^2 every 3 weeks when doxorubicin is used alone, or see local protocol

Pharmacokinetics

Molecular weight (daltons)	580
% Protein binding	80–85
% Excreted unchanged in urine	<15
Volume of distribution (L/kg)	21.5
Half-life – normal/ESRF (hrs)	35/unchanged

Dose in renal impairment GFR (mL/min)

20–50	Dose as in normal renal function
10–20	Dose as in normal renal function
<10	Dose as in normal renal function

Dose in patients undergoing renal replacement therapies

CAPD	Not dialysed. Dose as in normal renal function
HD	Not dialysed. Dose as in normal renal function
CAV/VVHD	Unknown dialysability. Dose as in normal renal function

Important drug interactions

POTENTIALLY HAZARDOUS INTERACTIONS WITH OTHER DRUGS

• Ciclosporin: increased risk of neurotoxicity

Administration

RECONSTITUTION

• Reconstitute with water for injection or sodium chloride 0.9%. 10 mg in 5 mL, 50 mg in 25 mL

ROUTE

• IV, intra-arterial, intravesical (bladder instillation)

RATE OF ADMINISTRATION

• IV: give via the tubing of a fast-running intravenous infusion of sodium chloride 0.9% or glucose 5%, taking 2–3 minutes over the injection

COMMENTS

• For bladder instillation: concentration of doxorubicin in bladder should be 50 mg per 50 mL. To avoid undue dilution in urine, the patient should be instructed not to drink any fluid in the 12 hours prior to instillation. This should limit urine production to approximately 50 mL per hour

Other information

• A cumulative dose of 450–550 mg/m^2 should only be exceeded with extreme caution. Above this level, the risk of irreversible congestive cardiac failure increases greatly

• Patients with impaired hepatic function have prolonged and elevated plasma concentrations of both the drug and its metabolites. Dose reduction is required

• Liposomal preparations available – up to 90 mg in 250 mL glucose 5%; if greater than 90 mg dilute in 500 mL glucose 5%

Doxycycline

Clinical use

Antibacterial agent, and prophylaxis/treatment of malaria

Dose in normal renal function

200 mg on day 1, then 100 mg daily;
severe infections 200 mg daily

Pharmacokinetics

Molecular weight (daltons)	463
% Protein binding	80–93
% Excreted unchanged in urine	33–45
Volume of distribution (L/kg)	0.75
Half-life – normal/ESRF (hrs)	15–24/18–25

Dose in renal impairment
GFR (mL/min)

20–50	Dose as in normal renal function
10–20	Dose as in normal renal function
<10	Dose as in normal renal function

Dose in patients undergoing renal replacement therapies

CAPD	Not dialysed. Dose as in normal renal function
HD	Not dialysed. Dose as in normal renal function
CAV/VVHD	Not dialysed. Dose as in normal renal function

Important drug interactions

POTENTIALLY HAZARDOUS INTERACTIONS WITH OTHER DRUGS

• Ciclosporin: possibly increases plasma-ciclosporin concentration

Administration

RECONSTITUTION
–

ROUTE

• Oral

RATE OF ADMINISTRATION
–

COMMENTS

• Do not take iron preparations, indigestion remedies or phosphate binders at the same time of day as doxycycline

Other information

–

Drotrecogin alfa

Clinical use

Treatment of adult patients with severe sepsis with multiple organ failure

Dose in normal renal function

24 micrograms/kg/hour for 96 hours

Pharmacokinetics

Molecular weight (daltons)	47,438.77
% Protein binding	–
% Excreted unchanged in urine	–
Volume of distribution (L/kg)	19.7 ± 11.5 litres
Half-life – normal/ESRF (hrs)	0.8/–

Dose in renal impairment GFR (mL/min)

20–50	Dose as in normal renal function
10–20	Dose as in normal renal function
<10	Dose as in normal renal function

Dose in patients undergoing renal replacement therapies

CAPD	Unknown dialysability. Dose as in normal renal function
HD	Unknown dialysability. Dose as in normal renal function
CAV/VVHD	Unknown dialysability. Dose as in normal renal function

Important drug interactions

POTENTIALLY HAZARDOUS INTERACTIONS WITH OTHER DRUGS

• Heparin (if >15 IU/kg/hour): enhanced effect
• Thrombolytic therapy: avoid for 3 days before administering drotrecogin
• Oral anticoagulants, antiplatelets: avoid for 7 days before administering drotrecogin

Administration

RECONSTITUTION

• Water for injection

ROUTE

• IV infusion

RATE OF ADMINISTRATION

• 24 micrograms/kg/hour

COMMENTS

• Further dilute with sodium chloride 0.9% to a concentration of 100–200 micrograms/mL

Other information

• No anticoagulation is required for haemofiltration as the drotrecogin acts as an anticoagulant
• Can be started 12 hours after major invasive procedures or surgery
• Clearance is reduced by 30% in renal impairment but no dose reduction is required
• It has a short half-life of 13 minutes and a β-half-life of 1.6 hours
• Plasma clearance
• Patients with sepsis: 40 L/hour
• Healthy subjects: 28 L/hour
• Haemodialysis patients: 30 L/hour
• Peritoneal dialysis patients: 23 L/hour

Efavirenz

Clinical use

Non-nucleoside reverse transcriptase inhibitor for progressive or advanced HIV infection in combination with other antiretroviral drugs

Dose in normal renal function

600 mg daily

Pharmacokinetics

Molecular weight (daltons)	315.7
% Protein binding	99.5–99.75
% Excreted unchanged in urine	<1
Volume of distribution (L/kg)	2–4
Half-life – normal/ESRF (hrs)	40–55 (multiple dosing) 52–76 (single dosing)

Dose in renal impairment GFR (mL/min)

20–50	Dose as in normal renal function
10–20	Dose as in normal renal function
<10	Dose as in normal renal function

Dose in patients undergoing renal replacement therapies

CAPD	Not dialysed. Dose as in normal renal function
HD	Not dialysed. Dose as in normal renal function
CAV/VVHD	Not dialysed. Dose as in normal renal function

Important drug interactions

POTENTIALLY HAZARDOUS INTERACTIONS WITH OTHER DRUGS

- Antidepressants: plasma concentration reduced by St John's Wort (avoid concomitant use)
- Antihistamines: increased risk of ventricular arrhythmias with terfenadine and mizolastine (avoid concomitant use)
- Anxiolytics and hypnotics: risk of prolonged sedation with midazolam (avoid concomitant use)
- Cisapride: avoid concomitant use
- Antivirals: lopinavir and ritonavir may require a dose increase when used with efavirenz; monitor LFTs when used in combination with ritonavir

Administration

RECONSTITUTION

–

ROUTE

- Oral

RATE OF ADMINISTRATION

–

COMMENTS

–

Other information

- Induces its own metabolism
- Metabolised by CYP 450 3A4 and 2B6 systems
- Monitor cholesterol levels as increases of 10–20% in total cholesterol has been reported
- Half-life of 10 hours in haemodialysis patients has been reported

Enalapril maleate

Clinical use

ACE inhibitor: hypertension, congestive heart failure

Dose in normal renal function

2.5–40 mg daily

Pharmacokinetics

Molecular weight (daltons)	493
% Protein binding	30–60
% Excreted unchanged in urine	43
Volume of distribution (L/kg)	1.7 ± 0.7
Half-life – normal/ESRF (hrs)	11–24/34–60

Dose in renal impairment GFR (mL/min)

20–50	Dose as in normal renal function
10–20	Start with 2.5 mg per day then dose according to response
<10	Start with 2.5 mg per day then dose according to response

Dose in patients undergoing renal replacement therapies

CAPD	Dialysed. Dose as in GFR = <10 mL/min
HD	Dialysed. Dose as in GFR = <10 mL/min
CAV/VVHD	Unknown dialysability. Dose as in GFR = 10–20 mL/min

Important drug interactions

POTENTIALLY HAZARDOUS INTERACTIONS WITH OTHER DRUGS

• Ciclosporin: possibly increases plasma-ciclosporin concentration
• Epoetin: increased risk of hyperkalaemia
• Lithium levels may be increased

• NSAIDs: antagonism of hypotensive effect; increased risk of hyperkalaemia and renal damage
• Diuretics: enhanced hypotensive effect; increased risk of hyperkalaemia with potassium-sparing diuretics
• Potassium supplements: increased risk of hyperkalaemia
• Anaesthetics: enhanced hypotensive effects

Administration

RECONSTITUTION
–

ROUTE
• Oral

RATE OF ADMINISTRATION
–

COMMENTS
–

Other information

• Side-effects, e.g. hyperkalaemia, metabolic acidosis are more common in patients with impaired renal function
• Close monitoring of renal function during therapy is necessary in those with renal insufficiency
• Renal failure has been reported in association with ACE inhibitors in patients with renal artery stenosis, post renal transplant, and in those with severe congestive heart failure
• A high incidence of anaphylactoid reactions has been reported in patients dialysed with high-flux polyacrylonitrile membranes and treated concomitantly with an ACE inhibitor – this combination should therefore be avoided
• ACE inhibitor cough may be helped by sodium cromoglycate inhalers
• Enalapril maleate is a pro-drug that requires hepatic conversion to enalaprilat, with a long half-life and as such is not suitable for use as an ACE inhibitor test dose agent
• Enalaprilat injection available on a 'named patient' basis

Enoxaparin (LMWH)

Clinical use

- Prophylaxis of thromboembolic disorders of venous origin
- Treatment of deep vein thrombosis (DVT) and pulmonary embolism (PE)
- Anticoagulation of the extra-corporeal circulation during haemodialysis
- Unstable angina

Dose in normal renal function

- Prophylaxis DVT: Low risk surgery – 20 mg SC once daily, 2 hours before surgery, thereafter for 7–10 days; High risk surgery – 40 mg SC once daily, 12 hours before surgery, thereafter for 7–10 days
- Treatment DVT and PE: 1.5 mg/kg (150 IU/kg) SC every 24 hours
- Unstable angina: 1 mg/kg every 12 hours for 2–8 days
- Anticoagulation of extra-corporeal circuits – see 'Other information'

Pharmacokinetics

Molecular weight (daltons)	Mean = 4500
% Protein binding	–
% Excreted unchanged in urine	–
Volume of distribution (L/kg)	7
Half-life – normal/ESRF (hrs)	4–5/–

Dose in renal impairment GFR (mL/min)

20–50	Dose as in normal renal function
10–20	Dose as in normal renal function for prophylaxis only – see 'Other information'
<10	Dose as in normal renal function for prophylaxis only – see 'Other information'

Dose in patients undergoing renal replacement therapies

CAPD	Not dialysed. Dose as in GFR < 10 mL/min
HD	Not dialysed. Dose as in GFR < 10 mL/min
CAV/VVHD	Not dialysed. Dose as in GFR = 10–20 mL/min

Important drug interactions

POTENTIALLY HAZARDOUS INTERACTIONS WITH OTHER DRUGS

- Use with care in patients receiving oral anticoagulants, platelet aggregation inhibitors, NSAIDs, aspirin or dextran
- Nitrates: GTN infusions increases the excretion of enoxaparin
- Ketorolac: increased risk of haemorrhage

Administration

RECONSTITUTION
–

ROUTE
- Deep SC injection

RATE OF ADMINISTRATION
–

COMMENTS
–

Other information

- In extra-corporeal circulation during haemodialysis, 1 mg/kg (100 IU/kg) enoxaparin is introduced into the arterial line of the circuit at the beginning of the session. The effect of this dose is usually sufficient for a 4-hour session, although if fibrin rings are found, a further dose of 500–1000 micrograms/kg (50–100 IU/kg) may be given. For patients with a high risk of haemorrhage, the dose should be reduced to 500 micrograms/kg for double vascular access or 750 micrograms/kg for single vascular access
- The dose of protamine to neutralise the effect of enoxaparin should equal the dose of enoxaparin: 100 anti-heparin units of protamine should neutralise the antifactor IIa activity generated by 1 mg (100 IU) of enoxaparin
- Rhone-Poulenc Rorer advise monitoring of the antifactor Xa activity, whatever the severity of the renal impairment, when treatment doses are being employed. They also advise monitoring patients if prolonged treatment using prophylactic doses are given
- Low molecular weight heparins are renally excreted and hence accumulate in severe renal impairment. While the doses recommended for prophylaxis against DVT and prevention of thrombus formation in extra-corporeal circuits are well tolerated in patients with ESRF, the doses recommended for treatment of DVT and PE have been associated with severe, sometimes fatal, bleeding episodes in such patients. Hence the use of unfractionated heparin would be preferable in these instances

Epirubicin

Clinical use

Antineoplastic agent: used for leukaemias, malignant lymphomas, multiple myeloma, and malignant neoplasms of breast, lung, ovary and gastric and colorectal cancers

Dose in normal renal function

60–90 mg/m^2 every 3 weeks, or see local protocol
Small-cell lung cancer: 120 mg/m^2 every 3 weeks
Non-small-cell lung cancer: 135 mg/m^2 every 3 weeks or 45 mg/m^2 on days 1, 2 and 3 every 3 weeks

Pharmacokinetics

Molecular weight (daltons)	580
% Protein binding	80–85
% Excreted unchanged in urine	9–10
Volume of distribution (L/kg)	23
Half-life – normal/ESRF (hrs)	30–40/unchanged

Dose in renal impairment GFR (mL/min)

20–50	Dose as in normal renal function
10–20	Dose as in normal renal function
<10	Dose as in normal renal function, but use lower dose

Dose in patients undergoing renal replacement therapies

CAPD	Removal unlikely. Dose as in normal renal function
HD	Removal unlikely. Dose as in normal renal function
CAV/VVHD	Unknown dialysability. Dose as in normal renal function

Important drug interactions

POTENTIALLY HAZARDOUS INTERACTIONS WITH OTHER DRUGS

• Ciclosporin: increased risk of neurotoxicity

Administration

RECONSTITUTION

• Reconstitute with water for injection or sodium chloride 0.9% (rapid dissolution only)

ROUTE

• IV, intravesical (bladder instillation), intrathecal

RATE OF ADMINISTRATION

• IV: give via the tubing of a fast-running intravenous infusion of sodium chloride 0.9% or glucose 5%, taking 3–5 minutes over the injection
• IV infusion: 30 minutes

COMMENTS

• For bladder instillation: concentration of epirubicin in bladder should be 50 mg per 50 mL. To avoid undue dilution in urine, the patient should be instructed not to drink any fluid in the 12 hours prior to instillation
• In the case of local toxicity dose is reduced to 30 mg per 50 mL

Other information

• A cumulative dose of 900–1000 mg/m^2 should only be exceeded with extreme caution. Above this level, the risk of irreversible congestive cardiac failure increases greatly
• Patients with impaired hepatic function have prolonged and elevated plasma concentrations of epirubicin. Dose reduction is required
• Epirubicin may make the urine red for 1–2 days after administration

Epoetin alfa (Eprex)

Clinical use

Management of anaemia associated with renal impairment in pre-dialysis and dialysis patients, and in patients receiving cancer chemotherapy

Dose in normal renal function

Renal: *Correction phase:* (to raise haemoglobin to target level) 50 units/kg three times weekly IV (increase according to response by 25 units/kg three times weekly at intervals of 4 weeks). Rise in haemoglobin should not exceed 2 g/100 mL/month (optimum rise in haemoglobin up to 1 g/100 mL/month to avoid hypertension). Target haemoglobin usually 10–12 g/100 mL *Maintenance phase:* adjust dose to maintain required haemoglobin level. The usual dose needed is 100–300 units/kg weekly in 2–3 divided doses

Cancer: initially 150 units/kg SC three times weekly and adjust according to response

Pharmacokinetics

Molecular weight (daltons)	30,400
% Protein binding	–
% Excreted unchanged in urine	–
Volume of distribution (L/kg)	0.03–0.05
Half-life – normal/ESRF (hrs)	IV: 4/unchanged SC: ≅ 24/unchanged

Dose in renal impairment GFR (mL/min)

20–50	Dose as in normal renal function
10–20	Dose as in normal renal function
<10	Dose as in normal renal function

Dose in patients undergoing renal replacement therapies

CAPD	Not dialysed. Dose as in normal renal function
HD	Not dialysed. Dose as in normal renal function
CAV/VVHD	Not dialysed. Dose as in normal renal function

Important drug interactions

POTENTIALLY HAZARDOUS INTERACTIONS WITH OTHER DRUGS

• Hyperkalaemia with ACE inhibitors and AT-II antagonists

Administration

RECONSTITUTION

• Ready reconstituted

ROUTE

• SC, cancer only (maximum 1 mL per injection site)/IV

RATE OF ADMINISTRATION

–

COMMENTS

• May also be given IV over 2 minutes, but higher doses normally needed to produce required response
• May be given intra-peritoneally, but larger doses needed

Other information

• Secondary to reports of pure red cell aplasia (PRCA), epoetin alfa is now only licensed for IV administration in renal patients
• There are reports of PRCA associated with epoetin therapy. This is a very rare condition and results in failure of the production of erythroid elements (i.e. red blood cell precursors) in the bone marrow, which in turn results in profound anaemia. This is possibly due to an immune response to the protein backbone of R-HuEPO. The antibodies formed as a result of this immune response render the patient unresponsive to the therapeutic effects of epoetin alfa, epoetin beta and darbepoetin
• Pre-treatment checks and appropriate correction/treatment needed for iron, folate and B$_{12}$ deficiency, infection, inflammation or aluminium toxicity to produce optimum response to therapy
• Concomitant iron therapy (200–300 mg elemental oral iron) needed daily. IV iron may be needed for patients with very low serum ferritins (<100 nanograms/mL)
• May increase heparin requirement during HD

Epoetin beta (Neorecormon)

Clinical use

Management of anaemia associated with renal impairment in pre-dialysis and dialysis patients, and in patients receiving cancer chemotherapy

Dose in normal renal function

Renal: *Correction phase:* (to raise haemoglobin to target level) 20 units/kg SC three times weekly for 4 weeks increasing, according to response, in steps of 20 units/kg three times weekly at monthly intervals. Maximum dose 720 units/kg weekly. Target haemoglobin usually 10–12 g/100 mL
Maintenance dose: (to maintain haemoglobin at target level) half correction phase dose, then adjust according to response at intervals of 1–2 weeks

Cancer: initially 450 units/kg weekly in 3–7 individual doses and adjust according to response

Pharmacokinetics

Molecular weight (daltons)	30,400
% Protein binding	–
% Excreted unchanged in urine	–
Volume of distribution (L/kg)	0.03–0.05
Half-life – normal/ESRF (hrs)	IV: 4–12/ unchanged SC: 13–28/ unchanged

Dose in renal impairment
GFR (mL/min)

20–50	Dose as in normal renal function
10–20	Dose as in normal renal function
<10	Dose as in normal renal function

Dose in patients undergoing renal replacement therapies

CAPD	Not dialysed. Dose as in normal renal function
HD	Not dialysed. Dose as in normal renal function
CAV/VVHD	Not dialysed. Dose as in normal renal function

Important drug interactions

POTENTIALLY HAZARDOUS INTERACTIONS WITH OTHER DRUGS

• Risk of hyperkalaemia with ACE inhibitors and AT-II antagonists

Administration

RECONSTITUTION

• Reconstitute using diluent provided only for multidose vial and penfill cartridges

ROUTE

• SC, IV

RATE OF ADMINISTRATION

–

COMMENTS

• May also be given IV over 2 minutes, but higher doses are needed to produce required response. (Does not represent cost-effective use.)

Other information

• Pre-treatment checks and appropriate correction/treatment needed for iron, folate and B_{12} deficiencies, infection, inflammation or aluminium toxicity to produce optimum response to therapy

• Concomitant iron therapy (200–300 mg elemental oral iron) needed daily. IV iron may be needed for patients with very low serum ferritins (<100 nanograms/mL)

• May increase heparin requirement during HD

• There are reports of pure red cell aplasia (PRCA) associated with epoetin therapy. This is a very rare condition and results in failure of the production of erythroid elements (i.e. red blood cell precursors) in the bone marrow, which in turn results in profound anaemia. This is possibly due to an immune response to the protein backbone of R-HuEPO. The antibodies formed as a result of this immune response render the patient unresponsive to the therapeutic effects of epoetin alfa, epoetin beta and darbepoetin

Epoprostenol (prostacyclin)

Clinical use

Vasodilator and inhibits platelet aggregation without prolonging bleeding time. Alternative to heparin to facilitate dialysis in patients with uraemic coagulopathy or disseminated intra-vascular coagulation. Also used in the treatment of peripheral vascular disease and pulmonary hypertension

Dose in normal renal function

2.5–10 nanograms/kg/minute. If used in DIC, sepsis, peripheral cyanosis or micro angiopathies, dose used is 5–20 nanograms/kg/minute

Pulmonary hypertension: usually 5–50 nanograms/kg/min, but can increase up to 300 nanograms/kg/min in severe cases

Pharmacokinetics

Molecular weight (daltons)	353
% Protein binding	–
% Excreted unchanged in urine	–
Volume of distribution (L/kg)	–
Half-life – normal/ESRF (hrs)	2–3 minutes/–

Dose in renal impairment GFR (mL/min)

20–50	Dose as in normal renal function
10–20	Dose as in normal renal function
<10	Dose as in normal renal function

Dose in patients undergoing renal replacement therapies

CAPD	Unknown dialysability. Dose as in normal renal function
HD	Unknown dialysability. Dose as in normal renal function
CAV/VVHD	Unknown dialysability. Dose as in normal renal function

Important drug interactions

POTENTIALLY HAZARDOUS INTERACTIONS WITH OTHER DRUGS

- Increased hypotensive effect with 'acetate' dialysis

Administration

RECONSTITUTION

- 500-microgram vial with diluent provided gives solution of 10,000 nanograms/mL. Can be diluted further

ROUTE

- IV or into blood supplying dialyser

RATE OF ADMINISTRATION

- Via CRIP

COMMENTS

- Complicated dosing schedule – check calculations carefully
- Infusion rate may be calculated by the following formula:

$$\text{Dose rate (mL/hr)} = \frac{\text{Dosage (nanogram/kg/min) x body weight (kg) x 60}}{\text{Concentration of infusion (nanogram/mL) (usually 10,000)}}$$

Other information

- Monitor BP and heart rate. Reduce dose if patient becomes hypotensive. Cardiovascular effects cease 30 minutes after stopping the infusion
- Some patients may exhibit allergic reaction to buffer solution used to reconstitute epoprostenol
- Solution retains 90% potency for 12 hours after dilution
- The concentrated solution should be filtered using the filter provided in the pack

Eprosartan

Clinical use

AT-II antagonist, used for hypertension

Dose in normal renal function

300–800 mg daily

Pharmacokinetics

Molecular weight (daltons)	520.6
% Protein binding	98
% Excreted unchanged in urine	<2 (as metabolites)
Volume of distribution (L/kg)	13 litres
Half-life – normal/ESRF (hrs)	5–9/unchanged

Dose in renal impairment GFR (mL/min)

20–50	Dose as in normal renal function
10–20	Dose as in normal renal function
<10	Dose as in normal renal function. Initially 300 mg daily

Dose in patients undergoing renal replacement therapies

CAPD	Unlikely dialysability. Dose as in normal renal function
HD	Not dialysed. Dose as in normal renal function
CAV/VVHD	Unlikely dialysability. Dose as in normal renal function

Important drug interactions

POTENTIALLY HAZARDOUS INTERACTIONS WITH OTHER DRUGS

• Ciclosporin: increased risk of hyperkalaemia and nephrotoxicity

• Epoetin: increased risk of hyperkalaemia; antagonism of hypotensive effect
• Lithium levels may be increased
• NSAIDs: antagonism of hypotensive effect; increased risk of hyperkalaemia and renal damage
• Diuretics: enhanced hypotensive effect; increased risk of hyperkalaemia with potassium-sparing diuretics
• Potassium supplements: increased risk of hyperkalaemia
• Anaesthetics: enhanced hypotensive effects
• Tacrolimus: increased risk of hyperkalaemia; antagonism of hypotensive effect

Administration

RECONSTITUTION

–

ROUTE

• Oral

RATE OF ADMINISTRATION

–

COMMENTS

–

Other information

• Side-effects, e.g. hyperkalaemia, metabolic acidosis are more common in patients with impaired renal function
• Close monitoring of renal function during therapy is necessary in those with renal insufficiency
• Renal failure has been reported in association with AT-II antagonists in patients with renal artery stenosis, post renal transplant, and in those with severe congestive heart failure

Erythromycin

Clinical use

Antibacterial agent

Dose in normal renal function

IV: mild to moderate infection – 25 mg/kg/day; severe infection or immunocompromised patients – 50 mg/kg/day (equivalent to 4 g per day for adults)

Oral: 250–500 mg every 6 hours or 0.5–1 g every 12 hours

Pharmacokinetics

Molecular weight (daltons)	734
% Protein binding	60–95
% Excreted unchanged in urine	15
Volume of distribution (L/kg)	0.78 (increases in ESRF)
Half-life – normal/ESRF (hrs)	1.4/5–6

Dose in renal impairment GFR (mL/min)

20–50	Dose as in normal renal function
10–20	Dose as in normal renal function
<10	50–75 % of normal dose, maximum 1.5 g daily

Dose in patients undergoing renal replacement therapies

CAPD	Removal unlikely. Dose as in GFR = <10 mL/min
HD	Not dialysed. Dose as in GFR = <10 mL/min
CAV/VVHD	Unknown dialysability. Dose as in normal renal function

Important drug interactions

POTENTIALLY HAZARDOUS INTERACTIONS WITH OTHER DRUGS

- Ciclosporin: markedly elevated ciclosporin blood levels – decreased levels on withdrawing drug. Monitor blood levels of ciclosporin carefully and adjust dose promptly as necessary

- Tacrolimus: markedly elevated tacrolimus blood levels – decreased levels on withdrawing drug. Monitor blood levels of tacrolimus carefully and adjust dose promptly as necessary

- Increased blood levels of: anticoagulants (e.g. warfarin), carbamazepine, digoxin, disopyramide, mizolastine, terfenadine, theophylline/aminophylline, phenytoin, amprenavir, midazolam, alfentanil, clozapine, zopiclone, rifabutin

- Avoid concomitant use with reboxetine, tolterodine, pimozide and ergotamine

- Risk of arrhythmias with terfenadine

- Lipid-lowering drugs: increased risk of myopathy

Administration

RECONSTITUTION

- 1 g with 20 mL water for injection, then dilute resultant solution further, e.g. 1 g in 200 mL (i.e. 5 mg/mL). [Some units use 50 mL with sodium chloride 0.9% (20 mg/mL).]

ROUTE

- IV

RATE OF ADMINISTRATION

- 1 hour using CRIP

COMMENTS

–

Other information

- May also give one-third of daily dose by infusion over 8 hours peripherally at concentration of 1 g/250 mL (4 mg/mL). Repeat 8-hourly, i.e. continuously

- Increased risk of ototoxicity in renal impairment

- Avoid peaks produced by oral twice-daily dosing, i.e. dose four times daily

- Monitor closely for thrombophlebitic reactions at site of infusion

Esomeprazole

Clinical use

Gastric acid suppression

Dose in normal renal function

20–40 mg daily

Pharmacokinetics

Molecular weight (daltons)	345
% Protein binding	97
% Excreted unchanged in urine	<1
Volume of distribution (L/kg)	0.22
Half-life – normal/ESRF (hrs)	1.3/unchanged

Dose in renal impairment GFR (mL/min)

20–50	Dose as in normal renal function
10–20	Dose as in normal renal function
<10	Dose as in normal renal function

Dose in patients undergoing renal replacement therapies

CAPD	Unlikely dialysability. Dose as in normal renal function
HD	Not dialysed. Dose as in normal renal function
CAV/VVHD	Unlikely dialysability. Dose as in normal renal function

Important drug interactions

POTENTIALLY HAZARDOUS INTERACTIONS WITH OTHER DRUGS

- Anti-epileptics: effects of phenytoin enhanced
- Anticoagulants: effect of warfarin possibly enhanced

Administration

RECONSTITUTION

–

ROUTE

- Oral

RATE OF ADMINISTRATION

–

COMMENTS

–

Other information

- Can be dispersed in half a glass of non-carbonated water. Stir well until it disintegrates; the liquid with pellets should be drunk immediately or within 30 minutes of preparation. The glass should then be rinsed with water which should also be drunk
- Do not crush or chew

Ethambutol

Clinical use

Antibacterial agent

Dose in normal renal function

15 mg/kg/day

Pharmacokinetics

Molecular weight (daltons)	204
% Protein binding	10–30
% Excreted unchanged in urine	75–90
Volume of distribution (L/kg)	3.9
Half-life – normal/ESRF (hrs)	4/7–15

Dose in renal impairment GFR (mL/min)

20–50	Dose as in normal renal function
10–20	15 mg/kg every 24–36 hours, or 7.5–15 mg/kg/day
<10	15 mg/kg every 48 hours, or 5–7.5 mg/kg/day

Dose in patients undergoing renal replacement therapies

CAPD	Dialysed. Dose as in GFR = <10 mL/min
HD	Dialysed. Dose as in GFR = <10 mL/min or on dialysis days only, give 25 mg/kg post-dialysis
CAV/VVHD	Dialysed. Dose as in GFR = 10–20 mL/min

Important drug interactions

POTENTIALLY HAZARDOUS INTERACTIONS WITH OTHER DRUGS

• None known

Administration

RECONSTITUTION

–

ROUTE

• Oral

RATE OF ADMINISTRATION

–

COMMENTS

–

Other information

• Monitor plasma levels. Dosages should be individually determined and adjusted according to measured levels and renal replacement therapy

• Baseline visual acuity tests should be performed prior to initiating ethambutol

• Daily dosing is preferred by some specialists to aid compliance and ensure maximum therapeutic effect

Ethosuximide

Clinical use

Epilepsy

Dose in normal renal function

500–1500 mg daily in divided doses

Pharmacokinetics

Molecular weight (daltons)	141
% Protein binding	10
% Excreted unchanged in urine	17–40
Volume of distribution (L/kg)	0.7
Half-life – normal/ESRF (hrs)	35–55/unchanged

Dose in renal impairment GFR (mL/min)

20–50	Dose as in normal renal function
10–20	Dose as in normal renal function
<10	Dose as in normal renal function

Dose in patients undergoing renal replacement therapies

CAPD	Dialysed. Dose as in normal renal function
HD	Dialysed. Dose as in normal renal function
CAV/VVHD	Unknown dialysability. Dose as in normal renal function

Important drug interactions

POTENTIALLY HAZARDOUS INTERACTIONS WITH OTHER DRUGS

• Isoniazid increases plasma concentrations
• Antidepressants and antipsychotics lower convulsive threshold
• Other anti-epileptics: concomitant administration may enhance toxicity

Administration

RECONSTITUTION

–

ROUTE

• Oral

RATE OF ADMINISTRATION

–

COMMENTS

–

Other information

–

Etidronate disodium

Clinical use

Bisphosphonate: Paget's disease of bone; hypercalcaemia of malignancy; treatment of vertebral osteoporosis (Didronel PMO)

Dose in normal renal function

Paget's disease and hypercalcaemia: 5–20 mg/kg daily

Vertebral osteoporosis: 400 mg daily for 14 days followed by 76 days of calcium carbonate 1.25 g (= 500 mg calcium)

Pharmacokinetics

Molecular weight (daltons)	250
% Protein binding	Depends on calcium concentration and pH
% Excreted unchanged in urine	40–60
Volume of distribution (L/kg)	0.3–1.3
Half-life – normal/ESRF (hrs)	2–6/–

Dose in renal impairment GFR (mL/min)

20–50	Maximum dose = 5 mg/kg/day
10–20	Maximum dose = 5 mg/kg/day – use with caution. (May also use Didronel PMO for osteoporosis)
<10	Maximum dose = 5 mg/kg/day – use with caution. (May also use Didronel PMO for osteoporosis)

Dose in patients undergoing renal replacement therapies

CAPD	Unknown dialysability. Dose as in GFR = <10 mL/min
HD	Unknown dialysability. Dose as in GFR = <10 mL/min
CAV/VVHD	Unknown dialysability. Dose as in GFR = 10–20 mL/min

Important drug interactions

POTENTIALLY HAZARDOUS INTERACTIONS WITH OTHER DRUGS

• See 'Comments'

Administration

RECONSTITUTION

–

ROUTE

• Oral. (Didronel IV no longer available in the UK)

RATE OF ADMINISTRATION

–

COMMENTS

• Take on an empty stomach. It is recommended that patients take the therapy with water at the midpoint of a 4-hour fast (i.e. 2 hours before and 2 hours after food)

• Do not give iron and mineral supplements, antacids or phosphate binders within 2 hours of an etidronate dose

• Oral bioavailability is very low. Only about 4% of dose is absorbed

Other information

• Hypercalcaemia may cause or exacerbate impaired renal function

• The renal clearance of etidronate is 1.2 mL/minute/kg, whilst the total body clearance is 2.2 mL/minute/kg. Elimination is likely to be reduced in patients with renal impairment and elderly with reduced renal function necessitating caution. Uptake of etidronate by bone represents non-renal clearance

• Occasional mild to moderate abnormalities in renal function (increased BUN and serum creatinine) have been observed when etidronate was given IV, as directed, to patients with hypercalcaemia of malignancy. These changes were reversible or remained stable without worsening after completion of the course of IV etidronate. In some patients with pre-existing renal impairment or in those who had received nephrotoxic drugs, further depression of renal function was seen. Appropriate monitoring of renal function is essential during treatment

Etodolac

Clinical use

NSAID: rheumatoid arthritis and osteoarthritis

Dose in normal renal function

600 mg once daily

Pharmacokinetics

Molecular weight (daltons)	287
% Protein binding	>99
% Excreted unchanged in urine	<5
Volume of distribution (L/kg)	0.4
Half-life – normal/ESRF (hrs)	5–7/unchanged

Dose in renal impairment GFR (mL/min)

20–50	Dose as in normal renal function, but avoid if possible
10–20	Dose as in normal renal function, but avoid if possible
<10	Dose as in normal renal function, but only use if ESRD on dialysis

Dose in patients undergoing renal replacement therapies

CAPD	Not dialysed. Dose as in normal renal function
HD	Not dialysed. Dose as in normal renal function
CAV/VVHD	Unlikely to be dialysed. Use lowest possible dose

Important drug interactions

POTENTIALLY HAZARDOUS INTERACTIONS WITH OTHER DRUGS

- Ciclosporin: increased risk of nephrotoxicity
- ACE inhibitors or AT-II antagonists: antagonism of hypotensive effect
- Other NSAIDs: increased side-effects
- Sulphonylureas: effect possibly enhanced
- Methotrexate: reduced excretion
- Lithium: reduced excretion
- Anticoagulants: enhanced effects
- Antibacterials: increased risk of convulsions with quinolones
- Tacrolimus: increased risk of nephrotoxicity

Administration

RECONSTITUTION

–

ROUTE

- Oral

RATE OF ADMINISTRATION

–

COMMENTS

- Take with or after food

Other information

- Inhibition of renal prostaglandin synthesis by NSAIDs may interfere with renal function, especially in the presence of existing renal disease. Avoid if possible; if not, check serum creatinine 48–72 hours after starting NSAID. If increased, discontinue therapy
- In patients with renal, cardiac or hepatic impairment, especially those taking diuretics, caution is required since the use of NSAIDs may result in deterioration of renal function. The dose should be kept as low as possible and renal function should be monitored
- Use normal doses in patients with ESRD on dialysis
- Use with caution in renal transplant recipients – can reduce intra-renal autocoid synthesis
- Accumulation of etodolac is unlikely in ARF, CRF or dialysis patients as it is metabolised in the liver

Etomidate

Clinical use

Intravenous induction of anaesthesia

Dose in normal renal function

0.3 mg/kg
High risk patients: 0.1 mg/kg/minute until
anaesthetised (about 3 minutes)

Pharmacokinetics

Molecular weight (daltons)	244
% Protein binding	75
% Excreted unchanged in urine	2
Volume of distribution (L/kg)	2–4.5
Half-life – normal/ESRF (hrs)	4–5/unchanged

Dose in renal impairment
GFR (mL/min)

20–50	Dose as in normal renal function
10–20	Dose as in normal renal function
<10	Dose as in normal renal function

Dose in patients undergoing renal replacement therapies

CAPD	Unknown dialysability. Dose as in normal renal function
HD	Unknown dialysability. Dose as in normal renal function
CAV/VVHD	Unknown dialysability. Dose as in normal renal function

Important drug interactions

POTENTIALLY HAZARDOUS INTERACTIONS WITH OTHER DRUGS

- Enhanced hypotensive effect with ACE inhibitors, AT-II antagonists, antihypertensives, antipsychotics, beta-blockers, calcium-channel blockers
- Increased risk of arrhythmias with dopaminergics and sympathomimetics

Administration

RECONSTITUTION

- 5–10 mL of infusion fluid or water for injection

ROUTE

- Intravenous injection only

RATE OF ADMINISTRATION

- 5 minutes to 3.5 hours

COMMENTS

- May be diluted with sodium chloride 0.9% or glucose 5%. Incompatible with Compound Sodium Lactate Infusion BP (Hartmann's solution)

Other information

- In cases of adrenocortical gland dysfunction and during very long surgical procedures, a prophylactic cortisol supplement may be required (e.g. 50–100 mg hydrocortisone)

Etoposide

Clinical use

Antineoplastic agent

Dose in normal renal function

IV: 60–120 mg/m^2 daily according to local protocol
Oral: twice the relevant IV dose should be given daily according to local protocol

Pharmacokinetics

Molecular weight (daltons)	589
% Protein binding	74–94
% Excreted unchanged in urine	20–60
Volume of distribution (L/kg)	0.17–0.5
Half-life – normal/ESRF (hrs)	4–8/19

Dose in renal impairment GFR (mL/min)

60	85% of dose
45–60	80% of dose and see 'Other information'
30–45	75% of dose and see 'Other information'
<30	Further dose reduction base on clinical response and see 'Other information'

Dose in patients undergoing renal replacement therapies

CAPD	Not dialysed. Dose as in GFR < 30 mL/min
HD	Not dialysed. Dose as in GFR < 30 mL/min
CAV/VVHD	Unknown dialysability. Dose as in GFR < 30 mL/min

Important drug interactions

POTENTIALLY HAZARDOUS INTERACTIONS WITH OTHER DRUGS

• Ciclosporin: 50% reduction in etoposide clearance

Administration

RECONSTITUTION

• Dilute with sodium chloride 0.9% to give a solution concentration of not more than 0.25 mg/mL of etoposide

ROUTE

• Oral or IV. Must not be given by intra-cavitary injection

RATE OF ADMINISTRATION

• IV infusion: not less than 30 minutes

COMMENTS

–

Other information

• Avoid skin contact
• One study suggested that patients with serum creatinine >130 micromol/L require a 30% dose reduction (Joel et al. (1991) Renal function and etoposide pharmacokinetics: is dose modification necessary? Am Soc Clin Oncol. 10: 103). This dose adjustment was calculated to result in equivalent total dose exposure in patients with reduced renal function. Furthermore, patients with a raised bilirubin and/or decreased albumin may have an increase in free etoposide and hence greater myelosuppression
• Reaches high concentration in kidney: possible accumulation in renal impairment
• Plasma clearance is reduced and Vd increased in renal impairment
• Kintzel et al. (1995) Cancer Treatment Reviews. 21: 33–64 provide dose modifications listed under 'Dose in renal impairment'
• Has been used in a haemodialysis patient at a dose increased gradually to 250 mg per treatment without any problems. (Holthius JJM et al. (1985) Pharmacokinetic evaluation of increased dosages of etoposide in a chronic haemodialysis patient. Cancer Treatment Rep. 69(11): 1279–82)
• BMS advise giving 75% of dose if GFR is 15–50 mL/min

Etoricoxib

Clinical use

NSAID: rheumatoid arthritis (RA) and
osteoarthritis (OA) and pain and inflammation
associated with acute gouty arthritis, dental pain
and dysmenorrhoea

Dose in normal renal function

RA: 90 mg once daily

OA and other indications: 60 mg once daily

Acute gouty arthritis or dental pain after surgery:
120 mg once daily (only for acute symptomatic
period)

Pharmacokinetics

Molecular weight (daltons)	358.8
% Protein binding	92
% Excreted unchanged in urine	<1
Volume of distribution (L/kg)	120 litres
Half-life – normal/ESRF (hrs)	22/unchanged

Dose in renal impairment
GFR (mL/min)

20–50	Dose as in normal renal function, but avoid if possible
10–20	Dose as in normal renal function, but avoid if possible
<10	Dose as in normal renal function, but only use if ESRD on dialysis

Dose in patients undergoing renal replacement therapies

CAPD	Unknown dialysability. Dose as in normal renal function
HD	Not dialysed. Dose as in normal renal function
CAV/VVHD	Unknown dialysability. Use lowest possible dose

Important drug interactions

POTENTIALLY HAZARDOUS INTERACTIONS WITH
OTHER DRUGS

• Ciclosporin: increased risk of nephrotoxicity
• ACE inhibitors and AT-II antagonists: antagonism
  of hypotensive effect
• Other NSAIDs: increased side-effects
• Sulphonylureas: effect possibly enhanced
• Methotrexate: reduced excretion
• Lithium: reduced excretion
• Anticoagulants: enhanced effects
• Antibacterials: increased risk of convulsions with
  quinolones
• Diuretics: increased risk of nephrotoxicity, may
  reduce effect of diuretics
• Tacrolimus: increased risk of nephrotoxicity
• Antivirals: increased risk of haematological
  toxicity with zidovudine; possibly increased
  plasma concentration by ritonavir

Administration

RECONSTITUTION

–

ROUTE

• Oral

RATE OF ADMINISTRATION

–

COMMENTS

• Take with or without food but onset of action is
  faster without food

Other information

• Clinical trials have shown renal effects similar to
  those observed with comparator NSAIDs.
  Monitor patient for deterioration in renal
  function and fluid retention
• Inhibition of renal prostaglandin synthesis by
  NSAIDs may interfere with renal function,
  especially in the presence of existing renal
  disease. Avoid if possible; if not, check serum
  creatinine 48–72 hours after starting NSAID.
  If raised, discontinue NSAID therapy
• Use normal doses in patients with ESRD on
  dialysis
• Use with caution in renal transplant recipients –
  can reduce intra-renal autocoid synthesis
• Etoricoxib should be used with caution in
  uraemic patients predisposed to GI bleeding or
  uraemic coagulopathies

Everolimus (unlicensed product)

Clinical use

Prophylaxis of acute rejection in allogenic renal and cardiac transplants, in combination with ciclosporin and prednisolone

Dose in normal renal function

0.75 mg twice daily

(titrate according to levels – see 'Other information')

Pharmacokinetics

Molecular weight (daltons)	958.2
% Protein binding	74
% Excreted unchanged in urine	<5
Volume of distribution (L/kg)	342 ± 107 litres
Half-life – normal/ESRF (hrs)	28 ± 7

Dose in renal impairment GFR (mL/min)

20–50	Dose as in normal renal function
10–20	Dose as in normal renal function
<10	Dose as in normal renal function

Dose in patients undergoing renal replacement therapies

CAPD	Unknown dialysability. Dose as in normal renal function
HD	Unknown dialysability. Dose as in normal renal function
CAV/VVHD	Unknown dialysability. Dose as in normal renal function

Important drug interactions

POTENTIALLY HAZARDOUS INTERACTIONS WITH OTHER DRUGS

- Ciclosporin: increases everolimus AUC by 168% and C_{max} by 82%
- Rifampicin: decreases everolimus levels by factor of 3. Increase dose x 3 and monitor levels
- Antifungals: fluconazole, ketoconazole, itraconazole increase everolimus blood levels
- Antibacterials: erythromycin, clarithromycin increase everolimus levels. Rifabutin, rifampicin decrease everolimus levels
- Anticonvulsants: carbamazepine, phenobarbital, phenytoin decrease everolimus levels
- St John's Wort: decreases everolimus levels
- Grapefruit juice: increases everolimus levels

Administration

RECONSTITUTION

–

ROUTE

- Oral

RATE OF ADMINISTRATION

–

COMMENTS

–

Other information

- None of the metabolites contribute significantly to the immunosuppressive activity of everolimus
- C_{max} and AUC are reduced by 60% and 16% respectively when everolimus is taken with a high-fat meal. Take doses consistently either with or without food to achieve consistent blood levels
- Patients achieving whole blood trough levels of ≥3.0 nanograms/mL have been found to have a lower incidence of biopsy-proven acute rejection

Ezetimibe

Clinical use

Hypercholesterolaemia either in combination with a statin or as monotherapy

Dose in normal renal function

10 mg daily

Pharmacokinetics

Molecular weight (daltons)	409.4
% Protein binding	99.7
% Excreted unchanged in urine	9 (as glucuronide)
Volume of distribution (L/kg)	No data
Half-life – normal/ESRF (hrs)	22/–

Dose in renal impairment GFR (mL/min)

20–50	Dose as in normal renal function
10–20	Dose as in normal renal function
<10	Dose as in normal renal function

Dose in patients undergoing renal replacement therapies

CAPD	Removal unlikely. Dose as in normal renal function
HD	Removal unlikely. Dose as in normal renal function
CAV/VVHD	Removal unlikely. Dose as in normal renal function

Important drug interactions

POTENTIALLY HAZARDOUS INTERACTIONS WITH OTHER DRUGS

- Ciclosporin: may increase ezetimibe levels, use with caution
- Colestyramine: reduces AUC of ezetimibe and therefore its efficacy
- Fibrates: avoid concomitant administration

Administration

RECONSTITUTION

–

ROUTE

- Oral

RATE OF ADMINISTRATION

–

COMMENTS

–

Other information

- When used with a statin LFTs should be performed before initiation of therapy and then according to recommendations of the statin
- If GFR < 30 mL/min there is a 1.5 increase in the AUC of ezetimibe but no dose adjustment is required

Famciclovir

Clinical use

Antiviral agent

Dose in normal renal function

Herpes zoster: 250 mg three times a day or 750 mg once daily for 7 days

First genital herpes infection: 250 mg three times a day for 5 days

Acute recurrent genital herpes: 125 mg twice a day for 5 days

Pharmacokinetics

Of penciclovir (active metabolite)

Molecular weight (daltons)	253
% Protein binding	<20
% Excreted unchanged in urine	43–75
Volume of distribution (L/kg)	1.5
Half-life – normal/ESRF (hrs)	1.6–2.9/3.8–25

Dose in renal impairment GFR (mL/min)

30–59	Herpes zoster and first episode genital herpes: 250 mg twice a day. Recurrent genital herpes: dose as in normal renal function
10–29	Herpes zoster and first episode genital herpes: 250 mg daily. Recurrent genital herpes: 125 mg daily
<10	Herpes zoster and first episode genital herpes: 250 mg on alternate days. Recurrent genital herpes: 125 mg on alternate days

Dose in patients undergoing renal replacement therapies

CAPD	Moderate dialysability likely. Dose as in GFR = <10 mL/min
HD	Dialysed. Dose as in GFR = <10 mL/min post dialysis on dialysis days
CAV/VVHD	Dialysability likely. Dose as in GFR = 10–29 mL/min

Important drug interactions

POTENTIALLY HAZARDOUS INTERACTIONS WITH OTHER DRUGS

• Probenecid: decreased excretion of famciclovir

• Increased famciclovir levels reported with MMF

Administration

RECONSTITUTION

–

ROUTE

• Oral

RATE OF ADMINISTRATION

–

COMMENTS

–

Other information

• Famciclovir is well absorbed after oral administration and is deacetylated and oxidised rapidly to form the potent and selective antiviral compound penciclovir

Famotidine

Clinical use

H_2-blocker: conditions associated with hyperacidity

Dose in normal renal function

20–800 mg daily (varies according to indication)

Pharmacokinetics

Molecular weight (daltons)	337
% Protein binding	15–22
% Excreted unchanged in urine	65–80
Volume of distribution (L/kg)	0.8–1.4
Half-life – normal/ESRF (hrs)	2.5–4/12–19

Dose in renal impairment GFR (mL/min)

20–50	Dose as in normal renal function
10–20	50% of normal dose
<10	20 mg at night (maximum)

Dose in patients undergoing renal replacement therapies

CAPD	Not dialysed. Dose as in GFR = <10 mL/min
HD	Not dialysed. Dose as in GFR = <10 mL/min
CAV/VVHD	Not dialysed. Dose as in GFR = 10–20 mL/min

Important drug interactions

POTENTIALLY HAZARDOUS INTERACTIONS WITH OTHER DRUGS

• None known

Administration

RECONSTITUTION

–

ROUTE

• Oral

RATE OF ADMINISTRATION

–

COMMENTS

–

Other information

–

Felodipine

Clinical use

Calcium-channel blocker: management of
hypertension, angina

Dose in normal renal function

5–10 mg once daily

Pharmacokinetics

Molecular weight (daltons)	384
% Protein binding	99
% Excreted unchanged in urine	<1
Volume of distribution (L/kg)	9–10
Half-life – normal/ESRF (hrs)	10–14/21–24

Dose in renal impairment
GFR (mL/min)

20–50	Dose as in normal renal function
10–20	Dose as in normal renal function
<10	Dose as in normal renal function

Dose in patients undergoing renal replacement therapies

CAPD	Not dialysed. Dose as in normal renal function
HD	Not dialysed. Dose as in normal renal function
CAV/VVHD	Not dialysed. Dose as in normal renal function

Important drug interactions

POTENTIALLY HAZARDOUS INTERACTIONS WITH
OTHER DRUGS

• Drugs which interfere with the CYP 450 enzyme
system may affect plasma concentrations of
felodipine: cimetidine, erythromycin, phenytoin,
carbamazepine, phenobarbital, antifungals

• Grapefruit juice should not be taken together
with felodipine

Administration

RECONSTITUTION

–

ROUTE

• Oral

RATE OF ADMINISTRATION

–

COMMENTS

–

Other information

–

Fenofibrate

Clinical use

Treatment of hyperlipidaemias types IIa, IIb, III, IV and V

Dose in normal renal function

Micronised preparation: 201–267 mg/day in 1–3 divided doses
M/R preparation: 160 mg daily

Pharmacokinetics

Molecular weight (daltons)	361
% Protein binding	99
% Excreted unchanged in urine	30–60
Volume of distribution (L/kg)	0.89
Half-life – normal/ESRF (hrs)	20/140–360

Dose in renal impairment
GFR (mL/min)

20–60	200 mg daily
10–20	100 mg daily
<10	Avoid

Dose in patients undergoing renal replacement therapies

CAPD	Unlikely to be dialysed. Avoid
HD	Unlikely to be dialysed. Avoid
CAV/VVHD	Unlikely to be dialysed. Dose as in GFR = 10–20 mL/min

Important drug interactions

POTENTIALLY HAZARDOUS INTERACTIONS WITH OTHER DRUGS

• Ciclosporin: ciclosporin levels appear to be unaffected, however it is recommended that concomitant therapy should be avoided because of the possibility of elevated serum creatinine levels
• In patients taking anticoagulants, the dose of anticoagulant should be reduced by one-third when treatment with fenofibrate is started, and then adjusted gradually if necessary
• Statins: increased risk of myopathy

Administration

RECONSTITUTION
–

ROUTE
• Oral

RATE OF ADMINISTRATION
–

COMMENTS
–

Other information

• A few studies have noted that the use of 'second generation' fibrates in transplant recipients is hampered by frequent rises in serum creatinine

Fenoprofen

Clinical use

NSAID: osteoarthritis, rheumatoid arthritis and
ankylosing spondylitis

Dose in normal renal function

300–600 mg four times a day

Pharmacokinetics

Molecular weight (daltons)	559
% Protein binding	>99
% Excreted unchanged in urine	2–5
Volume of distribution (L/kg)	0.10
Half-life – normal/ESRF (hrs)	2–3/unchanged

Dose in renal impairment
GFR (mL/min)

20–50	Start with low dose, but avoid if possible
10–20	Start with low dose, but avoid if possible
<10	Start with low dose, but only use if ESRD on dialysis

Dose in patients undergoing renal replacement therapies

CAPD	Unlikely to be dialysed. Start with low doses and increase according to response
HD	Unlikely to be dialysed. Start with low doses and increase according to response
CAV/VVHD	Unlikely to be dialysed. Dose as in GFR = 10–20 mL/min

Important drug interactions

POTENTIALLY HAZARDOUS INTERACTIONS WITH
OTHER DRUGS

• Ciclosporin: increased risk of nephrotoxicity
• ACE inhibitors and AT-II antagonists: increased risk of hyperkalaemia. Reduced hypotensive effect

• Anticoagulants: possible enhancement of effects of warfarin and acenocoumarol
• Sulphonylureas: effects possibly enhanced
• Methotrexate: excretion reduced
• Lithium: excretion reduced
• Anti-epileptics: effects of phenytoin enhanced
• Antibacterials: increased risk of convulsions with quinolones

Administration

RECONSTITUTION
–

ROUTE
• Oral

RATE OF ADMINISTRATION
–

COMMENTS
–

Other information

• Contra-indicated in patients with history of significantly impaired renal function
• Inhibition of renal prostaglandin synthesis by NSAIDs may interfere with renal function, especially in the presence of existing renal disease. Avoid use if possible. If not, check serum creatinine 48–72 hours after starting NSAID; if it has increased, discontinue therapy
• Possibility of decreased platelet aggregation
• Can use normal doses in patients with ESRD on dialysis
• Use with caution in renal transplant recipients – can reduce intra-renal autocoid synthesis
• Associated nephrotic syndrome, interstitial nephritis, hyperkalaemia, sodium retention

Fentanyl

Clinical use

Narcotic analgesic for short surgical procedures or use in ventilated patients, chronic intractable pain

Dose in normal renal function

Consult relevant data sheet

Pharmacokinetics

Molecular weight (daltons)	529
% Protein binding	79–87
% Excreted unchanged in urine	6–8
Volume of distribution (L/kg)	2–5
Half-life – normal/ESRF (hrs)	2–7/unchanged

Dose in renal impairment GFR (mL/min)

20–50	Dose as in normal renal function. Titrate according to response
10–20	75% of normal dose. Titrate according to response
<10	50% of normal dose. Titrate according to response

Dose in patients undergoing renal replacement therapies

CAPD	Not dialysed. Dose as in GFR = <10 mL/min
HD	Not dialysed. Dose as in GFR = <10 mL/min
CAV/VVHD	Not dialysed. Dose as in GFR = 10–20 mL/min

Important drug interactions

POTENTIALLY HAZARDOUS INTERACTIONS WITH OTHER DRUGS

- MAOIs: concurrent administration with MAOIs, or within 2 weeks of their discontinuation, is contra-indicated
- Non-selective CNS depressants may enhance or prolong respiratory depression
- Non-vagolytic muscle relaxants: bradycardia/asystole can occur

Administration

RECONSTITUTION

- Compatible with sodium chloride 0.9% and glucose 5%

ROUTE

- IV, IM (pre-med), topically (chronic pain)

RATE OF ADMINISTRATION

–

COMMENTS

–

Other information

- For short surgical procedures the degree of renal impairment is irrelevant
- For other indications, renal impairment may have a moderate effect on the elimination of the drug. However, as fentanyl is titrated to response the usual method of administration remains valid

Ferrous gluconate

Clinical use

Iron-deficiency anaemia. Prophylaxis and treatment of iron deficiency before and during epoetin therapy

Dose in normal renal function

Prophylaxis: 300 mg two times daily
Therapeutic: 300–600 mg 2–3 times daily

Pharmacokinetics

Molecular weight (daltons)	482
% Protein binding	–
% Excreted unchanged in urine	–
Volume of distribution (L/kg)	–
Half-life – normal/ESRF (hrs)	–

Dose in renal impairment
GFR (mL/min)

20–50	Dose as in normal renal function
10–20	Dose as in normal renal function
<10	Dose as in normal renal function

Dose in patients undergoing renal replacement therapies

CAPD	Not dialysed. Dose as in normal renal function
HD	Not dialysed. Dose as in normal renal function
CAV/VVHD	Not dialysed. Dose as in normal renal function

Important drug interactions

POTENTIALLY HAZARDOUS INTERACTIONS WITH OTHER DRUGS

• Reduced absorption of 4-quinolones

Administration

RECONSTITUTION
–

ROUTE
• Oral

RATE OF ADMINISTRATION
–

COMMENTS
–

Other information

• One 300 mg ferrous gluconate tablet contains 35 mg elemental iron. Best taken before food to aid absorption

• Phosphate-binding agents, e.g. calcium carbonate or magnesium carbonate reduce absorption of iron from the gut

• Monitor serum iron, transferrin saturation, ferritin levels (in line with local policy)

Ferrous sulphate

Clinical use

Iron-deficiency anaemia. Prophylaxis and treatment of iron deficiency before and during epoetin therapy

Dose in normal renal function

Prophylaxis: 200 mg daily
Therapeutic: 200 mg 2–3 times daily

Pharmacokinetics

Molecular weight (daltons)	278
% Protein binding	–
% Excreted unchanged in urine	–
Volume of distribution (L/kg)	–
Half-life – normal/ESRF (hrs)	–

Dose in renal impairment GFR (mL/min)

20–50	Dose as in normal renal function
10–20	Dose as in normal renal function
<10	Dose as in normal renal function

Dose in patients undergoing renal replacement therapies

CAPD	Not dialysed. Dose as in normal renal function
HD	Not dialysed. Dose as in normal renal function
CAV/VVHD	Not dialysed. Dose as in normal renal function

Important drug interactions

POTENTIALLY HAZARDOUS INTERACTIONS WITH OTHER DRUGS

• Decreases absorption of 4-quinolones

Administration

RECONSTITUTION
–

ROUTE
• Oral

RATE OF ADMINISTRATION
–

COMMENTS
–

Other information

• One 200 mg ferrous sulphate tablet contains 65 mg elemental iron
• Absorption of iron may be enhanced with concurrent administration of ascorbic acid
• Phosphate-binding agents, e.g. calcium carbonate or magnesium carbonate reduce absorption of iron from the gut
• Monitor: serum iron, transferrin saturation, ferritin levels (in line with local policy)

Fexofenadine

Clinical use

Antihistamine, used for symptomatic relief of rhinitis and urticaria

Dose in normal renal function

120–180 mg daily depending on condition

Pharmacokinetics

Molecular weight (daltons)	538
% Protein binding	60–70
% Excreted unchanged in urine	11
Volume of distribution (L/kg)	5.4–5.8
Half-life – normal/ESRF (hrs)	11–15/19–25

Dose in renal impairment GFR (mL/min)

20–50	Dose as in normal renal function. Use with care
10–20	Initial dose 60 mg once or twice daily. See 'Other information'
<10	Initial dose 60 mg once daily. See 'Other information'

Dose in patients undergoing renal replacement therapies

CAPD	Unlikely dialysability. Dose as in GFR = <10 mL/min
HD	Not dialysed. Dose as in GFR = <10 mL/min
CAV/VVHD	Unlikely dialysability. Dose as in GFR = 10–20 mL/min

Important drug interactions

POTENTIALLY HAZARDOUS INTERACTIONS WITH OTHER DRUGS

• Aluminium/magnesium-containing antacids: reduced absorption. Avoid for 2 hours

Administration

RECONSTITUTION

–

ROUTE

• Oral

RATE OF ADMINISTRATION

–

COMMENTS

• Take before food

Other information

• Less than 1.5% of a dose is metabolised via the CYP 450 3A4 system
• Larger doses may be used but increase carefully

Filgrastim

Clinical use

Recombinant human granulocyte-colony stimulating factor (rhG-CSF) – treatment of neutropenia

Dose in normal renal function

0.5–1.2 MU/kg/day according to indication and patient response

Pharmacokinetics

Molecular weight (daltons)	18,799
% Protein binding	Very high
% Excreted unchanged in urine	0
Volume of distribution (L/kg)	0.15
Half-life – normal/ESRF (hrs)	3.5/–

Dose in renal impairment
GFR (mL/min)

20–50	Dose as in normal renal function and titrate dose to response
10–20	Dose as in normal renal function and titrate dose to response
<10	Dose as in normal renal function and titrate dose to response

Dose in patients undergoing renal replacement therapies

CAPD	Not dialysed. Dose as in GFR = <10 mL/min
HD	Not dialysed. Dose as in GFR = <10 mL/min
CAV/VVHD	Not dialysed. Dose as in GFR = 10–20 mL/min

Important drug interactions

POTENTIALLY HAZARDOUS INTERACTIONS WITH OTHER DRUGS

• None known

Administration

RECONSTITUTION

–

ROUTE

• IV, SC

RATE OF ADMINISTRATION

• IV: over 30 minutes or continuous IV infusion over 24 hours

• SC: can give as continuous SC infusion over 24 hours

COMMENTS

• IV: dilute with glucose 5% only. Minimum concentration 0.2 MU per mL. Add Human Serum Albumin if concentration is less than 1.5 MU per mL

• SC: continuous infusion – dilute with 20 mL of glucose 5%

• Dilute Neupogen may be adsorbed to glass and plastic materials – follow recommendations for dilution

Other information

• One very small study (2–3 patients) concluded that body clearance of filgrastim was not affected by degree of renal impairment

Finasteride

Clinical use

Benign prostatic hypertrophy

Dose in normal renal function

5 mg daily

Pharmacokinetics

Molecular weight (daltons)	373
% Protein binding	≈93
% Excreted unchanged in urine	<0.05
Volume of distribution (L/kg)	1.07
Half-life – normal/ESRF (hrs)	6/–

Dose in renal impairment GFR (mL/min)

20–50	Dose as in normal renal function
10–20	Dose as in normal renal function
<10	Dose as in normal renal function

Dose in patients undergoing renal replacement therapies

CAPD	Unlikely to be dialysed. Dose as in normal renal function
HD	Unlikely to be dialysed. Dose as in normal renal function
CAV/VVHD	Unlikely to be dialysed. Dose as in normal renal function

Important drug interactions

POTENTIALLY HAZARDOUS INTERACTIONS WITH OTHER DRUGS

• None known

Administration

RECONSTITUTION

–

ROUTE

• Oral

RATE OF ADMINISTRATION

–

COMMENTS

–

Other information

• Data sheet states that no dosage adjustment is required in renally impaired patients whose creatinine clearance is as low as 9 mL/min. No studies have been done in patients with creatinine clearance of less than 9 mL/min

Flecainide

Clinical use

Class Ic anti-arrhythmic agent used for the treatment of ventricular arrhythmias and tachycardias

Dose in normal renal function

Supraventricular arrhythmias: 100–300 mg daily in two divided doses

Ventricular arrhythmias: 200–400 mg daily in two divided doses

IV bolus: 2 mg/kg over not less than 10 minutes

IV infusion: 2 mg/kg over 30 minutes, then

1st hour: 1.5 mg/kg/hour

Subsequently: 0.1–0.25 mg/kg/hour; maximum 600 mg in 24 hours

Pharmacokinetics

Molecular weight (daltons)	474
% Protein binding	52
% Excreted unchanged in urine	25
Volume of distribution (L/kg)	8.4–9.5
Half-life – normal/ESRF (hrs)	7–23/9–58

Dose in renal impairment GFR (mL/min)

20–50	See 'Other information'
10–20	See 'Other information'
<10	See 'Other information'

Dose in patients undergoing renal replacement therapies

CAPD	≈1% dialysed. Dose as in GFR = <10 mL/min
HD	≈1% dialysed. Dose as in GFR = <10 mL/min
CAV/VVHD	Minimal removal. Dose as in GFR = 10–20 mL/min

Important drug interactions

POTENTIALLY HAZARDOUS INTERACTIONS WITH OTHER DRUGS

• Other anti-arrhythmics: amiodarone increases plasma flecainide levels; increased risk of ventricular arrhythmias. Increased myocardial depression with any anti-arrhythmic

• Antidepressants: fluoxetine increases plasma flecainide levels; increased risk of ventricular arrhythmias with fluoxetine and tricyclics

• Antihistamines: increased risk of ventricular arrhythmias with mizolastine and terfenadine

• Anti-malarials: quinine increases plasma levels of flecainide

• Beta-blockers: increased myocardial depression and bradycardia

• Calcium-channel blocker: increased myocardial depression and asystole with verapamil

• Diuretics: cardiac toxicity increased if hypokalaemia occurs

• Antivirals: ritonavir increases plasma concentrations

Administration

RECONSTITUTION

–

ROUTE

• Oral, IV bolus, IV infusion

RATE OF ADMINISTRATION

• See 'Other information'

COMMENTS

• Infusion: dilute with glucose 5% infusion. If chloride-containing solutions are used the injection should be added to a volume of not less than 500 mL, otherwise a precipitate will form

• Plasma levels of 200–1000 nanogram/mL may be needed to obtain the maximum therapeutic effect. Plasma levels above 700–1000 nanogram/mL are associated with increased likelihood of adverse experiences

Other information

• Product information recommends reducing dosing recommendations for IV infusion by half in patients with severe renal impairment, defined as being a creatinine clearance of less than 35 mL/minute

• Product information recommends for patients with severe renal impairment as defined above, that the maximum initial oral dosage should be 100 mg daily (or 50 mg twice daily) with frequent plasma level monitoring strongly recommended

• Electrolyte disturbances should be corrected before using flecainide

• Plasma levels quoted in product information are trough levels. Sample prior to dose

Flucloxacillin

Clinical use

Antibacterial agent

Dose in normal renal function

Oral: 250–500 mg every 6 hours
IV/IM: 250 mg – 2 g every 6 hours

Pharmacokinetics

Molecular weight (daltons)	453
% Protein binding	95
% Excreted unchanged in urine	60–90
Volume of distribution (L/kg)	0–13 (altered in hypoalbumin-aemia and uraemia)
Half-life – normal/ESRF (hrs)	0.8–1.0/3.0

Dose in renal impairment GFR (mL/min)

20–50	Dose as in normal renal function
10–20	Dose as in normal renal function
<10	Dose as in normal renal function up to a total daily dose of 4 g

Dose in patients undergoing renal replacement therapies

CAPD	Not dialysed. Dose as in GFR = <10 mL/min
HD	Not dialysed. Dose as in GFR = <10 mL/min
CAV/VVHD	Not dialysed. Dose as in normal renal function

Important drug interactions

POTENTIALLY HAZARDOUS INTERACTIONS WITH OTHER DRUGS

• Reduces excretion of methotrexate

Administration

RECONSTITUTION

• IV: 250 mg and 500 mg in 5–10 mL water for injection; 1 g in 15–20 mL water for injection
• IM: 1.5 mL water for injection to 250 mg; 2 mL water for injection to 500 mg

ROUTE

• IV, IM, oral

RATE OF ADMINISTRATION

• 3–4 minutes – bolus
• 30–60 minutes – infusion

COMMENTS

• Compatible with various infusion fluids

Other information

• Monitor urine for protein at high doses
• Sodium content of injection 2.0 mmol/g
• Monitor LFTs in hypoalbuminaemic patients receiving high doses of flucloxacillin (e.g. CAPD patients)

Fluconazole

Clinical use

Antifungal agent

Dose in normal renal function

50–400 mg daily

Pharmacokinetics

Molecular weight (daltons)	306
% Protein binding	12
% Excreted unchanged in urine	70
Volume of distribution (L/kg)	0.7
Half-life – normal/ESRF (hrs)	22/98

Dose in renal impairment GFR (mL/min)

20–50	Dose as in normal renal function
10–20	Dose as in normal renal function
<10	50% of normal dose

Dose in patients undergoing renal replacement therapies

CAPD	Dialysed. Dose as in GFR = <10 mL/min
HD	Dialysed. Dose as in GFR = <10 mL/min. Give post dialysis
CAV/VVHD	Dialysed. Dose as in normal renal function

Important drug interactions

POTENTIALLY HAZARDOUS INTERACTIONS WITH OTHER DRUGS

- Ciclosporin: increases blood/serum ciclosporin levels
- Tacrolimus: increases blood/serum tacrolimus levels
- Potentiates effect of warfarin
- Increases phenytoin levels and effect
- Increases theophylline, rifabutin, zidovudine, sulphonylurea levels
- Metabolism accelerated by rifampicin

Administration

RECONSTITUTION

- IV preparation supplied as solution

ROUTE

- Oral, IV

RATE OF ADMINISTRATION

- IV: 5–10 mL/minute peripherally

COMMENTS

- Oral ≡ IV dose. Very high bioavailability

Other information

- Has been used as adjunct to IV amphotericin and IP flucytosine in CAPD peritonitis
- No dose adjustment is required for single-dose therapy
- Recurrent yeast peritonitis: flucytosine **2000 mg** orally stat, then 1000 mg daily in addition to fluconazole 150 mg IP or 200 mg orally on alternate days. Remove Tenchkoff after 4–7 days if no response
- 3 hours haemodialysis reduces blood levels by 50%

Flucytosine

Clinical use

Antifungal agent

Dose in normal renal function

Oral/IV: 200 mg/kg per day in four divided doses

Pharmacokinetics

Molecular weight (daltons)	129
% Protein binding	<10
% Excreted unchanged in urine	80–90
Volume of distribution (L/kg)	0.6
Half-life – normal/ESRF (hrs)	3–6/75–200

Dose in renal impairment GFR (mL/min)

20–40	50 mg/kg 12-hourly
10–20	50 mg/kg 24-hourly
<10	50 mg/kg then dose according to levels. Dose 500 mg – 1 g daily is usually adequate

Dose in patients undergoing renal replacement therapies

CAPD	Dialysed. Give 50 mg/kg daily in four divided doses. Monitor levels
HD	Dialysed. Dose as in GFR = <10 mL/min, given post dialysis. Monitor trough level pre-dialysis, and reduce post-dialysis dose accordingly
CAV/VVHD	Dialysed. Give dose as in GFR = 10–20 mL/min and monitor blood levels, pre-dose

Important drug interactions

POTENTIALLY HAZARDOUS INTERACTIONS WITH OTHER DRUGS

• Cytarabine: monitor flucytosine levels

Administration

RECONSTITUTION

–

ROUTE

• IV peripherally through a blood filter

RATE OF ADMINISTRATION

• 20–40 minutes

COMMENTS

–

Other information

• Monitor blood levels 24 hours after therapy commences. Pre-dose level 25–50 micrograms/mL is usually adequate. Do not exceed 80 micrograms/mL

• 250 mL intravenous flucytosine infusion contains 34.5 mmol sodium

• Bone marrow suppression more common in patients with renal impairment

• Tablets available on 'named patient' basis only

• Can be given IP at a dose of 50 mg/L

Fludarabine phosphate

Clinical use

B-cell chronic lymphocytic leukaemia

Dose in normal renal function

IV: 25 mg/m^2 daily for 5 days then repeated every 28 days

Oral: 40 mg/m^2 for 5 days every 28 days

Pharmacokinetics

Molecular weight (daltons)	365.2
% Protein binding	60
% Excreted unchanged in urine	40–60
Volume of distribution (L/kg)	2.4 ± 1.6
Half-life – normal/ESRF (hrs)	10–30/increased

Dose in renal impairment GFR (mL/min)

30–70	Reduce dose by 50–75%
10–30	50–75%. Use with care
<10	50%. Use with care

Dose in patients undergoing renal replacement therapies

CAPD	Unknown dialysability. Dose as in GFR = <10 mL/min
HD	Unknown dialysability. Dose as in GFR = <10 mL/min
CAV/VVHD	Unknown dialysability. Dose as in GFR = 10–30 mL/min

Important drug interactions

POTENTIALLY HAZARDOUS INTERACTIONS WITH OTHER DRUGS

• Other cytotoxics: increased pulmonary toxicity with pentostatin (unacceptably high incidence of fatalities); increases intracellular concentration of cytarabine

Administration

RECONSTITUTION

• Reconstitute each vial with 2 mL of water for injection to give a concentration of 25 mg/mL

ROUTE

• IV, oral

RATE OF ADMINISTRATION

• Infusion should be administered over 30 minutes

COMMENTS

• IV bolus in 10 mL of sodium chloride 0.9%
• IV infusion in 100 mL of sodium chloride 0.9%

Other information

• Administer up to achievement of response, usually six cycles then discontinue
• Patients with renal failure (GFR = 17–41 mL/min/m^2) receiving 20% of dose had a similar AUC as patients with normal renal function receiving the full dose

Fludrocortisone acetate

Clinical use

Replacement therapy in adrenal insufficiency

Dose in normal renal function

50–300 micrograms daily

Pharmacokinetics

Molecular weight (daltons)	422.5
% Protein binding	70–80
% Excreted unchanged in urine	80% (as metabolites)
Volume of distribution (L/kg)	widely distributed
Half-life – normal/ESRF (hrs)	3.5 (biological half-life 18–36 hours)

Dose in renal impairment GFR (mL/min)

20–50	Dose as in normal renal function
10–20	Dose as in normal renal function
<10	Dose as in normal renal function

Dose in patients undergoing renal replacement therapies

CAPD	Unknown dialysability. Dose as in normal renal function
HD	Unknown dialysability. Dose as in normal renal function
CAV/VVHD	Unknown dialysability. Dose as in normal renal function

Important drug interactions

POTENTIALLY HAZARDOUS INTERACTIONS WITH OTHER DRUGS

• Rifamycins: accelerate metabolism of corticosteroids
• Anticoagulants: altered effect of warfarin and acenocoumarol
• Anti-epileptics: accelerate metabolism of corticosteroids
• Antifungals: increased risk of hypokalaemia with amphotericin

Administration

RECONSTITUTION

–

ROUTE

• Oral

RATE OF ADMINISTRATION

–

COMMENTS

• Use for as short a time and as low a dose as possible

Other information

–

Flumazenil

Clinical use

Reversal of sedative effects of benzodiazepines in anaesthetic, intensive care and diagnostic procedures

Dose in normal renal function

Initially 200 micrograms over 15 seconds, then 100 micrograms at 60-second intervals if required; usual dose range 300–600 micrograms. Maximum dose: 1 mg, or 2 mg in intensive care situations. If drowsiness recurs, an IV infusion of 100–400 micrograms per hour may be given

Pharmacokinetics

Molecular weight (daltons)	303
% Protein binding	40–50
% Excreted unchanged in urine	<0.1
Volume of distribution (L/kg)	0.6–1.1
Half-life – normal/ESRF (hrs)	0.7–1.3/–

Dose in renal impairment GFR (mL/min)

20–50	Dose as in normal renal function
10–20	Dose as in normal renal function
<10	Dose as in normal renal function

Dose in patients undergoing renal replacement therapies

CAPD	Unknown dialysability. Dose as in normal renal function
HD	Unknown dialysability. Dose as in normal renal function
CAV/VVHD	Unknown dialysability. Dose as in normal renal function

Important drug interactions

POTENTIALLY HAZARDOUS INTERACTIONS WITH OTHER DRUGS

• None known

Administration

RECONSTITUTION

–

ROUTE

• IV injection, IV infusion

RATE OF ADMINISTRATION

• See 'Dose in normal renal function'

COMMENTS

• Infusion: suitable diluents include sodium chloride 0.9% infusion, glucose 5% IV infusion

Other information

• The half-life of flumazenil is shorter than those of diazepam and midazolam, hence patients should be closely monitored to avoid the risk of patients becoming resedated

Fluorouracil

Clinical use

Antineoplastic agent

Dose in normal renal function

IV infusion: 15 mg/kg/day to a total dose of
12–15 g

IV bolus: 12 mg/kg/day for 3 days, then 6 mg/kg on
alternate days or 15 mg/kg once a week

Intra-arterial infusion: 5.0–7.5 mg/kg by continuous
24-hour infusion

Maintenance: 5–15 mg/kg once a week
or consult relevant local chemotherapy protocol

Oral: 15 mg/kg weekly. Maximum 1 g in a day

Pharmacokinetics

Molecular weight (daltons)	130
% Protein binding	10
% Excreted unchanged in urine	15
Volume of distribution (L/kg)	0.25–0.5
Half-life – normal/ESRF (hrs)	0.1/unchanged

Dose in renal impairment
GFR (mL/min)

20–50	Dose as in normal renal function
10–20	Dose as in normal renal function
<10	Dose as in normal renal function

Dose in patients undergoing
renal replacement therapies

CAPD	Some removal likely. Dose as in GFR = <10 mL/min
HD	Dialysed. Dose as in GFR = <10 mL/min
CAV/VVHD	Dialysed. Dose as in GFR = 10–20 mL/min

Important drug interactions

POTENTIALLY HAZARDOUS INTERACTIONS WITH
OTHER DRUGS

• Metronidazole and cimetidine inhibit metabolism
(increased toxicity)

Administration

RECONSTITUTION

• Consult relevant local protocol

ROUTE

• IV infusion intermittent or continuous,
IV injection, intra-arterial, oral, topical

RATE OF ADMINISTRATION

• Consult relevant local protocol

COMMENTS

–

Other information

• Use ideal body-weight in patients showing
obesity, ascites, oedema

• Roche recommends decreasing the initial dose
by one-third to one-half in patients with impaired
hepatic or renal function

Fluoxetine

Clinical use

SSRI antidepressant: depressive illness, bulimia nervosa, obsessive compulsive disorder, premenstrual dysphoric disorder

Dose in normal renal function

20–60 mg daily depending on indication

Pharmacokinetics

Molecular weight (daltons)	346
% Protein binding	94.5
% Excreted unchanged in urine	<10
Volume of distribution (L/kg)	20–42
Half-life – normal/ESRF (hrs)	24–72/unchanged (acute dosing); 4–6 days/– (chronic dosing)

Dose in renal impairment GFR (mL/min)

20–50	Dose as in normal renal function
10–20	Dose as in normal renal function or on alternate days
<10	Dose as in normal renal function or on alternate days

Dose in patients undergoing renal replacement therapies

CAPD	Not dialysed. Dose as in GFR < 10 mL/min
HD	Not dialysed. Dose as in GFR < 10 mL/min
CAV/VVHD	Not dialysed. Dose as in GFR = 10–20 mL/min

Important drug interactions

POTENTIALLY HAZARDOUS INTERACTIONS WITH OTHER DRUGS

- Anticoagulants: effects of warfarin enhanced
- Other antidepressants: enhanced CNS effects of MAOIs and linezolid (increased risk of toxicity)
- Anti-epileptics: antagonism (lowered convulsive threshold). Plasma concentrations of carbamazepine and phenytoin increased
- Antipsychotics: plasma concentrations of haloperidol, clozapine and sertindole increased
- Dopaminergics: hypertension and CNS excitation
- Lithium: increased risk of CNS effects (lithium toxicity reported)
- Antihistamines: increased risk of arrhythmias with terfenadine
- Sibutramine: increased risk of CNS toxicity – avoid concomitant use

Administration

RECONSTITUTION

–

ROUTE

- Oral

RATE OF ADMINISTRATION

–

COMMENTS

–

Other information

- Accumulation may occur in patients with severe renal failure during chronic treatment (metabolites are excreted renally)
- Levy NB et al. (1996) General Hosp Psychiatry. 18: 8–13 studied seven patients undergoing haemodialysis and concluded that the process of HD does not alter the pharmacokinetics of fluoxetine or its major metabolite. All patients received fluoxetine 20 mg per day for 8 weeks

Flurbiprofen

Clinical use

NSAID: rheumatic disease and other
musculoskeletal disorders; dysmenorrhoea;
post-operative analgesia

Dose in normal renal function

Oral/PR: 150–200 mg daily in divided doses,
increased in acute conditions to 300 mg daily
Dysmenorrhoea: 50–100 mg every 4–6 hours

Pharmacokinetics

Molecular weight (daltons)	244
% Protein binding	99
% Excreted unchanged in urine	<20
Volume of distribution (L/kg)	0.10
Half-life – normal/ESRF (hrs)	3–5/unchanged

Dose in renal impairment
GFR (mL/min)

20–50	Dose as in normal renal function, but avoid if possible
10–20	Dose as in normal renal function but avoid if possible
<10	Dose as in normal renal function, but only if ESRD on dialysis

Dose in patients undergoing renal replacement therapies

CAPD	Removal very unlikely. Dose as in GFR = <10 mL/min
HD	Removal very unlikely. Dose as in GFR = <10 mL/min
CAV/VVHD	Removal very unlikely. Dose as in GFR = 10–20 mL/min

Important drug interactions

POTENTIALLY HAZARDOUS INTERACTIONS WITH
OTHER DRUGS

• Ciclosporin: increased risk of renal toxicity
• Tacrolimus: increased risk of renal toxicity
• Decreased excretion of lithium

• Cytotoxic agents: reduced excretion of methotrexate
• Antibacterials: increased risk of convulsions with quinolones
• Anticoagulants: effects of warfarin and acenocoumarol enhanced
• Antidiabetic agents: effects of sulphonylureas enhanced
• Anti-epileptic agents: effects of phenytoin enhanced
• ACE inhibitors and AT-II antagonists: antagonism of hypotensive effect; increased risk of hyperkalaemia and renal damage
• Uricosurics: probenecid delays excretion of NSAID

Administration

RECONSTITUTION

–

ROUTE

• Oral, PR

RATE OF ADMINISTRATION

–

COMMENTS

–

Other information

• NSAIDs have been reported to cause nephrotoxicity in various forms; interstitial nephritis, nephrotic syndrome and renal failure. In patients with renal, cardiac or hepatic impairment, caution is required since the use of NSAIDs may result in deterioration of renal function
• Inhibition of renal prostaglandin synthesis by NSAIDs may interfere with renal function, especially in the presence of existing renal disease. Avoid if possible; if not, check serum creatinine 48–72 hours after starting NSAID. If creatinine has increased, discontinue therapy
• Use normal doses in patients with ESRD on dialysis
• Use with caution in renal transplant recipients – can reduce intra-renal autocoid synthesis

Flutamide

Clinical use

Treatment of advanced prostate cancer

Dose in normal renal function

250 mg every 8 hours

Start 3 days before LHRH agonist

Pharmacokinetics

Molecular weight (daltons)	276.2
% Protein binding	>90
% Excreted unchanged in urine	45
Volume of distribution (L/kg)	No data
Half-life – normal/ESRF (hrs)	4–6

Dose in renal impairment GFR (mL/min)

20–50	Dose as in normal renal function
10–20	Dose as in normal renal function
<10	Dose as in normal renal function

Dose in patients undergoing renal replacement therapies

CAPD	Not dialysed. Dose as in normal renal function
HD	Not dialysed. Dose as in normal renal function
CAV/VVHD	Not dialysed. Dose as in normal renal function

Important drug interactions

POTENTIALLY HAZARDOUS INTERACTIONS WITH OTHER DRUGS

• Anticoagulants: effects of warfarin enhanced
• Avoid hepatoxic drugs
• Avoid excess alcohol consumption

Administration

RECONSTITUTION

–

ROUTE

• Oral

RATE OF ADMINISTRATION

–

COMMENTS

–

Other information

–

Fluvastatin

Clinical use

HMG CoA reductase inhibitor: primary
hypercholesterolaemia; slowing progression of
atherosclerosis; secondary prevention of coronary
events after percutaneous coronary intervention

Dose in normal renal function

Initially 20 mg daily in the evening; usual range
20–40 mg daily, adjusted at intervals of 4 weeks.
Maximum 40 mg twice daily

Slowing progression of atherosclerosis: 40 mg daily

Secondary prevention of coronary events after
percutaneous coronary intervention: 80 mg daily

XL: 80 mg daily

Pharmacokinetics

Molecular weight (daltons)	433.4
% Protein binding	>98
% Excreted unchanged in urine	<1
Volume of distribution (L/kg)	0.42
Half-life – normal/ESRF (hrs)	2.3–2.5/–

Dose in renal impairment GFR (mL/min)

20–50	Dose as in normal renal function
10–20	Dose as in normal renal function
<10	20 mg daily

Dose in patients undergoing renal replacement therapies

CAPD	Removal unlikely. Dose as in GFR < 10 mL/min
HD	Removal unlikely. Dose as in GFR < 10 mL/min
CAV/VVHD	Removal unlikely. Dose as in normal renal function

Important drug interactions

POTENTIALLY HAZARDOUS INTERACTIONS WITH
OTHER DRUGS

- Ciclosporin: concomitant treatment with
  ciclosporin may lead to risk of muscle toxicity
- Other lipid-lowering drugs and erythromycin:
  increased risk of serious muscle toxicity
- Antibacterials: rifampicin increases metabolism

Administration

RECONSTITUTION

–

ROUTE

- Oral

RATE OF ADMINISTRATION

–

COMMENTS

–

Other information

- The CSM has advised that rhabdomyolysis
  associated with lipid-lowering drugs, such as the
  fibrates and statins, appears to be rare (approx. 1
  case in every 100,000 treatment years), but may
  be increased in those with renal impairment and
  possibly in those with hypothyroidism
- Manufacturer's literature indicates fluvastatin is
  contra-indicated in patients with severe renal
  impairment (creatinine greater than or equal to
  160 micromol/L)

Folic acid

Clinical use

Folate deficient megaloblastic anaemia or supplement in HD patients

Dose in normal renal function

5 mg/day for 4 months, then weekly according to response

Pharmacokinetics

Molecular weight (daltons)	441.4
% Protein binding	70
% Excreted unchanged in urine	Varies with daily dose
Volume of distribution (L/kg)	–
Half-life – normal/ESRF (hrs)	2.5/–

Dose in renal impairment GFR (mL/min)

20–50	Dose as in normal renal function
10–20	Dose as in normal renal function
<10	Dose as in normal renal function

Dose for patients undergoing renal replacement therapies

CAPD	Dialysed. Dose as in normal renal function
HD	Dialysed. Dose as in normal renal function. Dose after HD
CAV/VVHD	Dialysed. Dose as in normal renal function

Important drug interactions

POTENTIALLY HAZARDOUS INTERACTIONS WITH OTHER DRUGS

• Reduces plasma phenytoin levels

Administration

RECONSTITUTION

–

ROUTE

• Oral

RATE OF ADMINISTRATION

–

COMMENTS

–

Other information

• If profusely folate deficient, give 10 mg/day for 1 month, then 5 mg/day

• Most nutritionists recommend 0.5–1 mg folic acid for patients on HD or CAPD; may accumulate in uraemic patients

• Dosage used by dialysis units varies from 5 mg daily to 5 mg once weekly

Folinic acid

Clinical use

Folinic acid rescue

Enhancement of 5-fluorouracil cytotoxicity in advanced colorectal cancer

Treatment of folate deficiency

Dose in normal renal function

Varies according to indication

Pharmacokinetics

Molecular weight (daltons)	511.5
% Protein binding	54
% Excreted unchanged in urine	–
Volume of distribution (L/kg)	17.5
Half-life – normal/ESRF (hrs)	32 minutes/–

Dose in renal impairment GFR (mL/min)

20–50	Dose as in normal renal function
10–20	Dose as in normal renal function
<10	Dose as in normal renal function

Dose in patients undergoing renal replacement therapies

CAPD	Some removal likely. Dose as in normal renal function
HD	Some removal likely. Dose as in normal renal function
CAV/VVHD	Some removal likely. Dose as in normal renal function

Important drug interactions

POTENTIALLY HAZARDOUS INTERACTIONS WITH OTHER DRUGS

• Folinic acid should not be administered simultaneously with a folic acid antagonist as this may nullify the effect of the antagonist

Administration

RECONSTITUTION

• For IV infusion compatible with: sodium chloride 0.9%, glucose 5%, compound sodium lactate

ROUTE

• IM, IV injection, IV infusion, oral

RATE OF ADMINISTRATION

• Because of the calcium content of leucovorin solutions, no more than 160 mg/minute should be injected IV

COMMENTS

–

Other information

–

Formoterol (eformoterol) fumarate

Clinical use

Long-acting selective beta-2 agonist

Dose in normal renal function

12 micrograms twice daily

Maximum dose: 24 micrograms twice daily

Turbohaler: 6–12 micrograms 1–2 times daily, maximum 72 micrograms daily

Pharmacokinetics

Molecular weight (daltons)	804.9
% Protein binding	61–64
% Excreted unchanged in urine	6.4–8
Volume of distribution (L/kg)	No data
Half-life – normal/ESRF (hrs)	2–3

Dose in renal impairment GFR (mL/min)

20–50	Dose as in normal renal function
10–20	Dose as in normal renal function
<10	Dose as in normal renal function

Dose in patients undergoing renal replacement therapies

CAPD	Not dialysed. Dose as in normal renal function
HD	Unlikely to be dialysed. Dose as in normal renal function
CAV/VVHD	Not dialysed. Dose as in normal renal function

Important drug interactions

POTENTIALLY HAZARDOUS INTERACTIONS WITH OTHER DRUGS

• None known

Administration

RECONSTITUTION

–

ROUTE

• Inhaled

RATE OF ADMINISTRATION

–

COMMENTS

–

Other information

–

Foscarnet

Clinical use

Antiviral agent: treatment of CMV retinitis (use for other forms of CMV and use in patients with serum creatinine >250 micromol/mL is *not* licensed)

Dose in normal renal function

60 mg/kg every 8 hours induction dose

Pharmacokinetics

Molecular weight (daltons)	192
% Protein binding	14–17
% Excreted unchanged in urine	85
Volume of distribution (L/kg)	0.22–0.78
Half-life – normal/ESRF (hrs)	2–6/>100

Dose in renal impairment GFR (mL/min)

Dose according to serum creatinine

20–50	28 mg/kg every 8 hours
10–20	15 mg/kg every 8 hours
<10	6 mg/kg every 8 hours

Dose in patients undergoing renal replacement therapies

CAPD	Dialysed. Dose in accordance with serum creatinine or as in GFR = <10 mL/min
HD	Dialysed. Dose in accordance with serum creatinine or as in GFR = <10 mL/min
CAV/VVHD	Dialysed. Dose in accordance with serum creatinine or as in GFR = 10–20 mL/min

Important drug interactions

POTENTIALLY HAZARDOUS INTERACTIONS WITH OTHER DRUGS

• None known

Administration

RECONSTITUTION

–

ROUTE

• Centrally (undiluted); peripherally (diluted)

RATE OF ADMINISTRATION

• Continuous infusion over 24 hours
• Or intermittent infusion over at least 60 minutes

COMMENTS

• If given peripherally dilute with glucose 5% to a concentration of 12 mg/mL or less
• If given peripherally, piggy-back to a glucose 5% infusion running at the same rate as the foscarnet solution

Other information

** Give 20 mg/kg over 30 minutes followed by daily dose as follows:

S-creatinine	Dose mg/kg/24 hours
<110	200
111–130	199–129
131–150	129–115
151–170	115–100
171–190	100–86
191–210	86–72
211–230	72–43
231–250	43–21
>250	Not recommended

Treatment usually continued for 2–3 weeks depending on response

• Some units dose by creatinine clearance/weight as follows:

Clearance mL/min/kg	Dose: mg/kg every 8 hours
1.6	60
1.5	57
1.4	53
1.3	49
1.2	46
1.1	42
1.0	39
0.9	35
0.8	32
0.7	28
0.6	25
0.5	21
0.4	18

• Maintain adequate hydration to prevent renal toxicity
• Monitor serum calcium and magnesium
• Some units use full-dose ganciclovir plus half-dose foscarnet concomitantly for treatment of resistant CMV disease

Fosinopril

Clinical use

ACE inhibitor: hypertension, congestive heart failure

Dose in normal renal function

10–40 mg once daily

Pharmacokinetics

Molecular weight (daltons)	586
% Protein binding	95
% Excreted unchanged in urine	<1
Volume of distribution (L/kg)	1.5
Half-life – normal/ESRF (hrs)	11.5–12/12–20

Dose in renal impairment GFR (mL/min)

20–50	Dose as in normal renal function
10–20	Dose as in normal renal function. Start with low dose
<10	Dose as in normal renal function. Start with low dose

Dose in patients undergoing renal replacement therapies

CAPD	Not dialysed. Dose as in GFR = <10 mL/min
HD	Not dialysed. Dose as in GFR = <10 mL/min
CAV/VVHD	Probably not dialysed. Dose as in GFR = 10–20 mL/min

Important drug interactions

POTENTIALLY HAZARDOUS INTERACTIONS WITH OTHER DRUGS

- Ciclosporin: increased risk of hyperkalaemia
- Antacids: reduced serum levels and urinary excretion of fosinoprilat

- Diuretics: hyperkalaemia with potassium-sparing diuretics, enhanced hypotensive effects
- Epoetin: increased risk of hyperkalaemia
- Lithium: reduced excretion. Possibility of enhanced lithium toxicity
- Potassium salts: increased risk of hyperkalaemia
- NSAIDs: antagonism of hypotensive effect, increased risk of hyperkalaemia and renal damage
- Anaesthetics: enhanced hypotensive effect

Administration

RECONSTITUTION

–

ROUTE

- Oral

RATE OF ADMINISTRATION

–

COMMENTS

–

Other information

- Any diuretic should preferably be discontinued for several days prior to beginning therapy with fosinopril to reduce the risk of an excessive hypotensive response
- Hepatobiliary elimination compensates for the diminished renal excretion
- Hyperkalaemia and other side-effects more common in patients with impaired renal function
- Close monitoring of renal function during therapy necessary in those with renal insufficiency
- Renal failure has been reported in association with ACE inhibitors in patients with renal artery stenosis, post renal transplant, or those with congestive heart failure
- A high incidence of anaphylactoid reactions has been reported in patients dialysed with high-flux polyacrylonitrile membranes and treated concomitantly with an ACE inhibitor – this combination should therefore be avoided

Fosphenytoin

Clinical use

Control of status epilepticus, seizures associated with neurosurgery or head injury when oral phenytoin is not possible

Dose in normal renal function

Treatment: 15 mg PE/kg (loading dose)

Maintenance: 4–5 mg PE/kg daily in 1–2 divided doses

Prophylaxis or treatment of seizures: 10–15 mg PE/kg then convert to phenytoin

Pharmacokinetics

Molecular weight (daltons)	406.2
% Protein binding	95–99
% Excreted unchanged in urine	1–5
Volume of distribution (L/kg)	4.3–10.8 litres
Half-life – normal/ESRF (hrs)	18.9 (IV), 41.2 (IM)/unchanged

Dose in renal impairment GFR (mL/min)

20–50	Reduce dose or rate by 10–25% and monitor carefully (except for status epilepticus)
10–20	Reduce dose or rate by 10–25% and monitor carefully (except for status epilepticus)
<10	Reduce dose or rate by 10–25% and monitor carefully (except for status epilepticus)

Dose in patients undergoing renal replacement therapies

CAPD	Unlikely to be dialysed. Dose as for GFR = <10 mL/min
HD	Not dialysed. Dose as for GFR = <10 mL/min
CAV/VVHD	Not dialysed. Dose as for GFR = 10–20 mL/min

Important drug interactions

POTENTIALLY HAZARDOUS INTERACTIONS WITH OTHER DRUGS

- Ciclosporin: increases ciclosporin metabolism so reduces blood levels

- Analgesics: some NSAIDs increase phenytoin levels
- Anti-arrhythmics: amiodarone increases phenytoin levels. Phenytoin reduces levels of disopyramide, mexiletine and quinidine
- Antibacterials: level increased by chloramphenicol,clarithromycin, cycloserine, isoniazid and metronidazole; level and antifolate effect increased by co-trimoxazole and trimethoprim; levels reduced by rifampicin; plasma concentration of doxycycline and telithromycin reduced; ciprofloxacin possibly alters phenytoin levels
- Anticoagulants: increased metabolism of acenocoumarol and warfarin (reduced effect)
- Antidepressants: antagonise anticonvulsant effect; fluoxetine, fluvoxamine and viloxazine increase phenytoin level; St John's Wort reduces phenytoin concentration; phenytoin reduces levels of mianserin, paroxetine and tricyclics
- Anti-epileptics: toxicity may be increased without enhanced effect
- Antifungals: levels increased by fluconazole and miconazole; plasma concentration of itraconazole and ketoconazole reduced
- Anti-malarials: mefloquine, chloroquine and hydroxychloroquine antagonises anticonvulsant effect; increased antifolate effect with pyrimethamine
- Antipsychotics: antagonise anticonvulsant effect
- Antivirals: plasma concentration of indinavir, lopinavir, nelfinavir and saquinavir possibly reduced; plasma phenytoin level reduced or increased by zidovudine
- Calcium-channel blockers: levels increased by diltiazem and nifedipine; effect of other calcium-channel blockers reduced
- Corticosteroids: metabolism of corticosteroids accelerated (effect reduced)
- Disulfiram: level of phenytoin increased
- Sex hormones: metabolism increased – reduced contraceptive effect
- Ulcer-healing drugs: cimetidine inhibits metabolism of phenytoin; sucralfate reduces absorption; omeprazole and esomeprazole enhances effect of phenytoin
- Uricosurics: sulfinpyrazone increases serum phenytoin levels

Administration

RECONSTITUTION

–

ROUTE

- IV, IM

RATE OF ADMINISTRATION

• Status epilepticus: 100–150 mg PE/min
• Treatment and prophylaxis of seizures:
  50–100 mg PE/min

COMMENTS

• Dilute further when using for IV infusion with
  sodium chloride 0.9% or glucose 5% to
  1.5–25 mg PE/ml

Other information

• 75 mg of fosphenytoin sodium is equivalent to
  50 mg of phenytoin
• 0.0037 mmol of phosphate/mg of fosphenytoin
• Never exceed 150 mg fosphenytoin per minute

• Decreased protein binding in renal failure
• Monitor ECG, BP and respiratory function during
  infusion
• IM route is contra-indicated in status epilepticus
• When substituting IV, IM use same dose and
  frequency as for oral phenytoin, administer at a
  rate of 50–100 mg PE/min
• May increase blood glucose in diabetic patients
• Some is dialysed out, as not all PE is bound to
  protein
• Half-life of fosphenytoin to phenytoin is
  15 minutes, more rapid in renal failure due
  to reduced protein binding

Furosemide (frusemide)

Clinical use

Loop diuretic

Dose in normal renal function

Oral: 20 mg – 2 g daily

IV: 20 mg – 1 g daily

Doses titrated to response

Pharmacokinetics

Molecular weight (daltons)	330.8
% Protein binding	95–99
% Excreted unchanged in urine	67
Volume of distribution (L/kg)	0.07–0.2
Half-life – normal/ESRF (hrs)	0.5–1.5/2–10

Dose in renal impairment GFR (mL/min)

20–50	Dose as in normal renal function
10–20	Dose as in normal renal function/ increased doses may be required
<10	Dose as in normal renal function/ increased doses may be required

Dose in patients undergoing renal replacement therapies

CAPD	Removal unlikely. Dose as in GFR = <10 mL/min
HD	Removal unlikely. Dose as in GFR = <10 mL/min
CAV/VVHD	Removal unlikely. Dose as in GFR = 10–20 mL/min

Important drug interactions

POTENTIALLY HAZARDOUS INTERACTIONS WITH OTHER DRUGS

• Ciclosporin: variable reports: increased nephrotoxicity, ototoxicity and hepatotoxicity

• Lithium: lithium excretion reduced
• ACE inhibitors: enhanced first-dose effect
• NSAIDs: increased risk of nephrotoxicity
• Aminoglycosides: increased risk of ototoxicity

Administration

RECONSTITUTION

–

ROUTE

• IV peripherally or centrally, IM, oral

RATE OF ADMINISTRATION

• 1 hour at not greater than 4 mg/minute

COMMENTS

• 250 mg to 50 mL sodium chloride 0.9% or undiluted via CRIP
• Increased danger of ototoxicity and nephrotoxicity if infused at faster rate than approximately 4 mg/minute
• Maximum dose by infusion: 1 g/24 hours
• Protect from light

Other information

• 500 mg orally ≡ 250 mg IV
• Excreted by tubular secretion, therefore in severe renal impairment (GFR 5–10 mL/min) higher doses may be required due to a reduction in the number of functioning nephrons
• Oliguria: start 250 mg daily, increasing 4–6 hourly to a maximum single dose of 2 g (rarely used)
• Furosemide acts within 1 hour of oral administration (after IV peak effect within 30 minutes), diuresis complete within 6 hours

Fusidic acid

Clinical use

Antibacterial agent

Dose in normal renal function

Oral: 480 mg every 8 hours (equivalent to 500 mg sodium fusidate every 8 hours)

IV: 480 mg every 8 hours (equivalent to 500 mg sodium fusidate every 8 hours)

Pharmacokinetics

Molecular weight (daltons)	526 (Na fusidate 538.7)
% Protein binding	95
% Excreted unchanged in urine	<10
Volume of distribution (L/kg)	6.79–14.73 litres
Half-life – normal/ESRF (hrs)	10–15/unchanged

Dose in renal impairment GFR (mL/min)

20–50	Dose as in normal renal function
10–20	Dose as in normal renal function
<10	Dose as in normal renal function

Dose in patients undergoing renal replacement therapies

CAPD	Not dialysed. Dose as in normal renal function
HD	Not dialysed. Dose as in normal renal function
CAV/VVHD	Not dialysed. Dose as in normal renal function

Important drug interactions

POTENTIALLY HAZARDOUS INTERACTIONS WITH OTHER DRUGS

• None known

Administration

RECONSTITUTION

• Use buffered solution provided, then dilute in 500 mL sodium chloride 0.9%

ROUTE

• IV peripherally, oral

RATE OF ADMINISTRATION

• 6 hours

COMMENTS

Unlicensed administration:

• 500 mg/10 mL buffered solution diluted to 100 mL and given via a central line over 2–6 hours

Other information

• 500 mg reconstituted with buffer contains 3.1 mmol sodium

• Can also be administered neat via central line (unlicensed)

Gabapentin

Clinical use

Anti-epileptic – adjunctive treatment of partial seizures with or without secondary generalisation
Neuropathic pain

Dose in normal renal function

300 mg on day 1, 300 mg twice daily on day 2, 300 mg three times daily on day 3, then increased according to response to 1.2 g daily (in three divided doses). If necessary may be further increased in steps of 300 mg daily to a maximum 2.4 g daily. Usual range 0.9–1.2 g daily; maximum period between doses should not exceed 12 hours

Neuropathic pain: loaded as above but maximum 1.8 g daily

Pharmacokinetics

Molecular weight (daltons)	171.2
% Protein binding	<3
% Excreted unchanged in urine	≈100
Volume of distribution (L/kg)	1.0
Half-life – normal/ESRF (hrs)	5–7/prolonged

Dose in renal impairment
GFR (mL/min)

60–90	400 mg three times daily
30–60	300 mg twice daily
15–30	300 mg once daily
<15	300 mg on alternate days

Dose in patients undergoing renal replacement therapies

CAPD	Probably dialysed. Dose as in GFR < 15 mL/min
HD	Dialysed. Loading dose of 300–400 mg in patients who have never received gabapentin. Maintenance dose of 200–300 mg after each HD session
CAV/VVHD	Dialysed. Dose as in GFR = 15–30 mL/min

Important drug interactions

POTENTIALLY HAZARDOUS INTERACTIONS WITH OTHER DRUGS

• Antacids reduce absorption
• Antidepressants: antagonism of anticonvulsive effect (convulsive threshold lowered)

Administration

RECONSTITUTION

–

ROUTE

• Oral

RATE OF ADMINISTRATION

–

COMMENTS

–

Other information

• Can cause false positive readings with some urinary protein tests
• In patients with moderate to severe renal impairment, start with the lowest possible dose and titrate upwards according to response

Ganciclovir

Clinical use

Antiviral agent

- IV: treatment of life- or sight-threatening cytomegalovirus (CMV) in immunocompromised people and for CMV prophylaxis in immunosuppressed patients secondary to organ transplantation
- Oral: maintenance treatment of CMV retinitis in AIDS patients (licensed), prophylaxis and maintenance against CMV infection in immunosuppressed patients (unlicensed use)

Dose in normal renal function

IV treatment:

Induction/Treatment of active CMV disease: 5 mg/kg 12-hourly for 14–21 days

Maintenance for CMV retinitis: 6 mg/kg per day for 5 days per week or 5 mg/kg per day 7 days per week

Prevention of CMV retinitis: as per treatment except induction length 7–14 days

Oral treatment:

Maintenance for CMV retinitis, or prophylaxis in immunosuppressed patients: 1000 mg three times per day

Pharmacokinetics

Molecular weight (daltons)	277
% Protein binding	<2
% Excreted unchanged in urine	90–100
Volume of distribution (L/kg)	0.47
Halflife-normal/ESRF (hrs)	2.9/30

Dose in renal impairment GFR (mL/min)

20–50	See 'Other information'
10–20	See 'Other Information'
<10	See 'Other Information'

Dose in patients undergoing renal replacement therapies

CAPD	Dialysed. Oral and IV: dose as in GFR = <10 mL/min
HD	Dialysed. IV: 1.25 mg/kg every day, given post dialysis on dialysis days. PO: 500 mg three times a week, given post dialysis on dialysis days
CAV/VVHD	Dialysed. IV: 2.5 mg/kg per day. PO: 500 mg once daily

Important drug interactions

POTENTIALLY HAZARDOUS INTERACTIONS WITH OTHER DRUGS

- Increased risk of myelosuppression with other myelosuppressive drugs
- Profound myelosuppression with zidovudine
- Generalised seizures reported with imipenem-cilastatin

Administration

RECONSTITUTION

- Reconstitute 1 vial (500 mg) with 10 mL water for injection (50 mg/mL)
- Then transfer dose to 100 mL sodium chloride 0.9%

ROUTE

- IV peripherally in fast-flowing vein or centrally – see below

RATE OF ADMINISTRATION

- Over 1 hour

COMMENTS

- May give 50% dose over 15 minutes after HD in washback (unlicensed)

Other information

IV dosage:

Creatinine clearance (mL/min)	Dose
>70	5 mg/kg 12-hourly
50–69	2.5 mg/kg 12-hourly
25–49	2.5 mg/kg 24-hourly
10–24	1.25 mg/kg 24-hourly
<10	1.25mg/kg 24-hourly, given after haemodialysis on dialysis days

Oral dose:

Creatinine clearance (mL/min)	Dose
>70	1000 mg three times a day
50–69	1500 mg daily
25–49	1000 mg daily
10–24	500 mg daily
<10	500 mg three times a week

- Monitor patient for myelosuppression, particularly in patients receiving prophylactic co-trimoxazole therapy
- Pre-dialysis therapeutic blood levels in range 5–12 mg/L
- Not to be infused in concentrations over 10 mg/mL peripherally
- Bioavailability of oral ganciclovir is 5%, so this should only be used for maintenance/prophylactic therapy

Gemcitabine hydrochloride

Clinical use

Palliative treatment, or first-line treatment with cisplatin, of locally advanced or metastatic non-small-cell lung cancer

Treatment of pancreatic cancer

Treatment of bladder cancer in combination with cisplatin

Dose in normal renal function

NSLC: 1000 mg/m^2 weekly for 3 weeks, I week rest then repeat

Pancreatic:1000 mg/m^2 weekly for 7 weeks, rest for I week then weekly for 3 weeks out of 4

Dose is reduced according to toxicity

Pharmacokinetics

Molecular weight (daltons)	299.7
% Protein binding	negligible
% Excreted unchanged in urine	<10
Volume of distribution (L/kg)	12.4 L/m^2 (women) 17.5 L/m^2 (men)
Half-life – normal/ESRF (hrs)	42–94 minutes

Dose in renal impairment GFR (mL/min)

20–50	Dose as in normal renal function
10–20	Use with caution. Reduce dose
<10	Avoid

Dose in patients undergoing renal replacement therapies

CAPD	Likely to be dialysed. Dose as in GFR = 10–20 mL/min
HD	Likely to be dialysed. Dose as in GFR = 10–20 mL/min
CAV/VVHD	Likely to be dialysed. Dose as in GFR = 10–20 mL/min

Important drug interactions

POTENTIALLY HAZARDOUS INTERACTIONS WITH OTHER DRUGS

• None known

Administration

RECONSTITUTION

• Reconstitute with sodium chloride 0.9%, 5 mL to 200 mg vial and 25 mL to I g vial

• Can be further diluted in sodium chloride 0.9% if required

ROUTE

• IV

RATE OF ADMINISTRATION

• 30 minutes

COMMENTS

–

Other information

• Gemcitabine causes reversible haematuria with or without proteinuria in about 50% of patients

• There is no evidence for cumulative renal toxicity with repeated dosing of gemcitabine

• Haemolytic uraemic syndrome (HUS) has been reported with a crude incidence rate of 0.015%

• A study looking at the use of gemcitabine 500–1000 mg/m^2 administered IV on days 1, 8 and 15 every 28 days in patients with renal dysfunction, concluded that this regimen was well tolerated in patients with a GFR as low as 30 mL/min

• Another study in patients with serum creatinines in the range 130–420 micromol/L at doses of 650–800 mg/m^2 weekly for 3 weeks out of a 4-week cycle, found dose-limiting toxicities, including neutropenia, fever, raised transaminases and increased serum creatinine. It was concluded that a reduced dose of gemcitabine may be appropriate in patients with established renal impairment

Gemfibrozil

Clinical use

Hyperlipidaemias of types IIa, IIb, III, IV and V

Dose in normal renal function

1.2 g daily, usually in two divided doses;
range 0.9–1.5 g daily

Pharmacokinetics

Molecular weight (daltons)	250
% Protein binding	95
% Excreted unchanged in urine	<5
Volume of distribution (L/kg)	–
Half-life – normal/ESRF (hrs)	1.5/1.5–2.4

Dose in renal impairment
GFR (mL/min)

20–50	Initially 900 mg daily
10–20	Initially 900 mg daily. Monitor carefully
<10	Initially 900 mg daily. Monitor carefully

Dose in patients undergoing renal replacement therapies

CAPD	Not dialysed. Dose as in GFR = <10 mL/min
HD	Not dialysed. Dose as in GFR = <10 mL/min
CAV/VVHD	Not dialysed. Dose as in GFR = 10–20 mL/min

Important drug interactions

POTENTIALLY HAZARDOUS INTERACTIONS WITH OTHER DRUGS

- Enhanced anticoagulant effect seen with acenocoumarol, phenindione and warfarin
- Ciclosporin: Parke-Davis have one report on file of an interaction with ciclosporin where serum ciclosporin levels were decreased. No effects on muscle were noted
- Statins: increased risk of myopathy

Administration

RECONSTITUTION

–

ROUTE

- Oral

RATE OF ADMINISTRATION

–

COMMENTS

–

Other information

- Adverse effects have not been reported in patients with renal disease, but such patients should start treatment at 900 mg daily, which may be increased after careful assessment of response and renal function
- Rare cases of rhabdomyolysis may be increased in those with renal impairment
- Approximately 60–70% is excreted in the urine as both conjugated and unconjugated drug
- Gemfibrozil alone has caused myalgia and myositis, but the effects appear to occur much more frequently and are more severe when an HMG CoA reductase inhibitor is also used. The combination is therefore not recommended

Gentamicin

Clinical use

Antibacterial agent

Dose in normal renal function

3–7 mg/kg (ideal body weight) daily (divided into 1–4 doses). CAPD peritonitis – see local policy and below

Pharmacokinetics

Molecular weight (daltons)	1418
% Protein binding	0–20
% Excreted unchanged in urine	95
Volume of distribution (L/kg)	0.23–0.26
Half-life – normal/ESRF (hrs)	2/20–60

Dose in renal impairment GFR (mL/min)

See 'Other information' for dosage for dialysis and for single daily dosing regimen

30–70	80 mg 12-hourly (60 mg if <60 kg)
10–30	80 mg 24-hourly (60 mg if <60 kg)
5–10	80 mg 48-hourly (60 mg if <60 kg) or post dialysis if on HD

Dose in patients undergoing renal replacement therapies

CAPD	Dialysed. CAPD clearance is about 3 mL/min. Dose as in GFR = 5–10 mL/min. Monitor levels
HD	Dialysed. Dose as in GFR = 5–10 mL/min. Give after dialysis
CAV/VVHD	Dialysed. Dose in GFR = 10–30 mL/min and measure levels

Important drug interactions

POTENTIALLY HAZARDOUS INTERACTIONS WITH OTHER DRUGS

- Ciclosporin: increased risk of nephrotoxicity
- Muscle relaxants: effect of tubocurarine enhanced
- Cytotoxics: increased risk of nephrotoxicity with cisplatin
- Cholinergics: antagonism of effect of neostigmine and pyridostigmine
- Botulinum toxin: neuromuscular block enhanced (risk of toxicity)

Administration

RECONSTITUTION

–

ROUTE

- Bolus IV injection or short infusion – maximum 100 mL

RATE OF ADMINISTRATION

- Bolus IV: over not less than 3 minutes. Short infusion: over not more than 20 minutes

COMMENTS

–

Other information

- *Adjustment for renal impairment:* Dialysis patients – 80 mg (or up to 2 mg/kg) post dialysis
- *Single daily dosing regimen:*
  GFR >80: 5.1 mg/kg every 24 hours
  GFR 60–80: 4.0 mg/kg every 24 hours
  GFR 40–60: 3.5 mg/kg every 24 hours
  GFR 30–40: 2.5 mg/kg every 24 hours
  GFR 20–30: 4.0 mg/kg every 48 hours
  GFR 10–20: 3.0 mg/kg every 48 hours
  GFR <10: 2.0 mg/kg every 48 hours
- Concurrent penicillins may result in sub-therapeutic blood levels
- Monitor blood levels. 1 hour post-dose, peak levels must not exceed 10 mg/L. Pre-dose trough levels should be less than 2 mg/L
- Empirical IP therapy for CAPD peritonitis in conjunction with vancomycin. A common regimen used is gentamicin 4–5 mg/L + vancomycin IP at dose of 1–2 g stat on days 1 and 7 of course. Monitoring of blood levels is advisable, as absorption is increased by inflamed peritoneum
- Potential nephrotoxicity of the drug may worsen residual renal function
- Long-term concurrent use of gentamicin with teicoplanin causes additive ototoxicity

Glibenclamide

Clinical use

Non-insulin-dependent diabetes mellitus

Dose in normal renal function

Initially 5 mg daily (elderly patients – 2.5 mg) adjusted according to response; maximum 15 mg daily

Pharmacokinetics

Molecular weight (daltons)	494
% Protein binding	98–99
% Excreted unchanged in urine	<5
Volume of distribution (L/kg)	0.15–0.2
Half-life – normal/ESRF (hrs)	5–10/–

Dose in renal impairment GFR (mL/min)

20–50	Initial dose of 1.25–2.5 mg once a day. Monitor closely
10–20	Initial dose of 1.25–2.5 mg once a day. Monitor closely
<10	Initial dose of 1.25–2.5 mg once a day. Use with caution with continuous monitoring

Dose in patients undergoing renal replacement therapies

CAPD	Not dialysed. Dose as in GFR = <10 mL/min
HD	Low dialysability. Dose as in GFR = <10 mL/min
CAV/VVHD	Unknown dialysability. Dose as in GFR = 10–20 mL/min

Important drug interactions

POTENTIALLY HAZARDOUS INTERACTIONS WITH OTHER DRUGS

• Analgesics: azapropazone, phenylbutazone and possibly other NSAIDs enhance effect
• Antibacterials: chloramphenicol, co-trimoxazole, 4-quinolones, sulphonamides and trimethoprim enhance effect
• Antifungals: fluconazole and miconazole increase glibenclamide plasma concentration
• Uricosurics: sulfinpyrazone enhances effect of glibenclamide

Administration

RECONSTITUTION

–

ROUTE

• Oral

RATE OF ADMINISTRATION

–

COMMENTS

• Take with breakfast

Other information

• The metabolites of glibenclamide are only weakly hypoglycaemic, this is not clinically relevant where renal and hepatic functions are normal. If CL_{CR} <10 mL/min, accumulation of metabolite and unchanged drug in plasma may cause prolonged hyperglycaemia
• Company information states that use is contra-indicated in severe renal impairment
• Compensatory excretion via bile in faeces occurs in renal impairment

Gliclazide

Clinical use

Non-insulin-dependent diabetes mellitus

Dose in normal renal function

Initially: 40–80 mg daily, adjusted according to response up to 160 mg as a single dose, with breakfast; higher doses divided. Maximum 320 mg daily

Pharmacokinetics

Molecular weight (daltons)	323
% Protein binding	85–95
% Excreted unchanged in urine	<5
Volume of distribution (L/kg)	0.24
Half-life – normal/ESRF (hrs)	8–11/prolonged

Dose in renal impairment GFR (mL/min)

20–50	Initially 20–40 mg daily. Use with caution and monitor
10–20	Initially 20–40 mg daily. Use with caution and monitor
<10	Initially 20–40 mg daily. Use with great caution and monitor closely

Dose in patients undergoing renal replacement therapies

CAPD	Unlikely dialysability. Dose as in GFR = <10 mL/min
HD	Unlikely dialysability. Dose as in GFR = <10 mL/min
CAV/VVHD	Unknown dialysability. Dose as in GFR = 10–20 mL/min

Important drug interactions

POTENTIALLY HAZARDOUS INTERACTIONS WITH OTHER DRUGS

- Analgesics: azapropazone, phenylbutazone and possibly other NSAIDs enhance effect
- Antibacterials: chloramphenicol, co-trimoxazole, 4-quinolones, sulphonamides and trimethoprim enhance effect
- Antifungals: fluconazole and miconazole increase gliclazide plasma concentration
- Uricosurics: sulfinpyrazone enhances effect

Administration

RECONSTITUTION

–

ROUTE

- Oral

RATE OF ADMINISTRATION

–

COMMENTS

–

Other information

- Care should be exercised in patients with hepatic and/or renal impairment and a small starting dose should be used with careful patient monitoring
- Company contra-indicates prescribing of Diamicron in severe renal impairment which they define as CL_{CR} below 40 mL/min

Glimepiride

Clinical use

Non-insulin-dependent diabetes mellitus

Dose in normal renal function

1–4 mg daily. Maximum 6 mg daily taken shortly
before or with first main meal

Pharmacokinetics

Molecular weight (daltons)	490.6
% Protein binding	>99
% Excreted unchanged in urine	58–60 (as metabolites)
Volume of distribution (L/kg)	8.8
Half-life – normal/ESRF (hrs)	5–9/prolonged

Dose in renal impairment GFR (mL/min)

20–50	Dose as in normal renal function
10–20	Dose as in normal renal function
<10	Contra-indicated

Dose in patients undergoing renal replacement therapies

CAPD	Unlikely dialysability. Dose as in GFR = <10 mL/min
HD	Unlikely dialysability. Dose as in GFR = <10 mL/min
CAV/VVHD	Unlikely dialysability. Dose as in GFR = 10–20 mL/min

Important drug interactions

POTENTIALLY HAZARDOUS INTERACTIONS WITH OTHER DRUGS

• Azapropazone, phenylbutazone and possibly other NSAIDs enhance effect of sulphonylureas
• Antibacterials: chloramphenicol, co-trimoxazole, 4-quinolones, sulphonamides and trimethoprim enhance effect
• Antifungals: fluconazole and miconazole increase sulphonylurea plasma concentration
• Sulfinpyrazone enhances effect

Administration

RECONSTITUTION
–

ROUTE
• Oral

RATE OF ADMINISTRATION
–

COMMENTS
–

Other information

–

Glipizide

Clinical use

Non-insulin-dependent diabetes mellitius

Dose in normal renal function

Initially 2.5–5 mg daily, adjusted according to response; maximum 20 mg daily; up to 15 mg may be given as a single dose before breakfast; higher doses divided

Pharmacokinetics

Molecular weight (daltons)	445
% Protein binding	97
% Excreted unchanged in urine	4.5–7
Volume of distribution (L/kg)	0.13–0.16
Half-life – normal/ESRF (hrs)	3–7/–

Dose in renal impairment GFR (mL/min)

20–50	Initially 2.5 mg daily. Use with caution
10–20	Initially 2.5 mg daily. Use with caution
<10	Contra-indicated

Dose in patients undergoing renal replacement therapies

CAPD	Dialysability insignificant, however contra-indicated if GFR <10 mL/min
HD	Dialysability insignificant, however contra-indicated if GFR <10 mL/min
CAV/VVHD	Dialysability insignificant. Dose as in GFR = 10–20 mL/min

Important drug interactions

POTENTIALLY HAZARDOUS INTERACTIONS WITH OTHER DRUGS

- Azapropazone, phenylbutazone and possibly other NSAIDs enhance effect of sulphonylureas
- Antibacterials: chloramphenicol, co-trimoxazole, 4-quinolones, sulphonamides and trimethoprim enhance effect
- Antifungals: fluconazole and miconazole increase glipizide plasma concentration
- Sulfinpyrazone enhances effect

Administration

RECONSTITUTION

–

ROUTE

- Oral

RATE OF ADMINISTRATION

–

COMMENTS

–

Other information

- Company does not recommend the use of Glibenese in patients with renal insufficiency
- Renal or hepatic insufficiency may cause elevated blood levels of glipizide (increased risk of serious hypoglycaemic reactions)

Granisetron

Clinical use

Prevention or treatment of nausea and vomiting induced by cytotoxic chemotherapy, radiotherapy or post-operative nausea and vomiting

Dose in normal renal function

Cytotoxic chemotherapy or radiotherapy:
PO: 1–2 mg within 1 hour before start of treatment, then 2 mg daily in 1–2 divided doses during treatment

IV: 3 mg before start of cytotoxic therapy, up to two additional 3 mg doses can be given within 24 hours no less than 10 minutes apart

Operative procedures: IV: 1 mg before induction of anaesthesia; treatment 1 mg (maximum 2 mg in one day)

Pharmacokinetics

Molecular weight (daltons)	312.4 (348.9 as hydrochloride)
% Protein binding	≈65
% Excreted unchanged in urine	<20
Volume of distribution (L/kg)	3
Half-life – normal/ESRF (hrs)	3.0–4.0/ unchanged

Dose in renal impairment GFR (mL/min)

20–50	Dose as in normal renal function
10–20	Dose as in normal renal function
<10	Dose as in normal renal function

Dose in patients undergoing renal replacement therapies

CAPD	Unknown dialysability. Dose as in normal renal function
HD	Unknown dialysability. Dose as in normal renal function. Company recommend timing HD for greater than 2 hours after granisetron dose
CAV/VVHD	Unknown dialysability. Dose as in normal renal function

Important drug interactions

POTENTIALLY HAZARDOUS INTERACTIONS WITH OTHER DRUGS

• None known

Administration

RECONSTITUTION

–

ROUTE

• Oral, IV bolus, IV infusion

RATE OF ADMINISTRATION

• IV bolus: diluted in 5 mL sodium chloride 0.9% over not less than 30 seconds
• IV infusion: 20–50 mL over 5 minutes

COMMENTS

• Compatible with sodium chloride 0.9%, sodium chloride 0.18% and glucose 4% solution, glucose 5%, Hartmann's solution, compound sodium lactate, 10% mannitol
• Maximum administered dose over 24 hours should not exceed 9 mg

Other information

• No special dosing adjustments necessary in patients with renal or hepatic failure

Griseofulvin

Clinical use

Antifungal agent: dermatophyte infections of the skin, scalp, hair and nails

Dose in normal renal function

500 mg daily, in divided doses or as a single dose
In severe infection dose may be doubled

Pharmacokinetics

Molecular weight (daltons)	353
% Protein binding	84
% Excreted unchanged in urine	1
Volume of distribution (L/kg)	1.6
Half-life – normal/ESRF (hrs)	9.5–21/20

Dose in renal impairment GFR (mL/min)

20–50	Dose as in normal renal function
10–20	Dose as in normal renal function
<10	Dose as in normal renal function

Dose in patients undergoing renal replacement therapies

CAPD	Not dialysed. Dose as in normal renal function
HD	Not dialysed. Dose as in normal renal function
CAV/VVHD	Not dialysed. Dose as in normal renal function

Important drug interactions

POTENTIALLY HAZARDOUS INTERACTIONS WITH OTHER DRUGS

• Anticoagulants: metabolism of acenocoumarol and warfarin accelerated (reduced anticoagulant effect)

• Metabolism of oral contraceptives accelerated (reduced contraceptive effect)

• Ciclosporin: griseofulvin possibly reduces plasma – ciclosporin concentration. (Two reports of such an interaction in literature.)

Administration

RECONSTITUTION

–

ROUTE

• Oral

RATE OF ADMINISTRATION

–

COMMENTS

–

Other information

• Use with extreme caution in patients with SLE

Haloperidol

Clinical use

Sedative in severe anxiety, intractable hiccup, nausea and vomiting, schizophrenia and other psychoses

Dose in normal renal function

Anxiety/hiccup: 1.5 mg three times daily

Nausea and vomiting: 0.5–2.0 mg daily

Schizophrenia: 1.5–5.0 mg two to three times daily, up to 120 mg daily in resistant cases

IM/IV: 2–10 mg initially, maximum 30 mg daily

Pharmacokinetics

Molecular weight (daltons)	375.9
% Protein binding	90–92
% Excreted unchanged in urine	1
Volume of distribution (L/kg)	14–30
Half-life – normal/ESRF (hrs)	10–40/–

Dose in renal impairment GFR (mL/min)

20–50	Dose as in normal renal function
10–20	Dose as in normal renal function
<10	Start with lower doses. For single doses use 100% of normal dose. Avoid repeated dosage because of accumulation

Dose in patients undergoing renal replacement therapies

CAPD	Not dialysed. Dose as in GFR = <10 mL/min
HD	Not dialysed. Dose as in GFR = <10 mL/min
CAV/VVHD	Not dialysed. Dose as in normal renal function

Important drug interactions

POTENTIALLY HAZARDOUS INTERACTIONS WITH OTHER DRUGS

- Anti-arrhythmics: increased risk of ventricular arrhythmias with amiodarone – avoid concomitant use
- Antibacterials: rifampicin increases the metabolism of haloperidol
- Anaesthetics: enhanced hypotensive effects
- Antidepressants: increased effect and side-effects
- Anti-epileptics: increased metabolism of haloperidol with carbamazepine; lowered seizure threshold
- Lithium: increased risk of neurotoxicity
- Sibutramine: increased risk of CNS toxicity – avoid concomitant use
- Terfenadine: increased risk of arrhythmias

Administration

RECONSTITUTION

–

ROUTE

- Oral, IM or IV (by slow bolus)

RATE OF ADMINISTRATION

–

COMMENTS

–

Other information

- May cause hypotension and excessive sedation
- Increased CNS sensitivity in renally impaired patients – start with small doses, metabolites may accumulate
- Equivalent IV/IM dose = 40% of oral dose

Heparin

Clinical use

Anticoagulant

Dose in normal renal function

Treatment of DVT and PE:

Loading dose: 5000–10,000 units then a continuous intravenous infusion of 15–25 units/kg/hour

Treatment of DVT:

15,000 units every 12 hours by subcutaneous injection, dose is adjusted according to laboratory monitoring or according to local protocols

Pharmacokinetics

Molecular weight (daltons)	3000–40,000
% Protein binding	>90
% Excreted unchanged in urine	None
Volume of distribution (L/kg)	0.06–0.1
Half-life – normal/ESRF (hrs)	0.3–2/slightly prolonged (half-life increases with dose)

Dose in renal impairment GFR (mL/min)

20–50	Dose as in normal renal function
10–20	Dose as in normal renal function
<10	Dose as in normal renal function

Dose in patients undergoing renal replacement therapies

CAPD	Not dialysed. Dose as in normal renal function
HD	Not dialysed. Dose as in normal renal function
CAV/VVHD	Not dialysed. Dose as in normal renal function

Important drug interactions

POTENTIALLY HAZARDOUS INTERACTIONS WITH OTHER DRUGS

• Analgesics: aspirin enhances anticoagulant effect; increased risk of haemorrhage with intravenous diclofenac and with ketorolac (avoid concomitant use, including low dose heparin). Possibly an increased risk of bleeding with NSAIDs

• Nitrates: GTN infusion increases excretion (reduced anticoagulant effect)

Administration

RECONSTITUTION

–

ROUTE

• IV infusion or bolus, SC

RATE OF ADMINISTRATION

• 15–25 units/kg/hour, or according to local protocol

COMMENTS

–

Other information

• The half-life is slightly prolonged in haemodialysis patients after intravenous administration

• Heparin is also used for the maintenance of extra-corporeal circuits in cardiopulmonary bypass and haemodialysis

• 1 mg protamine is required to neutralise 100 IU heparin. Give slowly over 10 minutes, and do not exceed a total dose of 50 mg

Hydralazine

Clinical use

Vasodilator antihypertensive agent

Dose in normal renal function

Oral: 25–50 mg twice daily. Maximum daily dose 100 mg in slow acetylators and women, 200 mg in fast acetylators

IV: Slow IV injection: 5–10 mg over 20 minutes. Repeat after 20–30 minutes if necessary

Infusion: 200–300 micrograms/minute initially reducing to 50–150 micrograms/minute

Pharmacokinetics

Molecular weight (daltons)	197
% Protein binding	87
% Excreted unchanged in urine	25
Volume of distribution (L/kg)	0.5–0.9
Half-life – normal/ESRF (hrs)	2–4.5/7–16

Dose in renal impairment GFR (mL/min)

20–50	Start with small dose and adjust in accordance with response
10–20	Start with small dose and adjust in accordance with response
<10	Start with small dose and adjust in accordance with response

Dose in patients undergoing renal replacement therapies

CAPD	Not dialysed. Dose as in GFR = <10 mL/min
HD	Not dialysed. Dose as in GFR = <10 mL/min
CAV/VVHD	Not dialysed. Dose as in GFR = 10–20 mL/min

Important drug interactions

POTENTIALLY HAZARDOUS INTERACTIONS WITH OTHER DRUGS

• Anaesthetics: increased hypotensive effects

Administration

RECONSTITUTION

• 20 mg with 1 mL water for injection **then dilute** with 10 mL sodium chloride 0.9% for IV injection or 500 mL sodium chloride 0.9% for IV infusion

ROUTE

• Oral, IV peripherally

RATE OF ADMINISTRATION

• As above

COMMENTS

–

Other information

• Avoid long-term use due to accumulation of metabolites, in severe renal insufficiency and dialysis patients

Hydrocortisone acetate

Clinical use

Corticosteroid: local inflammation of joints and soft tissue

Dose in normal renal function

5–50 mg according to joint size

Pharmacokinetics

Molecular weight (daltons)	404.5
% Protein binding	>90
% Excreted unchanged in urine	0
Volume of distribution (L/kg)	0.4–0.7
Half-life – normal/ESRF (hrs)	1.5–2.0/–

Dose in renal impairment GFR (mL/min)

20–50	Dose as in normal renal function
10–20	Dose as in normal renal function
<10	Dose as in normal renal function

Dose for patients undergoing renal replacement therapies

CAPD	Low dialysability. Dose as in normal renal function
HD	Low dialysability. Dose as in normal renal function
CAV/VVHD	Low dialysability. Dose as in normal renal function

Important drug interactions

POTENTIALLY HAZARDOUS INTERACTIONS WITH OTHER DRUGS

- Rifampicin: increased metabolism of hydrocortisone
- Anti-epileptics: increased metabolism of hydrocortisone

Administration

RECONSTITUTION

–

ROUTE

- Intra-articular, peri-articular

RATE OF ADMINISTRATION

–

COMMENTS

–

Other information

- Used for its local effects. Systemic absorption occurs slowly

Hydrocortisone sodium succinate

Clinical use

Corticosteroid: anti-inflammatory agent in respiratory, GI and endocrine disorders, and allergic states

Dose in normal renal function

100–500 mg, 3–4 times in 24 hours or as required

Pharmacokinetics

Molecular weight (daltons)	484.5
% Protein binding	90–95
% Excreted unchanged in urine	0
Volume of distribution (L/kg)	0.4–0.7
Half-life – normal/ESRF (hrs)	1.5–2/–

Dose in renal impairment GFR (mL/min)

20–50	Dose as in normal renal function
10–20	Dose as in normal renal function
<10	Dose as in normal renal function

Dose in patients undergoing renal replacement therapies

CAPD	Low dialysability. Dose as in normal renal function
HD	Low dialysability. Dose as in normal renal function
CAV/VVHD	Low dialysability. Dose as in normal renal function

Important drug interactions

POTENTIALLY HAZARDOUS INTERACTIONS WITH OTHER DRUGS

- Anticoagulants: anticoagulant effect of acenocoumarol and warfarin possibly altered
- Ciclosporin: convulsions reported with concurrent use
- Rifampicin accelerates metabolism of hydrocortisone
- Anti-epileptics: carbamazepine, phenobarbital, phenytoin and primidone accelerate metabolism
- Amphotericin: increased risk of hypokalaemia

Administration

RECONSTITUTION

- IV injection, IM injection: add 2 mL of sterile water for injection
- IV infusion: add not more than 2 mL water for injection, then add to 100–1000 mL (not less than 100 mL) glucose 5% or sodium chloride 0.9%

ROUTE

- IV injection, IV infusion, IM

RATE OF ADMINISTRATION

- IV bolus: 2–3 minutes

COMMENTS

–

Other information

- Non-plasma-protein bound hydrocortisone is removed by HD
- One study has shown that plasma clearance rates of hydrocortisone during haemodialysis were 30–63% higher than after dialysis. No recommendations exist to indicate dosing should be altered to take account of this

Hydromorphone hydrochloride

Clinical use

Relief of severe cancer pain

Dose in normal renal function

1.3 mg 4 hourly, increasing dose as required

SR: 4 mg 12 hourly, increasing dose as required

Pharmacokinetics

Molecular weight (daltons)	321.8
% Protein binding	7.1
% Excreted unchanged in urine	6
Volume of distribution (L/kg)	24.4 litres
Half-life – normal/ESRF (hrs)	2.5/–

Dose in renal impairment GFR (mL/min)

20–50	Dose as in normal renal function
10–20	Reduce dose – start with lowest dose and titrate according to response
<10	Reduce dose – start with lowest dose and titrate according to response

Dose in patients undergoing renal replacement therapies

CAPD	Unknown dialysability. Dose as in GFR < 10 mL/min
HD	Unknown dialysability. Dose as in GFR < 10 mL/min
CAV/VVHD	Unknown dialysability. Dose as in GFR = 10–20 mL/min

Important drug interactions

POTENTIALLY HAZARDOUS INTERACTIONS WITH OTHER DRUGS

- Anti-arrhythmics: delayed absorption of mexiletine
- Antipsychotics: enhanced sedative and hypotensive effect

Administration

RECONSTITUTION

–

ROUTE

- Oral

RATE OF ADMINISTRATION

–

COMMENTS

–

Other information

- 1.3 mg of hydromorphone is equivalent to 10 mg oral morphine
- Metabolised to mainly hydromorphone-3-glucuronide and some hydromorphone-6-glucuronide, which accumulate in renal failure. May cause neuroexcitation and cognitive impairment

Hydroxychloroquine sulphate

Clinical use

1 Treatment of rheumatoid arthritis, systemic lupus erythematosus
2 Dermatalogical conditions caused or aggravated by sunlight
3 Malaria (unlicensed in UK)

Dose in normal renal function

200–400 mg daily in divided doses, maximum of 6.5 mg/kg/day

Prophylaxis of malaria: 400 mg weekly

Pharmacokinetics

Molecular weight (daltons)	434
% Protein binding	50–55
% Excreted unchanged in urine	23–25
Volume of distribution (L/kg)	large
Half-life – normal/ESRF (hrs)	50 days (whole blood) 32 days (plasma)

Dose in renal impairment GFR (mL/min)

20–50	Maximum 75% of dose
10–20	Maximum 50% of dose
<10	Maximum 30% of dose – use with caution

Dose in patients undergoing renal replacement therapies

CAPD	Unknown dialysability. Dose as in GFR < 10 mL/min
HD	Unknown dialysability. Dose as in GFR < 10 mL/min
CAV/VVHD	Unknown dialysability. Dose as in GFR = 10–20 mL/min

Important drug interactions

POTENTIALLY HAZARDOUS INTERACTIONS WITH OTHER DRUGS

• Anti-arrhythmics: increased risk of ventricular arrhythmias with amiodarone
• Anti-epileptics: antagonism of anticonvulsant effect
• Other anti-malarials: increased risk of convulsions with mefloquine. Avoid concomitant use with artemether with lumefantrine
• Cardiac glycosides: may increase digoxin levels

Administration

RECONSTITUTION

–

ROUTE

• Oral

RATE OF ADMINISTRATION

–

COMMENTS

–

Other information

• Take with a meal or a glass of milk
• Excretory patterns are not well characterised, but hydroxychloroquine and its metabolites are slowly excreted via the kidneys
• Reduce dose only on prolonged use in mild to moderate renal failure
• In renal insufficiency need more than annual eye examinations

Hydroxyurea (hydroxycarbamide)

Clinical use

Antineoplastic agent

Dose in normal renal function

20–30 mg/kg daily, or 80 mg/kg every third day. Consult local protocol

Pharmacokinetics

Molecular weight (daltons)	76
% Protein binding	Minimal
% Excreted unchanged in urine	35–50
Volume of distribution (L/kg)	0.5
Half-life – normal/ESRF (hrs)	2–6/–

Dose in renal impairment GFR (mL/min)

20–50	100% of normal dose and titrate to response
10–20	50% of normal dose and titrate to response
<10	20% of normal dose and titrate to response

Dose in patients undergoing renal replacement therapies

CAPD	Probably dialysed. Dose as in GFR = <10 mL/min
HD	Probably dialysed. Dose as in GFR = <10 mL/min
CAV/VVHD	Probably dialysed. Dose as in GFR = 10–20 mL/min

Important drug interactions

POTENTIALLY HAZARDOUS INTERACTIONS WITH OTHER DRUGS

• None known

Administration

RECONSTITUTION

–

ROUTE

• Oral

RATE OF ADMINISTRATION

–

COMMENTS

–

Other information

• Full blood count, renal and hepatic function should be determined repeatedly during treatment

• Dosage should be based on the patient's actual or ideal weight, whichever is less

• Hydroxyurea has been associated with impairment of renal tubular function and accompanied by elevation in serum uric acid, BUN and creatinine levels

• The following formula can be used to determine the fraction of normal dose used for renally impaired patients: Fraction of normal dose = (normal dose) x { [f (k_f – 1)] + 1}. f = fraction of the original dose excreted as active or toxic moiety (f = 0.35 for hydroxyurea). k_f = patient's creatinine clearance (mL/min) divided by 120 mL/minute

• Administer with caution to patients with marked renal dysfunction; such patients may rapidly develop visual and auditory hallucinations and pronounced haematologic toxicity

Hydroxyzine

Clinical use

Antihistamine: pruritus

Dose in normal renal function

25 mg at night increasing as necessary to 3–4 times a day

Pharmacokinetics

Molecular weight (daltons)	448 (hydrochloride)
% Protein binding	–
% Excreted unchanged in urine	0
Volume of distribution (L/kg)	19.5
Half-life – normal/ESRF (hrs)	14–20/–

Dose in renal impairment GFR (mL/min)

20–50	Dose as in normal renal function
10–20	Start with small dose, e.g. 25 mg at night and increase to 2–3 times a day if necessary
<10	Start with small dose, e.g. 25 mg at night and increase to 2–3 times a day if necessary

Dose in patients undergoing renal replacement therapies

CAPD	Not dialysed. Dose as in GFR = <10 mL/min
HD	Not dialysed. Dose as in GFR = <10 mL/min
CAV/VVHD	Not dialysed. Dose as in GFR = 10–20 mL/min

Important drug interactions

POTENTIALLY HAZARDOUS INTERACTIONS WITH OTHER DRUGS

• None known

Administration

RECONSTITUTION

–

ROUTE

• Oral

RATE OF ADMINISTRATION

–

COMMENTS

–

Other information

• Increased possibility of side-effects, particularly drowsiness

Ibuprofen

Clinical use

NSAID: pain and inflammation in rheumatic disease and other musculoskeletal disorders; dysmenorrhoea; migraine

Dose in normal renal function

Initially: 1.2–1.8 g daily in 3–4 divided doses, after food. Maximum 2.4 g daily

Pharmacokinetics

Molecular weight (daltons)	206
% Protein binding	90–99
% Excreted unchanged in urine	<10
Volume of distribution (L/kg)	0.15–0.17
Half-life – normal/ESRF (hrs)	2–3.2/unchanged

Dose in renal impairment GFR (mL/min)

20–50	Dose as in normal renal function, but avoid if possible
10–20	Dose as in normal renal function, but avoid if possible
<10	Dose as in normal renal function, but only use if ESRD on dialysis

Dose in patients undergoing renal replacement therapies

CAPD	Not dialysed. Dose as in normal renal function
HD	Not dialysed. Dose as in normal renal function
CAV/VVHD	Not dialysed. Dose as in GFR = 10–20 mL/min

Important drug interactions

POTENTIALLY HAZARDOUS INTERACTIONS WITH OTHER DRUGS

- Ciclosporin: increased risk of nephrotoxicity
- Antibacterials: possibly increased risk of convulsions with quinolones
- Antivirals: increased risk of haematological toxicity with zidovudine
- Lithium: excretion reduced
- Cytotoxic agents: reduced excretion of methotrexate
- Diuretics: increased risk of nephrotoxicity, hyperkalaemia with potassium-sparing diuretics
- Anticoagulants: effects of warfarin and acenocoumarol enhanced
- Antidiabetic agents: effects of sulphonylureas enhanced
- Anti-epileptic agents: effects of phenytoin enhanced
- ACE inhibitors and AT-II antagonists: antagonism of hypotensive effect; increased risk of renal damage and hyperkalaemia
- Tacrolimus: increased risk of nephrotoxicity

Administration

RECONSTITUTION

–

ROUTE

- Oral

RATE OF ADMINISTRATION

–

COMMENTS

–

Other information

- Inhibition of renal prostaglandin synthesis by NSAIDs may interfere with renal function, especially in the presence of existing renal disease. Avoid if possible; if not, check serum creatinine 48–72 hours after starting NSAID. If raised, discontinue NSAID therapy
- Use normal doses in patients with ESRD on dialysis
- Use with caution in renal transplant recipients – can reduce intra-renal autocoid synthesis

Ifosfamide

Clinical use

Antineoplastic agent: tumours of lung, ovary, cervix, breast, testis and in soft tissue sarcoma

Dose in normal renal function

Usual total dose for each course is either 8–12 g/m², equally divided as single daily doses over 3–5 days, or, 5–6 g/m² (maximum 10 g) given as a 24-hour infusion

Pharmacokinetics

Molecular weight (daltons)	261
% Protein binding	0
% Excreted unchanged in urine	15
Volume of distribution (L/kg)	0.4–0.64
Half-life – normal/ESRF (hrs)	4–10/–

Dose in renal impairment GFR (mL/min)

20–50	75% of normal dose
10–20	75% of normal dose
<10	50% of normal dose

Dose in patients undergoing renal replacement therapies

CAPD	Dialysed. Dose as in GFR < 10 mL/min. Following dose do not perform CAPD exchange for 12 hours
HD	Dialysed. Dose as in GFR < 10 mL/min. Dose at minimum of 12 hours before HD session
CAV/VVHD	Dialysed. Dose as in GFR = 10–20 mL/min

Important drug interactions

POTENTIALLY HAZARDOUS INTERACTIONS WITH OTHER DRUGS

• Ifosfamide possibly enhances effect of warfarin

Administration

RECONSTITUTION

• Reconstitute 1-g vial with 12.5 mL water for injection. Reconstitute 2-g vial with 25 mL water for injection. The resultant solution of 8% ifosfamide should *not* be injected directly into the vein

ROUTE

• IV injection: dilute to less than a 4% solution
• IV infusion: dilute as detailed below

RATE OF ADMINISTRATION

• IV infusion – Either: (i) infuse in glucose 5% or sodium chloride 0.9% over 30–120 minutes; (ii) inject directly into a fast-running infusion; (iii) make up in 3 L of glucose 5% or sodium chloride 0.9%. Each litre should be given over 8 hours

COMMENTS

–

Other information

• Nephrotoxicity may occur with oliguria, raised uric acid, increased BUN and serum creatinine and decreased creatinine clearance
• Ifosfamide is known to be more nephrotoxic than cyclophosphamide hence greater caution is advised
• Data sheet contra-indicates the use of ifosfamide if serum creatinine >120 micromol/L
• If patient is anuric and on dialysis, neither the ifosfamide nor its metabolites nor mesna should appear in the urinary tract. The use of mesna may therefore be unnecessary, although this would be a clinical decision
• If the patient is passing urine, mesna should be given to prevent urothelial toxicity

Iloprost (unlicensed product)

Clinical use

Prostacyclin analogue for relief of pain, promotion of ulcer healing and limb salvage in patients with severe peripheral arterial ischaemia

Can also be used for treatment of pulmonary hypertension

Dose in normal renal function

Dose is adjusted according to individual tolerability within the range of 0.5–2.0 nanograms/kg/minute over 6 hours daily, or continuous infusions at a rate of 0.5–1.0 nanogram/kg/minute

Pulmonary hypertension: usually 1–12 nanograms/kg/min, but can use higher doses according to response

Pharmacokinetics

Molecular weight (daltons)	360.5
% Protein binding	≈60
% Excreted unchanged in urine	<5
Volume of distribution (L/kg)	0.7
Half-life – normal/ESRF (hrs)	0.3–0.5/–

Dose in renal impairment GFR (mL/min)

20–50	Dose as in normal renal function
10–20	Dose as in normal renal function
<10	50%–100% of dose

Dose in patients undergoing renal replacement therapies

CAPD	Unknown dialysability. Dose as in GFR < 10 mL/min
HD	Unknown dialysability. Dose as in GFR < 10 mL/min
CAV/VVHD	Unknown dialysability. Dose as in normal renal function

Important drug interactions

POTENTIALLY HAZARDOUS INTERACTIONS WITH OTHER DRUGS

• Beta-blockers, ACE inhibitors, vasodilators: additive antihypertensive effect

• Heparin, warfarin: increased risk of bleeding as iloprost inhibits platelet aggregation

• NSAIDs, phosphodiesterase inhibitors: additive inhibition of platelet aggregation

Administration

RECONSTITUTION

• Dilute 0.1 mg with 500 mL sodium chloride 0.9% or glucose 5%. Final concentration = iloprost 0.2 micrograms/mL

ROUTE

• IV infusion via peripheral vein or central venous catheter

RATE OF ADMINISTRATION

• Infuse 0.1 mg over 6 hours daily (see below)

COMMENTS

• Treatment should be started at an infusion rate of 10 mL/hour for 30 minutes, which corresponds to a dose of 0.5 nanograms/kg/minute for a patient of 65 kg. Then increase the dose in steps of 10 mL/hour every 30 minutes up to a rate of 40 mL/hour (50 mL/hour if patient's body weight is more than 75 kg). Depending on the occurrence of side-effects, such as headache and nausea, or an undesired drop in BP, the infusion rate should be reduced until the tolerable dose is found. If side-effects are severe, the infusion should be interrupted. For the rest of the treatment period, therapy should be continued with the dose found to be tolerated in the first 2–3 days

Other information

• BP and heart rate must be measured at the start of the infusion and after every increase in dose

• Duration of treatment is up to 4 weeks. Shorter treatment periods (3–5 days) are often sufficient in Raynaud's phenomenon

• Iloprost infusions can also be used to control blood pressure during a scleroderma hypertensive crisis

• For fluid-restricted patients, dilute 0.1 mg iloprost with 50 mL sodium chloride 0.9%, and run at a rate of 1–4 mL/hour

• Toxic by inhalation, contact with skin, and if swallowed

Imatinib

Clinical use

Treatment of chronic myeloid leukaemia in chronic phase, accelerated phase or blast crisis. Also used for Kit-positive unresectable or metastatic malignant GI stromal tumours

Dose in normal renal function

400–600 mg daily, increasing to a maximum of 800 mg daily

Pharmacokinetics

Molecular weight (daltons)	589.7
% Protein binding	95
% Excreted unchanged in urine	5
Volume of distribution (L/kg)	–
Half-life – normal/ESRF (hrs)	18/unknown

Dose in renal impairment GFR (mL/min)

20–50	Dose as in normal renal function
10–20	Dose as in normal renal function – see 'Other information'
<10	Dose as in normal renal function – see 'Other information'

Dose in patients undergoing renal replacement therapies

CAPD	Unknown dialysability – Dose as in GFR < 10 ml/min
HD	Unknown dialysability – Dose as in GFR < 10 ml/min
CAV/VVHD	Unknown dialysability – Dose as in GFR = 10–20 ml/min

Important drug interactions

POTENTIALLY HAZARDOUS INTERACTIONS WITH OTHER DRUGS

- Levels of imatinib increased by clarithromycin, erythromycin, itraconazole, ketoconazole
- Levels of imatinib decreased by phenytoin, carbamazepine, rifampicin, phenobarbital, dexamethasone, St John's Wort
- Imatinib increases levels of ciclosporin, tacrolimus, pimozide, simvastatin
- Imatinib enhances anticoagulant effects of warfarin

Administration

RECONSTITUTION

–

ROUTE

- Oral

RATE OF ADMINISTRATION

–

COMMENTS

–

Other information

- Half-life of main metabolite, the N-desmethyl derivative, which has similar potency to the parent compound, is 40 hours in normal renal function
- 68% of a dose and metabolites is recovered in the faeces, and 13% in the urine within 7 days
- Imatinib is associated with oedema and superficial fluid retention in 50–70% cases. This probability is increased in patients receiving higher doses, with age >65 years, and those with a prior history of cardiac disease. Severe fluid retention, e.g. pleural effusion, pericardial effusion, pulmonary oedema and ascites, has been reported in up to 16% of patients. This can be managed by diuretic therapy, and dose reduction or interruption of imatinib therapy
- Severe elevation of serum creatinine has been observed in approximately 1% of patients

Imidapril

Clinical use

ACE inhibitor, used for hypertension

Dose in normal renal function

2.5–20 mg once daily

Pharmacokinetics

Molecular weight (daltons)	441.9 (as hydrochloride)
% Protein binding	85
% Excreted unchanged in urine	9
Volume of distribution (L/kg)	–
Half-life – normal/ESRF (hrs)	2/increased (>24 hours as imidaprilat)

Dose in renal impairment GFR (mL/min)

30–50	Start with 2.5 mg and gradually increase and use with caution
<30	Start with 2.5 mg and gradually increase and use with caution

Dose in patients undergoing renal replacement therapies

CAPD	Probably dialysed. Start with 2.5 mg and gradually increase
HD	Dialysed. Start with 2.5 mg and gradually increase
CAV/VVHD	Probably dialysed. Start with 2.5 mg and gradually increase

Important drug interactions

POTENTIALLY HAZARDOUS INTERACTIONS WITH OTHER DRUGS

- Ciclosporin and tacrolimus: increased risk of hyperkalaemia and nephrotoxicity
- Epoetin: increased risk of hyperkalaemia; antagonism of hypotensive effect
- Lithium levels may be increased
- NSAIDs: antagonism of hypotensive effect; increased risk of hyperkalaemia and renal damage
- Diuretics: enhanced hypotensive effect; increased risk of hyperkalaemia with potassium-sparing diuretics
- Potassium supplements: increased risk of hyperkalaemia
- Anaesthetics: enhanced hypotensive effects

Administration

RECONSTITUTION

–

ROUTE

- Oral

RATE OF ADMINISTRATION

–

COMMENTS

–

Other information

- Imidapril is a pro-drug, rapidly converted to the active imidaprilat
- Hyperkalaemia and other side-effects are more common in patients with impaired renal function
- Close monitoring of renal function during therapy is necessary in those with renal insufficiency
- Renal failure has been reported in association with ACE inhibitors with renal artery stenosis, post renal transplant or congestive heart failure
- A high incidence of anaphylactoid reactions have been reported in patients dialysed with high-flux polyacrylonitrile membranes and treated concomitantly with an ACE inhibitor – this combination should therefore be avoided

Imipramine hydrochloride

Clinical use

Tricyclic antidepressant

Dose in normal renal function

25 mg up to three times daily increasing stepwise to 150–200 mg

Pharmacokinetics

Molecular weight (daltons)	317
% Protein binding	86–96
% Excreted unchanged in urine	<2
Volume of distribution (L/kg)	21
Half-life – normal/ESRF (hrs)	12–24/–

Dose in renal impairment GFR (mL/min)

20–50	Dose as in normal renal function
10–20	Dose as in normal renal function
<10	Dose as in normal renal function

Dose in patients undergoing renal replacement therapies

CAPD	Not dialysed. Dose as in normal renal function
HD	Not dialysed. Dose as in normal renal function
CAV/VVHD	Not dialysed. Dose as in normal renal function

Important drug interactions

POTENTIALLY HAZARDOUS INTERACTIONS WITH OTHER DRUGS

• Alcohol: enhanced sedative effect

• Anti-arrhythmics: increased risk of ventricular arrhythmias
• Other antidepressants: CNS excitation and hypertension with MAOIs and linezolid
• Anti-epileptics: convulsive threshold lowered
• Anti-malarials: avoid concomitant use with artemether with lumefantrine
• Antipsychotics: increased risk of ventricular arrhythmias with pimozide and thioridazine
• Beta-blockers: increased risk of ventricular arrhythmias
• Antihistamines: increased antimuscarinic and sedative effects. Increased risk of ventricular arrhythmias
• Antihypertensives: enhanced hypotensive effect
• Dopaminergics: avoid concomitant use with entacapone; CNS toxicity with selegiline
• Sibutramine: increased risk of CNS toxicity – avoid concomitant use
• Sympathomimetics: hypertension and arrhythmias

Administration

RECONSTITUTION

–

ROUTE

• Oral

RATE OF ADMINISTRATION

–

COMMENTS

–

Other information

• Imipramine metabolised to active metabolite desipramine, which has <1% urinary excretion

Indapamide

Clinical use

Essential hypertension

Dose in normal renal function

2.5–5 mg daily in the morning
Modified release: 1.5 mg daily in the morning

Pharmacokinetics

Molecular weight (daltons)	375
% Protein binding	76–79
% Excreted unchanged in urine	<5
Volume of distribution (L/kg)	0.3–1.3
Half-life – normal/ESRF (hrs)	14–18/unchanged

Dose in renal impairment GFR (mL/min)

20–50	Dose as in normal renal function
10–20	Dose as in normal renal function
<10	Dose as in normal renal function

Dose in patients undergoing renal replacement therapies

CAPD	Not dialysed. Dose as in normal renal function
HD	Not dialysed. Dose as in normal renal function
CAV/VVHD	Not dialysed. Dose as in normal renal function

Important drug interactions

POTENTIALLY HAZARDOUS INTERACTIONS WITH OTHER DRUGS

• Anti-arrhythmics: hypokalaemia leads to increased cardiac toxicity
• Antihistamines: increased risk of cardiac arrhythmias
• Antihypertensives: increased risk of hypotension
• Cardiac glycosides: risk of hypokalaemia
• Lithium: increased lithium levels
• NSAIDs: increased risk of nephrotoxicity of NSAIDs
• Antipsychotics: hypokalaemia increases the risk of ventricular arrhythmias with pimozide and thioridazine – avoid concomitant use

Administration

RECONSTITUTION

–

ROUTE

• Oral

RATE OF ADMINISTRATION

–

COMMENTS

–

Other information

• If pre-existing renal insufficiency is aggravated – stop indapamide
• Doses greater than 2.5 mg daily are not recommended
• Caution if hypokalaemia develops
• Ineffective in ESRF
• Studies in functionally anephric patients for one month undergoing chronic haemodialysis have not shown evidence of drug accumulation despite the fact that indapamide is not dialysable

Indinavir

Clinical use

Protease inhibitor, used for the treatment of HIV-infected patients with advanced or progressive immunodeficiency, in combination with a nucleoside reverse transcriptase inhibitor

Dose in normal renal function

800 mg every 8 hours

Pharmacokinetics

Molecular weight (daltons)	711.9
% Protein binding	60
% Excreted unchanged in urine	<20
Volume of distribution (L/kg)	–
Half-life – normal/ESRF (hrs)	1.8/unchanged

Dose in renal impairment GFR (mL/min)

20–50	Dose as in normal renal function. Monitor closely
10–20	Dose as in normal renal function. Monitor closely
<10	Dose as in normal renal function. Monitor closely

Dose in patients undergoing renal replacement therapies

CAPD	Unknown dialysability. Dose as for GFR < 10 mL/min
HD	Unknown dialysability. Dose as for GFR < 10 mL/min
CAV/VVHD	Unknown dialysability. Dose as for GFR = 10–20 mL/min

Important drug interactions

POTENTIALLY HAZARDOUS INTERACTIONS WITH OTHER DRUGS

• Antibacterials: rifampicin increases metabolism (avoid concomitant use); reduce dose of rifabutin by 50% and increase dose of indinavir

• Antidepressants: plasma concentration reduced by St John's Wort (avoid concomitant use)

• Antifungals: ketoconazole inhibits metabolism (reduce dose of indinavir to 600 mg every 8 hours); itraconazole increases plasma indinavir concentration

• Antihistamines: increased risk of arrhythmias with terfenadine

• Antipsychotics: possibly increased risk of arrhythmias with pimozide (avoid concomitant use); indinavir possibly increases plasma concentration of thioridazine

• Anxiolytics and hypnotics: increased risk of prolonged sedation with alprazolam and midazolam (avoid concomitant use)

• Ergotamine: risk of ergotism (avoid concomitant use)

• Lipid-regulating drugs: increased risk of myopathy with simvastatin (avoid concomitant use); and possibly with atorvastatin

• 5HT$_1$ agonists: plasma concentration of eletriptan increased (avoid concomitant use)

Administration

RECONSTITUTION

–

ROUTE

• Oral

RATE OF ADMINISTRATION

–

COMMENTS

–

Other information

• Give one hour before, or 2 hours after, or with a low-fat meal with water

• Adequate hydration is recommended. Drink 1.5 L of water in 24 hours

• If giving with didanosine leave 1 hour between each drug

• Mild renal insufficiency is usually due to crystalluria, but a case of interstitial nephritis has been reported

• If nephrolithiasis, including flank pain, with or without haematuria occur, temporarily stop therapy (e.g. for 1–3 days)

Insulin – soluble (Actrapid or Humulin S)

Clinical use

Emergency management of hyperkalaemia.
Hyperglycaemia, control of diabetes mellitus

Dose in normal renal function

Variable

Pharmacokinetics

Molecular weight (daltons)	5808
% Protein binding	5
% Excreted unchanged in urine	0
Volume of distribution (L/kg)	0.15
Half-life – normal/ESRF (hrs)	2–4/13

Dose in renal impairment GFR (mL/min)

20–50	Variable
10–20	Variable
<10	Variable

Dose in patients undergoing renal replacement therapies

CAPD	Not dialysed. Dose according to clinical response
HD	Not dialysed. Dose according to clinical response
CAV/VVHD	Not dialysed. Dose according to clinical response

Important drug interactions

POTENTIALLY HAZARDOUS INTERACTIONS WITH OTHER DRUGS

• None known

Administration

RECONSTITUTION

• Add 15–25 IU insulin to 50 mL 50% glucose

ROUTE

• IV via CRIP

RATE OF ADMINISTRATION

• Over 30 minutes

COMMENTS

• For maintenance infusion or sliding-scale infusion, add 50 IU insulin to 500 mL 10% glucose and adjust rate according to blood glucose levels
• Continue infusing insulin/glucose solution at rate of 10 mL/hour according to serum potassium

Other information

• Monitor blood glucose
• Prior to insulin/glucose infusion, give IV 20 mL 10% calcium gluconate to protect myocardium and 50–100 mL 8.4% sodium bicarbonate to correct acidosis
• Commence Calcium Resonium 15 g four times per day orally
• Insulin is metabolised renally: therefore requirements are reduced in ESRF

Interferon alfa-2a (Roferon A)

Clinical use

1 Hairy-cell leukaemia
2 AIDS-related Kaposi's sarcoma
3 Chronic myelogenous leukaemia
4 Cutaneous T-cell lymphoma
5 Chronic hepatitis B
6 Chronic hepatitis C
7 Follicular non-Hodgkin's lymphoma
8 Advanced renal cell carcinoma
9 Malignant melanoma

Dose in normal renal function

1 Hairy-cell leukaemia: 1.5–3 million IU three times per week
2 AIDS-related Kaposi's sarcoma: 3–36 million IU three times per week
3 Chronic myelogenous leukaemia: 9 million IU daily or three times per week
4 Cutaneous T-cell lymphoma: 3–18 million IU daily or three times per week
5 Chronic hepatitis B: 2.5–5 million IU/m^2 three times per week
6 Chronic hepatitis C: 3–4.5 million IU three times per week
7 Follicular non-Hodgkin's lymphoma: 6 million IU/m^2 on days 22–26 of each 28-day cycle
8 Advanced renal cell carcinoma: 9–18 million IU three times per week
9 Malignant melanoma: 1.5–3 million IU three times a week

Pharmacokinetics

Molecular weight (daltons)	15,000–21,000
% Protein binding	–
% Excreted unchanged in urine	Negligible
Volume of distribution (L/kg)	0.4
Half-life – normal/ESRF (hrs)	3.7–8.5

Dose in renal impairment GFR (mL/min)

20–50	Dose as in normal renal function – monitor renal function closely
10–20	Dose as in normal renal function – monitor renal function closely
<10	Use with great caution – see 'Other information'

Dose in patients undergoing renal replacement therapies

CAPD	Not dialysed – dose as in GFR < 10 mL/min
HD	Not dialysed – dose as in GFR < 10 mL/min
CAV/VVHD	Not dialysed – dose as in GFR = 10–20 mL/min

Important drug interactions

POTENTIALLY HAZARDOUS INTERACTIONS WITH OTHER DRUGS

• Immunosuppressants, e.g. ciclosporin, tacrolimus, sirolimus may have an antagonistic effect

Administration

RECONSTITUTION
–

ROUTE
• SC, IM

RATE OF ADMINISTRATION
–

COMMENTS
–

Other information

• Interferon up-regulates the cell surface presentation of class II histocompatibility antigens, which raises the possibility of drug-induced allograft rejection. There are numerous clinical reports of allograft rejection, ARF and graft loss after interferon therapy. Hence extreme care should be exercised in the use of interferon after renal transplantation

• Interferon is metabolised primarily in the kidney. It is excreted in the urine, but is reabsorbed by the tubules where it undergoes lysosomal degradation in these cells. With regard to patients undergoing haemodialysis, the interferon molecule is too large to be dialysed, so we can assume in these patients interferon may accumulate as it will not undergo the proteolytic degradation associated with reabsorption. Hence, the dose may need to be adjusted accordingly

• Several small controlled trials have examined the efficacy of low-dose interferon therapy (3 MIU three times a week given after dialysis) for chronic hepatitis C in patients on haemodialysis. Treatment appears to have been remarkably effective; it is possible that reduced renal clearance of interferon results in higher and more sustained levels of the drug

Interferon alfa-2b (IntronA)

Clinical use

1 Chronic hepatitis B
2 Chronic hepatitis C
3 Hairy-cell leukaemia
4 Multiple myeloma
5 Carcinoid tumour
6 Chronic myelogenous leukaemia
7 Follicular lymphoma
8 Malignant melanoma

Dose in normal renal function

1 Chronic hepatitis B: 5–10 million IU/m^2 three times a week
2 Chronic hepatitis C: 3 million IU three times a week
3 Hairy-cell leukaemia: 2 million IU three times a week
4 Multiple myeloma: 3 million IU three times a week
5 Carcinoid tumour: 3–9 million IU/m^2 three times a week
6 Chronic myelogenous leukaemia: 4–5 million IU three times a week
7 Follicular lymphoma: 5 million IU three times a week
8 Malignant melanoma: 20 million IU/m^2 daily, decreasing to 10 million IU/m^2 three times a week

Pharmacokinetics

Molecular weight (daltons)	15,000–21,000
% Protein binding	–
% Excreted unchanged in urine	–
Volume of distribution (L/kg)	0.4
Half-life – normal/ESRF (hrs)	2–7

Dose in renal impairment GFR (mL/min)

20–50	Dose as in normal renal function – monitor renal function closely
10–20	Dose as in normal renal function – monitor renal function closely
<10	Use with great caution – see 'Other information'

Dose in patients undergoing renal replacement therapies

CAPD	Not dialysed – dose as in GFR < 10 mL/min
HD	Not dialysed – dose as in GFR < 10 mL/min
CAV/VVHD	Not dialysed – dose as in GFR = 10–20 mL/min

Important drug interactions

POTENTIALLY HAZARDOUS INTERACTIONS WITH OTHER DRUGS

• Immunosuppressants, e.g. ciclosporin, tacrolimus, sirolimus may have an antagonistic effect
• Administration of interferon in combination with other chemotherapeutic agents, e.g. cytarabine, cyclophosphamide, doxorubicin, teniposide, may lead to increased risk of severe toxicity

Administration

RECONSTITUTION
–

ROUTE
• IM, SC

RATE OF ADMINISTRATION
–

COMMENTS
–

Other information

• Interferon up-regulates the cell surface presentation of class II histocompatibility antigens, which raises the possibility of drug-induced allograft rejection. There are numerous clinical reports of allograft rejection, ARF and graft loss after interferon therapy. Hence extreme care should be exercised in the use of interferon after renal transplantation

• Interferon is metabolised primarily in the kidney. It is excreted in the urine, but is reabsorbed by the tubules where it undergoes lysosomal degradation in these cells. With regard to patients undergoing haemodialysis, the interferon molecule is too large to be dialysed, so we can assume in these patients interferon may accumulate as it will not undergo the proteolytic degradation associated with reabsorption. Hence, the dose may need to be adjusted accordingly

• Several small controlled trials have examined the efficacy of low-dose interferon therapy (3 MIU three times a week given after dialysis) for chronic hepatitis C in patients on haemodialysis. Treatment appears to have been remarkably effective; it is possible that reduced renal clearance of interferon results in higher and more sustained levels of the drug

Interferon alfa-2b (Viraferon)

Clinical use

Chronic hepatitis B
Chronic hepatitis C

Dose in normal renal function

Chronic hepatitis B: 5–10 million IU three times a week

Chronic hepatitis C: 3 million IU three times a week

Pharmacokinetics

Molecular weight (daltons)	15,000–21,000
% Protein binding	–
% Excreted unchanged in urine	Negligible – see 'Other information'
Volume of distribution (L/kg)	–
Half-life – normal/ESRF (hrs)	2–7

Dose in renal impairment GFR (mL/min)

20–50	Dose as in normal renal function – monitor renal function closely
10–20	Dose as in normal renal function – monitor renal function closely
<10	Use with great caution – see 'Other information'

Dose in patients undergoing renal replacement therapies

CAPD	Not dialysed. Dose as in GFR < 10 mL/min
HD	Not dialysed. Dose as in GFR < 10 mL/min
CAV/VVHD	Not dialysed. Dose as in GFR = 10–20 mL/min

Important drug interactions

POTENTIALLY HAZARDOUS INTERACTIONS WITH OTHER DRUGS

• Ciclosporin: may have an antagonistic effect
• Tacrolimus: may have an antagonistic effect

Administration

RECONSTITUTION

–

ROUTE

• SC, IV

RATE OF ADMINISTRATION

• 20 minutes

COMMENTS

• Add to sodium chloride 0.9% in PVC bags or glass bottles

Other information

• Interferon up-regulates the cell surface presentation of class II histocompatibility antigens, which raises the possibility of drug-induced allograft rejection. There are numerous clinical reports of allograft rejection, ARF and graft loss after interferon therapy. Hence extreme care should be exercised in the use of interferon after renal transplantation

• Interferon is metabolised primarily in the kidney. It is excreted in the urine, but is reabsorbed by the tubules where it undergoes lysosomal degradation in these cells. With regard to patients undergoing haemodialysis, the interferon molecule is too large to be dialysed, so we can assume in these patients interferon may accumulate as it will not undergo the proteolytic degradation associated with reabsorption. Hence, the dose may need to be adjusted accordingly

• Several small controlled trials have examined the efficacy of low-dose interferon therapy (3 MIU three times a week given after dialysis) for chronic hepatitis C in patients on haemodialysis. Treatment appears to have been remarkably effective; it is possible that reduced renal clearance of interferon results in higher and more sustained levels of the drug

Interferon beta-1a

Clinical use

Treatment of relapsing-remitting multiple sclerosis

Dose in normal renal function

Avonex: 6 million IU (30 micrograms) once a week
Rebif: 22–44 micrograms three times a week

Pharmacokinetics

Molecular weight (daltons)	15,000–21,000
% Protein binding	–
% Excreted unchanged in urine	Negligible – see 'Other information'
Volume of distribution (L/kg)	–
Half-life – normal/ESRF (hrs)	10

Dose in renal impairment GFR (mL/min)

20–50	Dose as in normal renal function – monitor renal function
10–20	Dose as in normal renal function – monitor renal function
<10	Use with caution due to risk of accumulation and monitor renal function

Dose in patients undergoing renal replacement therapies

CAPD	Not dialysed. Use with caution with close monitoring
HD	Not dialysed. Use with caution with close monitoring
CAV/VVHD	Not dialysed. Use with caution with close monitoring

Important drug interactions

POTENTIALLY HAZARDOUS INTERACTIONS WITH OTHER DRUGS

• Administer with caution with drugs with a narrow therapeutic window and cleared by cytochrome CYP 450

Administration

RECONSTITUTION

• With diluent provided

ROUTE

• IM (Avonex), SC (Rebif)

RATE OF ADMINISTRATION

–

COMMENTS

• Stable for 6 hours at 2–8°C once reconstituted

Other information

• Pre-treatment with paracetamol is recommended to reduce incidence of flu-like symptoms
• Vary the site of injection each week
• Rare cases of lupus erythematosus syndrome have occurred
• Transient increases in creatinine, potassium, urea, nitrogen and urinary calcium may occur

Interferon beta-1b (Betaferon)

Clinical use

Treatment of relapsing-remitting and secondary progressive multiple sclerosis

Dose in normal renal function

8 million IU every second day

Pharmacokinetics

Molecular weight (daltons)	15,000–21,000
% Protein binding	No data
% Excreted unchanged in urine	Negligible – see 'Other information'
Volume of distribution (L/kg)	No data
Half-life – normal/ESRF (hrs)	5–10

Dose in renal impairment GFR (mL/min)

20–50	No data on use in renal impairment. Dose as in normal renal function and monitor renal function carefully
10–20	No data on use in renal impairment. Dose as in normal renal function and monitor renal function carefully
<10	No data on use in renal impairment. Use with caution and monitor renal function carefully

Dose in patients undergoing renal replacement therapies

CAPD	Not dialysed. Dose as in GFR < 10 mL/min
HD	Not dialysed. Dose as in GFR < 10 mL/mm
CAV/VVHD	Unlikely dialysability. Dose as in GFR = 10–20 ml/min

Important drug interactions

POTENTIALLY HAZARDOUS INTERACTIONS WITH OTHER DRUGS

* Ciclosporin and tacrolimus: interferon reported to reduce the activity of hepatic CYP 450 enzymes

Administration

RECONSTITUTION

* With 1.2 mL of diluent provided

ROUTE

* SC

RATE OF ADMINISTRATION

–

COMMENTS

–

Other information

* Pre-treatment with paracetamol is recommended to reduce incidence of flu-like symptoms

* Interferon up-regulates the cell surface presentation of class II histocompatibility antigens, which raises the possibility of drug-induced allograft rejection. There are numerous clinical reports of allograft rejection, ARF and graft loss after interferon therapy. Hence extreme care should be exercised in the use of interferon after renal transplantation

* Interferon is metabolised primarily in the kidney. It is excreted in the urine, but is reabsorbed by the tubules where it undergoes lysosomal degradation in these cells. With regard to patients undergoing haemodialysis, the interferon molecule is too large to be dialysed, so we can assume in these patients interferon may accumulate as it will not undergo the proteolytic degradation associated with reabsorption. Hence, the dose may need to be adjusted accordingly

Interferon gamma-1b (Immukin)

Clinical use

Adjunct to antibiotics to reduce the frequency of serious infections in patients with chronic granulomatous disease

Dose in normal renal function

50 micrograms/m^2 three times a week
or 1.5 micrograms/kg three times a week if
BSA < 0.5 m^2

Pharmacokinetics

Molecular weight (daltons)	15,000–21,000
% Protein binding	No data
% Excreted unchanged in urine	Negligible
Volume of distribution (L/kg)	12.4
Half-life – normal/ESRF (hrs)	5.9

Dose in renal impairment GFR (mL/min)

20–50	No data on use in renal impairment – dose as for normal renal function and monitor renal function closely
10–20	No data on use in renal impairment – dose as for normal renal function and monitor renal function closely
<10	Use with caution due to risk of accumulation – monitor renal function closely

Dose in patients undergoing renal replacement therapies

CAPD	Not dialysed. Dose as in GFR < 10 mL/min
HD	Not dialysed. Dose as in GFR < 10 mL/min
CAV/VVHD	Unlikely dialysability. Dose as in GFR = 10–20 ml/min

Important drug interactions

POTENTIALLY HAZARDOUS INTERACTIONS WITH OTHER DRUGS

• None known

Administration

RECONSTITUTION

–

ROUTE

• SC

RATE OF ADMINISTRATION

–

COMMENTS

–

Other information

• Pre-treatment with paracetamol is recommended to reduce incidence of flu-like symptoms

• Interferon up-regulates the cell surface presentation of class II histocompatibility antigens, which raises the possibility of drug-induced allograft rejection. There are numerous clinical reports of allograft rejection, ARF and graft loss after interferon therapy. Hence extreme care should be exercised in the use of interferon after renal transplantation

• Interferon is metabolised primarily in the kidney. It is excreted in the urine, but is reabsorbed by the tubules where it undergoes lysosomal degradation in these cells. With regard to patients undergoing haemodialysis, the interferon molecule is too large to be dialysed, so we can assume in these patients interferon may accumulate as it will not undergo the proteolytic degradation associated with reabsorption. Hence, the dose may need to be adjusted accordingly

Ipratropium bromide

Clinical use

Anticholinergic bronchodilator: reversible airways obstruction, particularly in chronic bronchitis

Dose in normal renal function

Depends on presentation used.

Nebuliser solution: 100–500 micrograms up to 4 times daily

Inhaler: 20–80 micrograms 3–4 times daily

Pharmacokinetics

Molecular weight (daltons)	430
% Protein binding	20
% Excreted unchanged in urine	2.8
Volume of distribution (L/kg)	4.6
Half-life – normal/ESRF (hrs)	1.6–3.8/–

Dose in renal impairment GFR (mL/min)

20–50	Dose as in normal renal function
10–20	Dose as in normal renal function
<10	Dose as in normal renal function

Dose in patients undergoing renal replacement therapies

CAPD	Unknown dialysability. Dose as in normal renal function
HD	Unknown dialysability. Dose as in normal renal function
CAV/VVHD	Unknown dialysability. Dose as in normal renal function

Important drug interactions

POTENTIALLY HAZARDOUS INTERACTIONS WITH OTHER DRUGS

• None known

Administration

RECONSTITUTION

• Nebuliser: the dose of nebuliser solution may need to be diluted in order to obtain a final volume suitable for the nebuliser. Sterile sodium chloride 0.9% should be used if dilution is required

ROUTE

• Inhaled

RATE OF ADMINISTRATION

• Nebuliser: according to nebuliser

COMMENTS

–

Other information

• Following inhalation, only a small amount of ipratropium reaches the systemic circulation. Any swallowed drug is poorly absorbed from the GI tract

Irbesartan

Clinical use

AT-II receptor antagonist, used for hypertension, diabetic nephropathy

Dose in normal renal function

75–300 mg daily

Pharmacokinetics

Molecular weight (daltons)	428.5
% Protein binding	96
% Excreted unchanged in urine	<2
Volume of distribution (L/kg)	53–93 litres
Half-life – normal/ESRF (hrs)	11–15/unchanged

Dose in renal impairment GFR (mL/min)

20–50	Dose as in normal renal function
10–20	Dose as in normal renal function
<10	Dose as in normal renal function

Dose in patients undergoing renal replacement therapies

CAPD	Not dialysed. Initial dose 75 mg daily and gradually increase
HD	Not dialysed. Initial dose 75 mg daily and gradually increase
CAV/VVHD	Unknown dialysability. Initial dose 75 mg daily and gradually increase

Important drug interactions

POTENTIALLY HAZARDOUS INTERACTIONS WITH OTHER DRUGS

- Ciclosporin and tacrolimus: increased risk of hyperkalaemia and nephrotoxicity
- Anaesthetics: enhanced hypotensive effect
- Analgesics: antagonism of hypotensive effect and increased risk of renal impairment with NSAIDs; hyperkalaemia with ketorolac and other NSAIDs
- Diuretics: enhanced hypotensive effect; hyperkalaemia with potassium-sparing diuretics
- Lithium: reduced excretion. Possibility of enhanced lithium toxicity
- Potassium salts: increased risk of hyperkalaemia

Administration

RECONSTITUTION

–

ROUTE

- Oral

RATE OF ADMINISTRATION

–

COMMENTS

–

Other information

- Hyperkalaemia and other side-effects are more common in patients with impaired renal function
- Renal failure has been reported in association with AT-II antagonists in patients with renal artery stenosis, post renal transplant, or in those with congestive heart failure
- Close monitoring of renal function during therapy is necessary in those with renal insufficiency

Irinotecan hydrochloride

Clinical use

Treatment of metastatic colorectal cancer resistant to fluorouracil, or in conjunction with fluorouracil (5-FU)

Dose in normal renal function

Without 5-FU: 350 mg/m^2 every 3 weeks

With 5-FU: 180 mg/m^2 every 2 weeks

Pharmacokinetics

Molecular weight (daltons)	677.2
% Protein binding	65
% Excreted unchanged in urine	20
Volume of distribution (L/kg)	157 litres
Half-life – normal/ESRF (hrs)	14/–

Dose in renal impairment GFR (mL/min)

20–50	Dose as in normal renal function and monitor closely
10–20	Dose as in normal renal function and monitor closely
<10	Reduce dose and monitor closely

Dose in patients undergoing renal replacement therapies

CAPD	Unlikely dialysability. Dose as in GFR < 10 mL/min
HD	Unlikely dialysability. Dose as in GFR < 10 mL/min
CAV/VVHD	Unlikely dialysability. Dose as in GFR = 10–20 mL/min

Important drug interactions

POTENTIALLY HAZARDOUS INTERACTIONS WITH OTHER DRUGS

• None known

Administration

RECONSTITUTION

–

ROUTE

• IV infusion

RATE OF ADMINISTRATION

• Over 30–90 minutes

COMMENTS

• Dilute in 250 mL sodium chloride 0.9% or glucose 5%

Other information

• Manufacturer advises avoiding use in renal impairment due to lack of data

• Infrequent reports of renal insufficiency due to inadequate hydration

• Transient, mild to moderate increase in serum creatinine reported in 7.3% patients

Iron dextran 5% solution

Clinical use

Prophylaxis (when oral treatment is not effective or contra-indicated) or treatment of iron deficiency during epoetin therapy especially if serum ferritin is very low (<50 nanograms/mL)

Dose in normal renal function

Total iron infusion: Dose of iron dextran (mg) = weight(kg) x [target Hb(g/L) – actual Hb(g/L)] x 0.24 + 500 mg iron for iron stores (if body weight >35 kg)

20 mg/kg (up to a maximum of 1 g) as a single dose

Target haemoglobin level = 11 g/dL for renal patients as a guide

or

100–200 mg two or three times a week depending on haemoglobin

- **A test dose is essential.** Give 0.5 mL or 25 mg iron slowly and observe for 60 minutes for anaphylaxis. Have resuscitative equipment and drugs at hand (adrenaline, chlorphenamine and hydrocortisone)

Pharmacokinetics

Molecular weight (daltons)	165,000
% Protein binding	0
% Excreted unchanged in urine	<0.2
Volume of distribution (L/kg)	0.031–0.055
Half-life – normal/ESRF (hrs)	20/–

Dose in renal impairment GFR (mL/min)

20–50	Dose as in normal renal function
10–20	Dose as in normal renal function
<10	Dose as in normal renal function

Dose in patients undergoing renal replacement therapies

CAPD	Not dialysed. Dose as in normal renal function
HD	Not dialysed. Dose as in normal renal function
CAV/VVHD	Not dialysed. Dose as in normal renal function

Important drug interactions

POTENTIALLY HAZARDOUS INTERACTIONS WITH OTHER DRUGS

- Oral iron: reduced absorption of oral iron

Administration

RECONSTITUTION

–

ROUTE

- IV peripherally

RATE OF ADMINISTRATION

- Infusion: not more than 100 mL in 30 minutes (first 25 mg over 15 mins)
- Bolus: 25 mg over 1–2 mins, if no adverse reactions within 15 minutes administer the rest of the dose
- Total dose infusion: over 4–6 hours, first 25 mg over 15 mins (increase rate of infusion to 45–60 drops per minute)

COMMENTS

- Infusion: dilute 100–200 mg in 100 mL sodium chloride 0.9% or glucose 5%
- Bolus: dilute in 10–20 mL sodium chloride 0.9% or glucose 5%
- Total dose infusion in 500 mL sodium chloride 0.9% or glucose 5%
- Keep under strict supervision during and for 1 hour after infusion

Other information

- Do not give to patients with history of asthma
- If patients with a history of allergy are prescribed iron dextran, give adequate antihistamine cover prior to administration
- The dose of iron dextran varies widely from 100 mg per dialysis session for 6–10 sessions, to single doses of 500 mg to 1 g
- The incidence of anaphylaxis with the Cosmofer brand of iron dextran is significantly lower than with the old Imferon brand, since the iron is complexed to a much shorter dextran chain than was used previously

Iron III hydroxide sucrose complex

Clinical use

Prophylaxis (when oral treatment is not effective or contra-indicated) or treatment of iron deficiency during epoetin therapy especially if serum ferritin is very low (<50 nanograms/mL)

Iron-deficiency anaemia

Dose in normal renal function

According to local protocol – see 'Other information'

Pharmacokinetics

Molecular weight (daltons)	43,000
% Protein binding	–
% Excreted unchanged in urine	<5
Volume of distribution (L/kg)	8 litres
Half-life – normal/ESRF (hrs)	6

Dose in renal impairment GFR (mL/min)

20–50	Dose as in normal renal function
10–20	Dose as in normal renal function
<10	Dose as in normal renal function

Dose in patients undergoing renal replacement therapies

CAPD	Not dialysed. Dose as in normal renal function
HD	Not dialysed. Dose as in normal renal function
CAV/VVHD	Not dialysed. Dose as in normal renal function

Important drug interactions

POTENTIALLY HAZARDOUS INTERACTIONS WITH OTHER DRUGS

• Do not administer with oral iron

Administration

RECONSTITUTION

–

ROUTE

• IV

RATE OF ADMINISTRATION

• Bolus: 1 mL/minute

• Infusion: in sodium chloride 0.9% at a concentration of 1 mg/mL over 20–30 minutes per 100 mg

COMMENTS

• A test dose is required before administration

• Doses can be administered via the venous limb of the dialysis machine

• Stable for 24 hours at room temperature

Other information

Some regimens are:

• 50–300 mg weekly

• 100 mg once or twice monthly

• 20–40 mg with each dialysis

• Oral iron can be restarted 5 days after completion of the course of IV iron

Isoniazid

Clinical use

Antibacterial agent: treatment of, and prophylaxis of, tuberculosis in 'at risk' immunocompromised patients

Dose in normal renal function

300 mg daily

Pharmacokinetics

Molecular weight (daltons)	137
% Protein binding	4–30
% Excreted unchanged in urine	5–30
Volume of distribution (L/kg)	0.75
Half-life – normal/ESRF (hrs)	0.7–4/8–17 (depends on acetylator status)

Dose in renal impairment GFR (mL/min)

20–50	Dose as in normal renal function
10–20	Dose as in normal renal function
<10	200–300 mg daily

Dose in patients undergoing renal replacement therapies

CAPD	Dialysed. Dose as in GFR < 10 mL/min
HD	Dialysed. Dose as in GFR < 10 mL/min. Give dose post dialysis
CAV/VVHD	Probably dialysed. Dose as in normal renal function

Important drug interactions

POTENTIALLY HAZARDOUS INTERACTIONS WITH OTHER DRUGS

• Anti-epileptics: metabolism of carbamazepine, ethosuximide and phenytoin inhibited (enhanced effect); also with carbamazepine, isoniazid hepatotoxicity possibly increased

Administration

RECONSTITUTION

• Dilute with water for injection if required

ROUTE

• Oral, IM, IV, intrapleural or intrathecal

RATE OF ADMINISTRATION

• Not critical. Give by slow IV bolus

COMMENTS

–

Other information

• Adjust dose accordingly if hepatic illness, slow/fast acetylator status identified
• Pyridoxine hydrochloride 25 mg daily has been recommended for prophylaxis of peripheral neuritis

Isosorbide dinitrate

Clinical use

Vasodilator: prophylaxis and treatment of angina; left ventricular failure

Dose in normal renal function

Sublingual: 5–10 mg

Oral: angina, 30–120 mg daily in divided doses; LVF: up to 240 mg daily

IV: 2–10 mg/hour

Pharmacokinetics

Molecular weight (daltons)	236
% Protein binding	16–40
% Excreted unchanged in urine	<2
Volume of distribution (L/kg)	1.4–8.6
Half-life – normal/ESRF (hrs)	0.5–1/–

Dose in renal impairment GFR (mL/min)

20–50	Dose as in normal renal function
10–20	Dose as in normal renal function
<10	Dose as in normal renal function

Dose in patients undergoing renal replacement therapies

CAPD	Not dialysed. Dose as in normal renal function
HD	Not dialysed. Dose as in normal renal function
CAV/VVHD	Unknown dialysability. Dose as in normal renal function

Important drug interactions

POTENTIALLY HAZARDOUS INTERACTIONS WITH OTHER DRUGS

• Sildenafil: hypotensive effect significantly enhanced – avoid concomitant use

Administration

RECONSTITUTION

• Dilute using sodium chloride 0.9% or glucose 5% to 1 mg/10 mL or 2 mg/10 mL. Final volume 500 mL

ROUTE

• Oral, sublingual, IV infusion

RATE OF ADMINISTRATION

• 1 mg/10 mL; 60 mL/hour ≡ 6 mg/hour
• 2 mg/10 mL; 30 mL/hour ≡ 6 mg/hour

COMMENTS

• The use of PVC giving sets and containers should be avoided since significant losses of the active ingredient by absorption can occur

Other information

• Isosorbide dinitrate undergoes extensive first-pass metabolism, mainly in the liver. The major metabolites are isosorbide-2-mononitrate and isosorbide-5-mononitrate; both possess vasodilatory activity and may contribute to the activity of the parent compound. Both metabolites have longer half-lives than the parent compound

Isosorbide mononitrate

Clinical use

Vasodilator: treatment and prophylaxis of angina.
Adjunct in congestive heart failure

Dose in normal renal function

20–120 mg/day in divided doses

Pharmacokinetics

Molecular weight (daltons)	191
% Protein binding	72
% Excreted unchanged in urine	10–20
Volume of distribution (L/kg)	1.5–4
Half-life – normal/ESRF (hrs)	0.15–0.5/4

Dose in renal impairment
GFR (mL/min)

20–50	Dose as in normal renal function
10–20	Dose as in normal renal function
<10	Dose as in normal renal function

Dose in patients undergoing renal replacement therapies

CAPD	Not dialysed. Dose as in normal renal function
HD	Dialysed. Dose as in normal renal function. Dose after haemodialysis on dialysis days
CAV/VVHD	Probably dialysed. Dose as in normal renal function

Important drug interactions

POTENTIALLY HAZARDOUS INTERACTIONS WITH OTHER DRUGS

• Sildenafil: hypotensive effect significantly enhanced – avoid concomitant use

Administration

RECONSTITUTION

–

ROUTE

• Oral

RATE OF ADMINISTRATION

–

COMMENTS

–

Other information

• Tolerance may develop. This may be minimised by having 'nitrate free' periods

Isotretinoin

Clinical use

Treatment of nodulo-cystic and conglobate acne and severe acne which has failed to respond to an adequate course of systemic antibiotic

Dose in normal renal function

0.5 mg/kg daily in 1–2 divided doses initially.
Range: 0.1–1 mg/kg/day

Topically: 1–2 times daily

Pharmacokinetics

Molecular weight (daltons)	300
% Protein binding	99.5
% Excreted unchanged in urine	50
Volume of distribution (L/kg)	1.5
Half-life – normal/ESRF (hrs)	10–20/–

Dose in renal impairment GFR (mL/min)

<50   Contra-indicated. See 'Other information'

Dose in patients undergoing renal replacement therapies

CAPD	Not dialysed. Dose as in GFR = <50 mL/min
HD	Not dialysed. Dose as in GFR = <50 mL/min
CAV/VVHD	Not dialysed. Dose as in GFR = <50 mL/min

Important drug interactions

POTENTIALLY HAZARDOUS INTERACTIONS WITH OTHER DRUGS

• Rare cases of benign intracranial hypertension have been reported with isotretinoin and tetracyclines. Supplementary treatment with tetracyclines is therefore contra-indicated

Administration

RECONSTITUTION

–

ROUTE

• Oral, topical (0.5% gel)

RATE OF ADMINISTRATION

–

COMMENTS

–

Other information

• Patients on haemodialysis have been treated successfully on 10–20 mg daily or 20 mg on alternate days

• Since the drug is highly protein bound, it is not expected to be significantly removed by dialysis

Ispaghula husk (Fybogel & Fybogel Orange)

Clinical use

Treatment of constipation and of patients requiring a high-fibre regimen

Dose in normal renal function

One sachet (3.5 g) in water twice daily

Pharmacokinetics

Molecular weight (daltons)	–
% Protein binding	0
% Excreted unchanged in urine	0
Volume of distribution (L/kg)	Not absorbed
Half-life – normal/ESRF (hrs)	Not absorbed

Dose in renal impairment GFR (mL/min)

20–50	Dose as in normal renal function
10–20	Dose as in normal renal function
<10	Dose as in normal renal function

Dose in patients undergoing renal replacement therapies

CAPD	Not dialysed. Dose as in normal renal function
HD	Not dialysed. Dose as in normal renal function
CAV/VVHD	Not dialysed. Dose as in normal renal function

Important drug interactions

POTENTIALLY HAZARDOUS INTERACTIONS WITH OTHER DRUGS

• None known

Administration

RECONSTITUTION

–

ROUTE

• Oral

RATE OF ADMINISTRATION

–

COMMENTS

• Fybogel should be stirred into 150 mL water and taken as quickly as possible, preferably after meals
• Additional fluid intake should be maintained

Other information

• Fybogel is low in sodium and potassium, containing approximately 0.4 mmol sodium and 0.7 mmol potassium per sachet
• Fybogel is sugar and gluten free
• Fybogel contains aspartame (contributes to the phenylalanine intake and may affect control of phenylketonuria)
• Fluid restrictions for dialysis patients can render this treatment inappropriate

Ispaghula husk (Regulan)

Clinical use

Treatment of constipation and of patients requiring a high-fibre regimen

Dose in normal renal function

One sachet in water 1–3 times daily

Pharmacokinetics

Molecular weight (daltons)	–
% Protein binding	0
% Excreted unchanged in urine	0
Volume of distribution (L/kg)	Not absorbed
Half-life – normal/ESRF (hrs)	Not absorbed

Dose in renal impairment GFR (mL/min)

20–50	Dose as in normal renal function
10–20	Dose as in normal renal function
<10	Dose as in normal renal function

Dose in patients undergoing renal replacement therapies

CAPD	Not dialysed. Dose as in normal renal function
HD	Not dialysed. Dose as in normal renal function
CAV/VVHD	Not dialysed. Dose as in normal renal function

Important drug interactions

POTENTIALLY HAZARDOUS INTERACTIONS WITH OTHER DRUGS

• None known

Administration

RECONSTITUTION

–

ROUTE

• Oral

RATE OF ADMINISTRATION

–

COMMENTS

• The measured dose of Regulan should be stirred into 150 mL cool water and taken immediately
• Additional fluid intake should be maintained

Other information

• Orange and lemon/lime flavours contain: 3.4 g ispaghula husk BP, 0.23 mmol sodium, <1 mmol potassium per sachet and are gluten and sugar free
• They also contain aspartame (contributes to the phenylalanine intake and may affect control of phenylketonuria)
• Fluid restrictions in dialysis patients can render this treatment inappropriate

Isradipine

Clinical use

Calcium-channel blocker: essential hypertension

Dose in normal renal function

Initially 2.5 mg twice daily, increased if necessary after 3–4 weeks to 5 mg twice daily

Pharmacokinetics

Molecular weight (daltons)	371
% Protein binding	95
% Excreted unchanged in urine	<5
Volume of distribution (L/kg)	3–4
Half-life – normal/ESRF (hrs)	1.9–4.8/10–11

Dose in renal impairment GFR (mL/min)

20–50	Dose as in normal renal function
10–20	Dose as in normal renal function
<10	Dose as in normal renal function

Dose in patients undergoing renal replacement therapies

CAPD	Not dialysed. Dose as in normal renal function
HD	Not dialysed. Dose as in normal renal function
CAV/VVHD	Not dialysed. Dose as in normal renal function

Important drug interactions

POTENTIALLY HAZARDOUS INTERACTIONS WITH OTHER DRUGS

- Anaesthetics: isoflurane enhances hypotensive effect of isradipine
- Antibacterials: rifampicin possibly increases the metabolism of isradipine
- Anti-epileptics: effect of isradipine reduced by carbamazepine, phenobarbital, phenytoin and primidone
- Antihypertensives: enhanced hypotensive effect
- Ritonavir: possibly increased levels of isradipine
- Theophylline: possible increase in theophylline levels

Administration

RECONSTITUTION

–

ROUTE

- Oral

RATE OF ADMINISTRATION

–

COMMENTS

–

Other information

- In elderly patients, or where hepatic or renal function is impaired, initial dose should be 1.25 mg twice daily. Dose should be increased according to the requirements of the individual patient

Itraconazole

Clinical use

Antifungal agent

Dose in normal renal function

100–200 mg every 12–24 hours according to indication

Pharmacokinetics

Molecular weight (daltons)	706
% Protein binding	99.8
% Excreted unchanged in urine	<0.03
Volume of distribution (L/kg)	10.7
Half-life – normal/ESRF (hrs)	20–25/25

Dose in renal impairment GFR (mL/min)

20–50	Dose as in normal renal function
10–20	Dose as in normal renal function
<10	Dose as in normal renal function

Dose in patients undergoing renal replacement therapies

CAPD	Not dialysed. Dose as in normal renal function
HD	Not dialysed. Dose as in normal renal function
CAV/VVHD	Not dialysed. Dose as in normal renal function

Important drug interactions

POTENTIALLY HAZARDOUS INTERACTIONS WITH OTHER DRUGS

- Ciclosporin: metabolism of ciclosporin inhibited (increased plasma ciclosporin levels)
- Anti-arrhythmics: plasma concentration of quinidine increased, increased risk of ventricular arrhythmias
- Antibacterials: rifampicin accelerates metabolism of itraconazole
- Anticoagulants: effect of warfarin and acenocoumarol enhanced
- Antidepressants: avoid concomitant use with reboxetine
- Anti-epileptics: plasma concentrations of itraconazole reduced by phenytoin
- Antihistamines: itraconazole inhibits terfenadine metabolism (avoid concomitant use – cardiac toxicity reported)
- Antipsychotics: increased risk of ventricular arrhythmias with pimozide – avoid concomitant use
- Antivirals: plasma concentration of indinavir increased
- Anxiolytics and hypnotics: plasma concentration of midazolam increased by itraconazole
- Calcium-channel blockers: metabolism of felodipine inhibited
- Cardiac glycosides: plasma concentrations of digoxin increased
- Lipid-lowering drugs: itraconazole increases risk of myopathy with simvastatin. Avoid
- Sirolimus: plasma concentration increased by itraconazole
- Tacrolimus: possibly increased tacrolimus levels

Administration

RECONSTITUTION

–

ROUTE

- Oral, IV infusion

RATE OF ADMINISTRATION

- Over 60 minutes

COMMENTS

- Add 250-mg vial to 50 mL sodium chloride 0.9%, administer 60 mL (increased volume due to large displacement value)

Other information

- The oral bioavailability of itraconazole may be lower in some patients with renal insufficiency, e.g. those receiving CAPD. Monitoring of itraconazole plasma levels and dose adaptation are advisable. Janssen-Cilag offer no guidelines for dose alteration
- Janssen-Cilag advise no dose alterations required in renal impairment as drug is extensively metabolised in the liver and pharmacokinetics are unchanged in patients with ESRF compared to normal

Ketoprofen

Clinical use

NSAID: Pain and mild inflammation in rheumatic disease and other musculo-skeletal disorders; acute gout, dysmenorrhoea

Dose in normal renal function

100–200 mg daily in 2–4 divided doses

Pharmacokinetics

Molecular weight (daltons)	254
% Protein binding	94–99
% Excreted unchanged in urine	<1
Volume of distribution (L/kg)	0.11
Half-life – normal/ESRF (hrs)	1.5–4/unchanged

Dose in renal impairment GFR (mL/min)

20–50	Dose as in normal renal function, but avoid if possible
10–20	Dose as in normal renal function, but avoid if possible
<10	Dose as in normal renal function, but only use if ESRD on dialysis

Dose in patients undergoing renal replacement therapies

CAPD	Unlikely to be dialysed. Dose as in GFR < 10 mL/min
HD	Unlikely to be dialysed. Dose as in GFR < 10 mL/min
CAV/VVHD	Unlikely to be dialysed. Dose as in GFR = 10–20 mL/min

Important drug interactions

POTENTIALLY HAZARDOUS INTERACTIONS WITH OTHER DRUGS

- Ciclosporin: increased risk of nephrotoxicity
- ACE inhibitors and AT-II antagonists: antagonism of hypotensive effect. Increased risk of renal damage and hyperkalaemia
- Antibacterials: possibly increased risk of convulsions with quinolones
- Anticoagulants: effects of warfarin and acenocoumarol enhanced
- Antidiabetics: effects of sulphonylureas enhanced
- Anti-epileptics: effect of phenytoin enhanced
- Antivirals: increased risk of haematological toxicity with zidovudine
- Diuretics: increased risk of nephrotoxicity, hyperkalaemia with potassium-sparing diuretics
- Methotrexate: excretion reduced
- Lithium: excretion reduced
- Tacrolimus: increased risk of nephrotoxicity

Administration

RECONSTITUTION

–

ROUTE

- Oral, IM, rectal. (The injection must not be given by the IV route)

RATE OF ADMINISTRATION

–

COMMENTS

- IM: maximum 200 mg in 24 hours. Injection should not be used for longer than 3 days. Dose 50–100 mg every 4 hours (see maximum). Administer by deep IM injection into the upper, outer quadrant of the buttock

Other information

- Combined oral and rectal treatment, maximum total daily dose 200 mg
- Inhibition of renal prostaglandin synthesis by NSAIDs may interfere with renal function, especially in the presence of existing renal disease. Avoid if possible; if not, check serum creatinine 48–72 hours after starting NSAID. If raised, discontinue NSAID therapy
- Use normal doses in patients with ESRD on dialysis
- Use with caution in renal transplant recipients – can reduce intra-renal autocoid synthesis
- NSAIDs decrease platelet aggregation
- Associated with nephrotic syndrome, interstitial nephritis, hyperkalaemia and sodium retention

Ketorolac trometamol

Clinical use

Short-term management of moderate to severe
acute post-operative pain

Dose in normal renal function

Post-operative:
• Oral: 10 mg every 4–6 hours (elderly every
6–8 hours); maximum 40 mg daily; maximum
duration 7 days
• IM/IV: initially 10 mg, then 10–30 mg when
required every 4–6 hours (every 2 hours in initial
post-operative period). Maximum 90 mg daily
(elderly and patients less than 50 kg: maximum
60 mg daily). Maximum duration 2 days

Pharmacokinetics

Molecular weight (daltons)	376
% Protein binding	>99
% Excreted unchanged in urine	5–10
Volume of distribution (L/kg)	0.13–0.25
Half-life – normal/ESRF (hrs)	IM dose: 3.5–9.2/5.9–19.2

Dose in renal impairment
GFR (mL/min)

20–50	Maximum 60 mg daily
10–20	Avoid if possible. Use small doses and monitor closely
<10	Avoid if possible. Use small doses and monitor closely

Dose in patients undergoing renal replacement therapies

CAPD	Unlikely dialysability. Dose as in GFR < 10 mL/min
HD	Unlikelydialysability. Dose as in GFR < 10 mL/min
CAV/VVHD	Unknown dialysability. Dose as in GFR = 10–20 mL/min

Important drug interactions

POTENTIALLY HAZARDOUS INTERACTIONS WITH
OTHER DRUGS

• Ciclosporin: increased risk of nephrotoxicity
• ACE inhibitors and AT-II antagonists: increased
risk of renal damage and increased risk of
hyperkalaemia, antagonism of hypotensive effect
• Other NSAIDs: avoid concomitant administration
of two or more NSAIDs
• Antibacterials: possibly increased risk of
convulsions with quinolones
• Anticoagulants: effect of warfarin and
acenocoumarol possibly enhanced, increased risk
of haemorrhage with parenteral ketorolac
• Antidiabetics: effects of sulphonylureas possibly
enhanced
• Antivirals: increased risk of haematological
toxicity with zidovudine
• Diuretics: increased risk of nephrotoxicity,
hyperkalaemia with potassium-sparing diuretics
• Methotrexate: excretion of methotrexate
reduced
• Lithium: excretion of lithium reduced
(avoid concomitant use)
• Probenecid: delays excretion of ketorolac
• Pentoxifylline: risk of ketorolac-associated
bleeding increased
• Anti-epileptics: effect of phenytoin possibly
enhanced
• Tacrolimus: increased risk of nephrotoxicity

Administration

RECONSTITUTION

• Compatible with sodium chloride 0.9%, glucose
5%, compound sodium lactate or Plasmalyte
solutions

ROUTE

• IM, IV, oral. (IV/IM preparation is not for epidural
or spinal administration)

RATE OF ADMINISTRATION

• IV: administer IV bolus over no less than
15 seconds

COMMENTS

–

Other information

• Drugs that inhibit prostaglandin biosynthesis (including NSAIDs) have been reported to cause nephrotoxicity, including, but not limited to, glomerular nephritis, interstitial nephritis, renal papillary necrosis, nephrotic syndrome and acute renal failure. In patients with renal, cardiac or hepatic impairment, caution is required since the use of NSAIDs may result in deterioration of renal function

• Ketorolac and its metabolites are excreted primarily by the kidney

• Reported renal side-effects include increased urinary frequency, oliguria, acute renal failure, hyponatraemia, hyperkalaemia, haemolytic uraemic syndrome, flank pain (with or without haematuria), raised serum urea and creatinine and interstitial nephritis

Klean-Prep

Clinical use

Colonic lavage prior to diagnostic examination or surgical procedures requiring a clean colon

Dose in normal renal function

4 sachets, each reconstituted in 1 litre of water, at a rate of 250 mL every 10–15 minutes

Pharmacokinetics

Molecular weight (daltons)	–
% Protein binding	N/A
% Excreted unchanged in urine	N/A
Volume of distribution (L/kg)	N/A
Half-life – normal/ESRF (hrs)	N/A

Dose in renal impairment GFR (mL/min)

20–50	Dose as in normal renal function
10–20	Dose as in normal renal function
<10	Dose as in normal renal function

Dose in patients undergoing renal replacement therapies

CAPD	Not absorbed. Dose as in normal renal function
HD	Not absorbed. Dose as in normal renal function
CAV/VVHD	Not absorbed. Dose as in normal renal function

Important drug interactions

POTENTIALLY HAZARDOUS INTERACTIONS WITH OTHER DRUGS

• None known

Administration

RECONSTITUTION

• Each sachet in 1 litre of water

ROUTE

• Oral

RATE OF ADMINISTRATION

• 250 mL every 15–30 minutes
• If given via naso-gastric tube, rate is 20–30 mL/minute

COMMENTS

• Klean-Prep is formulated to be hyperosmotic and draw water into the bowel. None is absorbed systemically

Other information

Each sachet of Klean-Prep contains:
• Polyethylene glycol 3350 – 59.0 g
• Anhydrous sodium sulphate – 5.685 g
• Sodium bicarbonate – 1.685 g
• Sodium chloride – 1.465 g
• Potassium chloride – 0.7425 g

The electrolyte content of 1 sachet when made up in 1 litre of water is:
• Sodium – 125 mmol
• Sulphate – 40 mmol
• Chloride – 35 mmol
• Bicarbonate – 20 mmol
• Potassium – 10 mmol

Labetalol

Clinical use

Beta-adrenoceptor blocker: hypertensive crisis, hypertension

Dose in normal renal function

Oral: 100–800 mg 2–3 times daily. Usual dose 200 mg twice a day

IV: 15 mg/hour – 120 mg/hour according to medication

Pharmacokinetics

Molecular weight (daltons)	365 (hydrochloride)
% Protein binding	50
% Excreted unchanged in urine	5
Volume of distribution (L/kg)	5.6
Half-life – normal/ESRF (hrs)	3–9/unchanged

Dose in renal impairment GFR (mL/min)

20–50	Dose as in normal renal function
10–20	Dose as in normal renal function
<10	Dose as in normal renal function

Dose in patients undergoing renal replacement therapies

CAPD	Not dialysed. Dose as in normal renal function
HD	Not dialysed. Dose as in normal renal function
CAV/VVHD	Probably not dialysed. Dose as in normal renal function

Important drug interactions

POTENTIALLY HAZARDOUS INTERACTIONS WITH OTHER DRUGS

- Anaesthetics: enhanced hypotensive effect
- Anti-arrhythmics: increased risk of myocardial depression and bradycardia. Amiodarone: increased risk of bradycardia and AV block
- Antidepressants: enhanced hypotensive effect with MAOIs
- Antihypertensives: enhanced hypotensive effect
- Calcium-channel blockers: increased risk of bradycardia and AV block with diltiazem. Care if used with nifedipine. Asystole, severe hypotension and heart failure with verapamil
- Moxisylyte: possibly severe postural hypotension
- Sympathomimetics: severe hypertension

Administration

RECONSTITUTION

–

ROUTE

- Oral, IV peripherally

RATE OF ADMINISTRATION

- 2 mg/minute initially then titrate according to response or according to medication

COMMENTS

- 200 mg labetalol (40 mL) to 200 mL glucose 5%
- *Bolus dosing in crisis*: 50 mg IV over 1 minute. Repeat at 5-minute intervals to maximum 200 mg

Other information

- No adverse effects on renal function
- No accumulation in renal impairment
- Hypoglycaemia can occur in dialysis patients

Lacidipine

Clinical use

Calcium-channel blocker: hypertension

Dose in normal renal function

Initially 2 mg as a single daily dose, increased after 3–4 weeks to 4 mg daily, then if necessary to 6 mg daily

Pharmacokinetics

Molecular weight (daltons)	456
% Protein binding	>95
% Excreted unchanged in urine	0
Volume of distribution (L/kg)	0.9–2.3
Half-life – normal/ESRF (hrs)	13–19/–

Dose in renal impairment GFR (mL/min)

20–50	Dose as in normal renal function
10–20	Dose as in normal renal function
<10	Dose as in normal renal function

Dose in patients undergoing renal replacement therapies

CAPD	Unknown dialysability. Dose as in normal renal function
HD	Unknown dialysability. Dose as in normal renal function
CAV/VVHD	Unknown dialysability. Dose as in normal renal function

Important drug interactions

POTENTIALLY HAZARDOUS INTERACTIONS WITH OTHER DRUGS

- Ciclosporin: 10 kidney transplant patients on ciclosporin, prednisone and azathioprine were given 4 mg lacidipine daily. A very small increase in the trough serum levels (+6%) and AUC (+14%) of the ciclosporin occurred
- Anaesthetics: isoflurane enhances hypotensive effect of lacidipine
- Antihypertensives: enhanced hypotensive effect
- Anti-epileptics: effects decreased by carbamazepine, phenobarbital, phenytoin and primidone
- Theophylline: effect of theophylline possibly enhanced

Administration

RECONSTITUTION

–

ROUTE

- Oral

RATE OF ADMINISTRATION

–

COMMENTS

–

Other information

–

Lactulose

Clinical use

Constipation, hepatic encephalopathy

Dose in normal renal function

Constipation: 15–30 mL twice daily

Hepatic encephalopathy: 30–50 mL three times daily adjusted to produce 2–3 soft stools daily

Pharmacokinetics

Molecular weight (daltons)	342
% Protein binding	–
% Excreted unchanged in urine	<3
Volume of distribution (L/kg)	N/A. Not absorbed
Half-life – normal/ESRF (hrs)	–

Dose in renal impairment GFR (mL/min)

20–50	Dose as in normal renal function
10–20	Dose as in normal renal function
<10	Dose as in normal renal function

Dose in patients undergoing renal replacement therapies

CAPD	Not dialysed. Dose as in normal renal function
HD	Not dialysed. Dose as in normal renal function
CAV/VVHD	Not dialysed. Dose as in normal renal function

Important drug interactions

POTENTIALLY HAZARDOUS INTERACTIONS WITH OTHER DRUGS

• None known

Administration

RECONSTITUTION

–

ROUTE

• Oral

RATE OF ADMINISTRATION

–

COMMENTS

–

Other information

• May take up to 72 hours to work
• Not significantly absorbed from the GI tract
• Safe for diabetics – lactulose is converted to malic, formic and acetic acid in the bowel
• Osmotic and bulking effect

Lamivudine

Clinical use

Nucleoside reverse transcriptase inhibitor for combination treatment of HIV infection with progressive immunodeficiency. (CD4+ count <500 cells/mm³)

Treatment of chronic hepatitis B in adults

Dose in normal renal function

HIV: 150 mg twice daily or 300 mg daily

Hepatitis B: 100 mg daily

Pharmacokinetics

Molecular weight (daltons)	229.3
% Protein binding	<36
% Excreted unchanged in urine	70
Volume of distribution (L/kg)	1.3
Half-life – normal/ESRF (hrs)	5–7/increased 3–4-fold

Dose in renal impairment GFR (mL/min)

See 'Other information'

30–50	HIV: 150 mg daily Hepatitis B: 100 mg stat then 50 mg daily
15–30	HIV: 150 mg stat then 100 mg daily Hepatitis B: 100 mg stat then 25 mg daily
5–15	HIV: 150 mg stat then 50 mg daily Hepatitis B: 35 mg stat then 15 mg daily
<5	HIV: 50 mg stat then 25 mg daily Hepatitis B: 35 mg stat then 10 mg daily

Dose in patients undergoing renal replacement therapies

CAPD	Unlikely dialysability. Dose as in GFR = <5 mL/min
HD	Not dialysed. Dose as in GFR = <5 mL/min
CAV/VVHD	Unknown dialysability. Dose as in GFR = 5–15 mL/min

Important drug interactions

POTENTIALLY HAZARDOUS INTERACTIONS WITH OTHER DRUGS

• Trimethoprim: inhibits excretion of lamivudine – avoid concomitant use of high-dose co-trimoxazole

• Other antivirals: avoid concomitant use with IV ganciclovir and foscarnet

Administration

RECONSTITUTION

–

ROUTE

• Oral

RATE OF ADMINISTRATION

–

COMMENTS

• Administer with or without food

Other information

• 15 mL of oral suspension contains 3 g of sucrose

• Dose from Bennett:

GFR = >50 mL/min: 100% of dose

GFR = 10–50 mL/min: 150 mg loading dose then 50–150 mg daily

GFR = <10 mL/min + HD: 50–150 mg loading dose then 25–50 mg daily

• Hills AE, Fish DN (1998) Dosage adjustments of antiretroviral agents in patients with organ dysfunction. Am J Health-Syst Pharm. **55**: 2528–33

Lamotrigine

Clinical use

Monotherapy and adjunctive treatment of partial seizures and primary and secondary generalised tonic-clonic seizures

Dose in normal renal function

25–200 mg daily in divided doses, according to clinical indication. Maximum 500 mg daily

Pharmacokinetics

Molecular weight (daltons)	256
% Protein binding	55
% Excreted unchanged in urine	<10
Volume of distribution (L/kg)	0.92–1.22
Half-life – normal/ESRF (hrs)	24–35/50

Dose in renal impairment GFR (mL/min)

20–50	Caution. Start with low doses and monitor closely
10–20	Caution. Start with low doses and monitor closely
<10	Caution. Start with low doses and monitor closely

Dose in patients undergoing renal replacement therapies

CAPD	Unlikely dialysability. Dose as in GFR < 10 mL/min
HD	Not dialysed. Dose as in GFR < 10 mL/min
CAV/VVHD	Unknown dialysability. Dose as in GFR = 10–20 mL/min

Important drug interactions

POTENTIALLY HAZARDOUS INTERACTIONS WITH OTHER DRUGS

- Other anti-epileptics: concomitant administration of two or more anti-epileptics may enhance toxicity without a corresponding increase in anti-epileptic effect; moreover, interactions between individual anti-epileptics can complicate monitoring of treatment
- Antidepressants: antagonism of anticonvulsant effect

Administration

RECONSTITUTION

–

ROUTE

- Oral

RATE OF ADMINISTRATION

–

COMMENTS

–

Other information

- There is no experience of treatment with lamotrigine in patients with renal failure. Pharmacokinetic studies using single doses in subjects with renal failure indicate that lamotrigine pharmacokinetics are little affected, but plasma concentrations of the major glucuronide metabolite increase almost 8-fold due to reduced renal clearance
- The 2-N-glucuronide is inactive and accounts for 75–90% of the drug metabolised present in the urine. Although the metabolite is inactive the consequences of accumulation are unknown; hence the company advise caution with the use of lamotrigine in renal impairment
- The half-life of lamotrigine is affected by other drugs, it is reduced to 14 hours when given with enzyme-inducing drugs, e.g. carbamazepine and phenytoin, and is increased to approximately 70 hours when co-administered with sodium valproate alone

Lansoprazole

Clinical use

Benign gastric ulcer, duodenal ulcer, duodenal ulcer or gastritis associated with *H. pylori,* reflux oesophagitis

Dose in normal renal function

15–30 mg daily in the morning; duration dependent on indication

Pharmacokinetics

Molecular weight (daltons)	369
% Protein binding	99.8
% Excreted unchanged in urine	0
Volume of distribution (L/kg)	16–32 litres
Half-life – normal/ESRF (hrs)	1–2/unchanged

Dose in renal impairment GFR (mL/min)

20–50	Dose as in normal renal function
10–20	Dose as in normal renal function
<10	Dose as in normal renal function

Dose in patients undergoing renal replacement therapies

CAPD	Unlikely removal. Dose as in normal renal function
HD	Not dialysed. Dose as in normal renal function
CAV/VVHD	Unknown dialysability, probably not removed. Dose as in normal renal function

Important drug interactions

POTENTIALLY HAZARDOUS INTERACTIONS WITH OTHER DRUGS

• Ciclosporin: theoretical, interaction unlikely – little information available

Administration

RECONSTITUTION

–

ROUTE

• Oral

RATE OF ADMINISTRATION

–

COMMENTS

–

Other information

• Lansoprazole is metabolised substantially by the liver; no dose adjustment is necessary in renal impairment. The recommended dose should not be exceeded

Lanthanum carbonate (unlicensed product)

Clinical use

Phosphate binder in patients with ESRD

Dose in normal renal function

675–3000 mg daily in divided doses, with meals

Pharmacokinetics

Molecular weight (daltons)	Lanthanum – atomic weight 139
% Protein binding	Not absorbed
% Excreted unchanged in urine	Not absorbed
Volume of distribution (L/kg)	Not absorbed
Half-life – normal/ESRF (hrs)	Not absorbed

Dose in renal impairment GFR (mL/min)

20–50	Dose as in normal renal function
10–20	Dose as in normal renal function
<10	Dose as in normal renal function

Dose in patients undergoing renal replacement therapies

CAPD	Not dialysed. Dose as in normal renal function
HD	Not dialysed. Dose as in normal renal function
CAV/VVHD	Not dialysed. Dose as in normal renal function

Important drug interactions

POTENTIALLY HAZARDOUS INTERACTIONS WITH OTHER DRUGS

• None known

Administration

RECONSTITUTION

–

ROUTE

• Oral

RATE OF ADMINISTRATION

–

COMMENTS

–

Other information

• Following ingestion, lanthanum carbonate is converted in the GI tract to the insoluble lanthanum phosphate, which is not readily absorbed into the blood

• Bioavailability of drugs administered concomitantly may be reduced due to binding by lanthanum carbonate

Leflunomide

Clinical use

Disease-modifying agent for active rheumatoid arthritis

Dose in normal renal function

Loading dose: 100 mg daily for 3 days then 10–20 mg daily

Pharmacokinetics

Molecular weight (daltons)	270.2
% Protein binding	>99
% Excreted unchanged in urine	nil
Volume of distribution (L/kg)	11 litres
Half-life – normal/ESRF (hrs)	2 weeks (metabolite)/ unchanged

Dose in renal impairment GFR (mL/min)

20–50	Dose as in normal renal function
10–20	Use with caution. See 'Other information'
<10	Use with caution. See 'Other information'

Dose in patients undergoing renal replacement therapies

CAPD	Not dialysed. Use with caution
HD	Not dialysed. Use with caution
CAV/VVHD	Not dialysed. Use with caution

Important drug interactions

POTENTIALLY HAZARDOUS INTERACTIONS WITH OTHER DRUGS

- Hepatotoxic or haematotoxic drugs: increased risk of toxicity
- Anion-exchange resin: colestyramine significantly decreases effect of leflunomide
- Live vaccines: not recommended
- Drugs metabolised by CYP 2C9: use with caution

Administration

RECONSTITUTION

–

ROUTE

- Oral

RATE OF ADMINISTRATION

–

COMMENTS

- Administer with food

Other information

- Contra-indicated by manufacturer due to insufficient evidence
- Protein binding is variable in CRF
- US licence says it can be used in renal impairment with caution
- Half-life is reduced after haemodialysis

Lepirudin

Clinical use

Anticoagulant for people with heparin-associated thrombocytopenia

Dose in normal renal function

0.4 mg/kg bolus followed by 0.15 mg/kg/hour (max 16.5 mg/hour) infusion adjusted according to APTT usually for 2–10 days (max body weight 110 kg)

Pharmacokinetics

Molecular weight (daltons)	6979.4
% Protein binding	No data
% Excreted unchanged in urine	35
Volume of distribution (L/kg)	No data
Half-life – normal/ESRF (hrs)	10 mins (initial half-life) 1.3 (terminal)/48

Dose in renal impairment GFR (mL/min)

45–60	Reduce bolus to 0.2 mg/kg and infusion rate by 50%
30–44	Reduce bolus to 0.2 mg/kg and infusion rate to 30% of normal
15–29	Reduce bolus to 0.2 mg/kg and infusion rate to 15% of normal
<15	Avoid, or if APTT is below lower therapeutic limit, then 0.1 mg/kg on alternate days as an IV bolus

Dose in patients undergoing renal replacement therapies

CAPD	Probably dialysed. Dose as for GFR = <15 mL/min
HD	Dialysed. Dose as for GFR = <15 mL/min
CAV/VVHD	Dialysed. Dose as for GFR = 15–29 mL/min

Important drug interactions

POTENTIALLY HAZARDOUS INTERACTIONS WITH OTHER DRUGS

- Thrombolytics: may increase risk of bleeding complications; enhance effect of lepirudin
- Antiplatelets and anticoagulants: increased risk of bleeding complications

Administration

RECONSTITUTION

- Reconstitute using 1 mL water for injection or sodium chloride 0.9%

ROUTE

- IV

RATE OF ADMINISTRATION

- 0.15 mg/kg/hour

COMMENTS

- Further dilute with sodium chloride 0.9% or glucose 5% if for infusion
- Warm to room temperature before using
- Bolus concentration should be 5 mg/mL and infusion 2 mg/mL
- Change syringe at least every 12 hours after start of infusion

Other information

- Dialysed out if used with high-flux polysulfone dialysers
- Lepirudin may also be used for the prevention of clotting in the extra-corporeal circulation during haemodialysis and haemofiltration. *Non-licensed indication*
- Dose for dialysis anticoagulation if <4.5-hour session is 0.14–0.15 mg/kg as an IV bolus pre-dialysis
- Nowak G et al. (1997) Anticoagulation with r-hirudin in regular haemodialysis with heparin-induced thrombocytopenia (HIT II). Wien Klin Wochenschr. 109(10): 354–8
- Van Wyk V et al. (1995) A comparison between the use of recombinant hirudin and heparin during haemodialysis. Kidney International. 48: 1338–43
- Alternative is 0.01 mg/kg IV bolus followed by a continuous infusion of 0.01 mg/kg/hour, adjust to APTT 1.5–2 times normal. 0.005 mg/kg/hour was adequate. (Schneider T et al. (2000) Continuous haemofiltration with r-hirudin (lepirudin) as anticoagulant in a patient with heparin-induced thrombocytopenia. Wien Klin Wochenschr. 112(12): 552–5)
- Recent reports of seven cases of severe anaphylactic reactions resulting in five fatalities and at least six of the cases were after re-exposure. In some cases it was used outside its therapeutic indication
- Use with great caution, as it cannot be reversed. Results from studies in pigs have found that von Willebrand factor 66 IU/kg can reduce bleeding time

Lercanidipine

Clinical use

Calcium-channel blocker, used for mild to moderate hypertension

Dose in normal renal function

10–20 mg daily

Pharmacokinetics

Molecular weight (daltons)	648.2
% Protein binding	>98
% Excreted unchanged in urine	50 (as metabolites)
Volume of distribution (L/kg)	No data
Half-life – normal/ESRF (hrs)	8–10/increased

Dose in renal impairment GFR (mL/min)

20–50	Use small doses and titrate to response
10–20	Use small doses and titrate to response
<10	Use small doses and titrate to response

Dose in patients undergoing renal replacement therapies

CAPD	Unlikely dialysability. Dose as in GFR = <10 mL/min
HD	Unlikely dialysability. Dose as in GFR = <10 mL/min
CAV/VVHD	Unlikely dialysability. Dose as in GFR = 10–20 mL/min

Important drug interactions

POTENTIALLY HAZARDOUS INTERACTIONS WITH OTHER DRUGS

• Anaesthetics: isoflurane enhances hypotensive effect
• Antihypertensives: enhanced hypotensive effect; increased risk of first-dose hypotensive effect of post-synaptic alpha-blockers such as prazosin
• Beta-blockers: may enhance hypotensive effect of propranolol and metoprolol
• Theophylline levels may increase
• Antivirals: ritonavir possibly increases plasma levels

Administration

RECONSTITUTION

–

ROUTE

• Oral

RATE OF ADMINISTRATION

–

COMMENTS

–

Other information

• Grapefruit juice may increase plasma levels of lercanidipine
• Take before food
• Avoid in severe renal failure due to risk of accumulation

Letrozole

Clinical use

Treatment of advanced breast cancer in post-menopausal women in whom other anti-oestrogen therapy or tamoxifen has failed

Pre-operative treatment in post-menopausal women with localised hormone-receptor-positive breast cancer to allow later breast-conserving surgery

Dose in normal renal function

2.5 mg daily

Pharmacokinetics

Molecular weight (daltons)	285.3
% Protein binding	60
% Excreted unchanged in urine	6
Volume of distribution (L/kg)	1.87
Half-life – normal/ESRF (hrs)	48/unchanged

Dose in renal impairment GFR (mL/min)

20–50	Dose as in normal renal function
10–20	Dose as in normal renal function
<10	Use with caution

Dose in patients undergoing renal replacement therapies

CAPD	Probably dialysed. Use with caution
HD	Dialysed. Use with caution
CAV/VVHD	Probably dialysed. Use with caution

Important drug interactions

POTENTIALLY HAZARDOUS INTERACTIONS WITH OTHER DRUGS

• None known

Administration

RECONSTITUTION

–

ROUTE

• Oral

RATE OF ADMINISTRATION

–

COMMENTS

–

Other information

–

Leuprorelin acetate

Clinical use

Treatment of endometriosis and advanced prostate cancer

Dose in normal renal function

11.25 mg every 3 months (SC depot injection, prostate cancer only)

Or 3.75 mg every 4 weeks

Endometriosis: 3.75 mg every month for maximum 6 months (not to be repeated)

Pharmacokinetics

Molecular weight (daltons)	1269.5
% Protein binding	No data
% Excreted unchanged in urine	No data
Volume of distribution (L/kg)	27.36–36.01 litres
Half-life – normal/ESRF (hrs)	3/increased

Dose in renal impairment GFR (mL/min)

20–50	Dose as in normal renal function
10–20	Dose as in normal renal function
<10	Dose as in normal renal function. Monitor closely

Dose in patients undergoing renal replacement therapies

CAPD	Unlikely dialysability. Dose as in normal renal function
HD	Unlikely dialysability. Dose as in normal renal function
CAV/VVHD	Unlikely dialysability. Dose as in normal renal function

Important drug interactions

POTENTIALLY HAZARDOUS INTERACTIONS WITH OTHER DRUGS

• None known

Administration

RECONSTITUTION

• With diluent provided

ROUTE

• IM, SC depot

RATE OF ADMINISTRATION

–

COMMENTS

–

Other information

• Women on dialysis may be at greater risk of ovarian hyperstimulation possibly because dialysis affects circulating leuprorelin concentration so endogenous gonadotrophins were still excreted. Or haemodialysis patients may have increased responsiveness to endogenous gonadotrophins

Levamisole (unlicensed product)

Clinical use

Treatment of roundworm (*Ascaris lumbricoides*)

Dose in normal renal function

120–150 mg as a single dose

Pharmacokinetics

Molecular weight (daltons)	240.8
% Protein binding	19–26
% Excreted unchanged in urine	5
Volume of distribution (L/kg)	100–120 litres
Half-life – normal/ESRF (hrs)	3–4 (16 for metabolites)

Dose in renal impairment GFR (mL/min)

20–50	Dose as in normal renal function
10–20	Dose as in normal renal function
<10	Dose as in normal renal function

Dose in patients undergoing renal replacement therapies

CAPD	Unknown dialysability. Dose as in normal renal function, for single dose only
HD	Unknown dialysability. Dose as in normal renal function, for single dose only
CAV/VVHD	Unknown dialysability. Dose as in normal renal function

Important drug interactions

POTENTIALLY HAZARDOUS INTERACTIONS WITH OTHER DRUGS

- Alcohol: may produce a disulfiram-like reaction
- Phenytoin: increased levels of phenytoin have been reported
- Warfarin: enhanced INR

Administration

RECONSTITUTION

–

ROUTE

- Oral

RATE OF ADMINISTRATION

–

COMMENTS

–

Other information

- Available on a 'named patient' basis from IDIS
- Avoid in patients with pre-existing blood disorders
- Has been used to treat relapsing nephrotic syndrome in children (*Lancet.* (1991) **337**: 1555–7)
- Has also been used in haemodialysis patients to enhance response to hepatitis B vaccine (*Artif Organs.* (2002) **26**(6): 492–6)

Levetiracetam

Clinical use

Anti-epileptic agent

Dose in normal renal function

500 mg – 1.5 g twice daily

Pharmacokinetics

Molecular weight (daltons)	170.21
% Protein binding	<10
% Excreted unchanged in urine	66 (95% drug + metabolite)
Volume of distribution (L/kg)	0.5–0.7
Half-life – normal/ESRF (hrs)	6–8/25

Dose in renal impairment GFR (mL/min)

50–79	500 mg – 1 g twice daily
30–49	250–750 mg twice daily
<30	250–500 mg twice daily

Dose in patients undergoing renal replacement therapies

CAPD	Likely dialysability. 750 mg loading dose then 500 mg – 1 g daily
HD	Dialysed. 750 mg loading dose then 500 mg – 1 g once daily
CAV/VVHD	Likely dialysability. Dose as in GFR = 30–49 mL/min

Important drug interactions

POTENTIALLY HAZARDOUS INTERACTIONS WITH OTHER DRUGS

- Antidepressants: antagonism of anticonvulsant effect (convulsive threshold lowered)
- Anti-malarials: mefloquine antagonises anticonvulsant effect; chloroquine and hydroxychloroquine occasionally reduce seizure threshold

Administration

RECONSTITUTION

–

ROUTE

- Oral

RATE OF ADMINISTRATION

–

COMMENTS

–

Other information

- 51% of the dose is removed with 4 hours of haemodialysis
- The inactive metabolite ucb L057 accumulates in renal failure

Levocetirizine

Clinical use

Treatment of symptoms associated with allergic conditions

Dose in normal renal function

5 mg daily

Pharmacokinetics

Molecular weight (daltons)	388.9
% Protein binding	90
% Excreted unchanged in urine	85.4 (includes metabolites)
Volume of distribution (L/kg)	0.4
Half-life – normal/ESRF (hrs)	7.9 ± 1.9

Dose in renal impairment GFR (mL/min)

20–50	5 mg every 48 hours
10–20	5 mg every 72 hours
<10	5 mg every 72 hours. See 'Other information'

Dose in patients undergoing renal replacement therapies

CAPD	Unlikely dialysability. Dose as in GFR < 10 mL/min
HD	Not dialysed. Dose as in GFR < 10 mL/min
CAV/VVHD	Unlikely dialysability. Dose as in GFR = 10–20 mL/min

Important drug interactions

POTENTIALLY HAZARDOUS INTERACTIONS WITH OTHER DRUGS

• None known

Administration

RECONSTITUTION

–

ROUTE

• Oral

RATE OF ADMINISTRATION

–

COMMENTS

–

Other information

• Data sheet recommends avoid, but anecdotally it has been used in haemodialysis patients

• Less than 10% is removed during a 4-hour haemodialysis session

• Has been used at a dose of 5 mg daily for treatment of angioedema in a haemodialysis patient

Levodopa

Clinical use

Treatment of parkinsonism

Dose in normal renal function

125–500 mg daily in divided doses after meals, increased according to response

Pharmacokinetics

Molecular weight (daltons)	197.2
% Protein binding	5–8
% Excreted unchanged in urine	11
Volume of distribution (L/kg)	0.9–1.6
Half-life – normal/ESRF (hrs)	1–3/unknown

Dose in renal impairment GFR (mL/min)

20–50	Dose as in normal renal function
10–20	Dose as in normal renal function
<10	Dose as in normal renal function

Dose in patients undergoing renal replacement therapies

CAPD	Unknown dialysability. Dose as in normal renal function
HD	Unknown dialysability. Dose as in normal renal function
CAV/VVHD	Unknown dialysability. Dose as in normal renal function

Important drug interactions

POTENTIALLY HAZARDOUS INTERACTIONS WITH OTHER DRUGS

- Bupropion: increased risk of side-effects
- Anaesthetics: risk of arrythmias with volatile liquid anaesthetics such as halothane
- Antidepressants: hypertensive crisis with MAOIs and linezolid (including moclobemide) – avoid for at least 2 weeks after stopping MAOI
- Ferrous sulphate: reduces AUC of levodopa by 30–50%, clinically significant in some but not all patients

Administration

RECONSTITUTION

–

ROUTE

- Oral

RATE OF ADMINISTRATION

–

COMMENTS

–

Other information

–

Levofloxacin

Clinical use

Antibacterial agent

Dose in normal renal function

250–500 mg once or twice a day (varies depending on indication)

Pharmacokinetics

Molecular weight (daltons)	361.4
% Protein binding	30–40
% Excreted unchanged in urine	>85
Volume of distribution (L/kg)	1.25
Half-life – normal/ESRF (hrs)	6–8/35

Dose in renal impairment GFR (mL/min)

20–50	Initial dose 250–500 mg then reduce dose by 50%
10–20	Initial dose 250–500 mg then 125 mg 12–48-hourly
<10	Initial dose 250–500 mg then 125 mg 24–48-hourly

Dose in patients undergoing renal replacement therapies

CAPD	Not dialysed. Dose as in GFR = <10 mL/min
HD	Not dialysed. Dose as in GFR = <10 mL/min
CAV/VVHD	Not dialysed. Dose as in GFR = 10–20 mL/min

Important drug interactions

POTENTIALLY HAZARDOUS INTERACTIONS WITH OTHER DRUGS

- Ciclosporin: half-life of ciclosporin increased by 33%; increased risk of nephrotoxicity
- Analgesics: possibly increased risk of convulsions with NSAIDs
- Anti-malarials: manufacturer advises avoid concomitant use with artemether and lumefantrine

Administration

RECONSTITUTION

–

ROUTE

- Oral, IV

RATE OF ADMINISTRATION

- 30 minutes per 250 mg

COMMENTS

–

Other information

- Dose and frequency depend on indication

Linezolid

Clinical use

Antibacterial agent

Dose in normal renal function

400–600 mg twice daily

Pharmacokinetics

Molecular weight (daltons)	337.3
% Protein binding	31
% Excreted unchanged in urine	30–55
Volume of distribution (L/kg)	50 litres
Half-life – normal/ESRF (hrs)	5–7/–

Dose in renal impairment GFR (mL/min)

20–50	Dose as for normal renal function
10–20	Dose as for normal renal function
<10	Dose as for normal renal function but monitor closely

Dose in patients undergoing renal replacement therapies

CAPD	Likely to be dialysed. Dose as in GFR = <10 mL/min
HD	Dialysed. Dose as in GFR = <10 mL/min
CAV/VVHD	Dialysed. Dose as in GFR = 10–20 mL/min

Important drug interactions

POTENTIALLY HAZARDOUS INTERACTIONS WITH OTHER DRUGS

• Phenylpropanolamine and pseudoephedrine: enhance increase in blood pressure
• MAOIs: avoid concomitant administration

Administration

RECONSTITUTION

–

ROUTE

• Oral, IV

RATE OF ADMINISTRATION

• Over 30–120 mins

COMMENTS

–

Other information

• 30% of dose is removed by haemodialysis
• Two metabolites accumulate in renal failure which have MAOI activity but no antibacterial activity therefore monitor patients closely
• There is 5 mmol sodium per 300 mL infusion
• Linezolid is a weak reversible non-selective inhibitor of MAO therefore can be used with drugs not normally given with MAOIs, e.g. SSRIs but monitor closely

Liothyronine (tri-iodothyronine)

Clinical use

Hypothyroidism

Dose in normal renal function

Oral: 20 micrograms daily increased to
60 micrograms in 2–3 divided doses

IV: 5–20 micrograms every 4–12 hours, or
50 micrograms initially then 25 micrograms every
8 hours reducing to 25 micrograms twice a day

Pharmacokinetics

Molecular weight (daltons)	651
% Protein binding	<99
% Excreted unchanged in urine	2.5
Volume of distribution (L/kg)	0.1–0.2
Half-life – normal/ESRF (hrs)	16–48/–

Dose in renal impairment GFR (mL/min)

<50	Dose as in normal renal function

Dose in patients undergoing renal replacement therapies

CAPD	Not dialysed. Dose as in normal renal function
HD	Not dialysed. Dose as in normal renal function
CAV/VVHD	Not dialysed. Dose as in normal renal function

Important drug interactions

POTENTIALLY HAZARDOUS INTERACTIONS WITH OTHER DRUGS

• Anticoagulants: it is likely that the effect of acenocoumarol, phenindione and warfarin are enhanced

Administration

RECONSTITUTION

• Dissolve with 1–2 mL water for injection

ROUTE

• IV, oral

RATE OF ADMINISTRATION

• Slow bolus

COMMENTS

• Alkaline solution – may cause irritation if given IM

Other information

• Protein-losing states, such as nephrotic syndrome, will result in a decrease in total T_3 and T_4

• Thyroxine (T_4) is the drug of choice in hypothyroidism, but liothyronine T_4 can be used due to its rapid onset of action

• Elderly patients should receive smaller initial doses

Lisinopril

Clinical use

ACE inhibitor: hypertension, congestive heart failure, following myocardial infarction in haemodynamically stable patients, diabetic nephropathy

Dose in normal renal function

Hypertension and congestive heart failure: initially 2.5 mg daily; maintenance dose depends on indication, maximum 40 mg daily

Pharmacokinetics

Molecular weight (daltons)	441
% Protein binding	0–10
% Excreted unchanged in urine	80–90
Volume of distribution (L/kg)	1.3–1.5
Half-life – normal/ESRF (hrs)	11–12/40–50

Dose in renal impairment GFR (mL/min)

20–50	50–75% of the normal dose
10–20	50–75% of the normal dose and titrate according to response
<10	25–50% of the normal dose and titrate according to response

Dose in patients undergoing renal replacement therapies

CAPD	Unknown dialysability. Dose as in GFR < 10 mL/min. Adjust according to response
HD	Dialysed. Dose as in GFR < 10 mL/min. Adjust according to response
CAV/VVHD	Unknown dialysability. Dose as in GFR = 10–20 mL/min. Adjust according to response

Important drug interactions

POTENTIALLY HAZARDOUS INTERACTIONS WITH OTHER DRUGS

- Ciclosporin: increased risk of hyperkalaemia
- Anaesthetics: enhanced hypotensive effect
- NSAIDs: antagonism of hypotensive effect; hyperkalaemia. Increased risk of renal damage
- Diuretics: enhanced hypotensive effect; hyperkalaemia with potassium-sparing diuretics
- Epoetin: increased risk of hyperkalaemia
- Lithium: ACE inhibitors reduce excretion of lithium
- Potassium salts: increased risk of hyperkalaemia

Administration

RECONSTITUTION

–

ROUTE

- Oral

RATE OF ADMINISTRATION

–

COMMENTS

–

Other information

- Close monitoring of renal function during therapy is necessary in those with renal insufficiency
- Renal failure has been reported in association with ACE inhibitors and has been mainly in patients with severe congestive heart failure, renal artery stenosis, or post renal transplant
- A high incidence of anaphylactoid reactions has been reported in patients dialysed with high-flux polyacrylonitrile membranes and treated concomitantly with an ACE inhibitor. This combination should therefore be avoided
- Hyperkalaemia and other side-effects are more common in patients with impaired renal function

Lithium carbonate

Clinical use

Treatment and prophylaxis of mania, manic depressive illness, and recurrent depression; aggressive or self-mutilating behaviour

Dose in normal renal function

See individual preparations. Adjust according to lithium plasma concentrations

Pharmacokinetics

Molecular weight (daltons)	74
% Protein binding	0
% Excreted unchanged in urine	95
Volume of distribution (L/kg)	0.5–0.9
Half-life – normal/ESRF (hrs)	14–28/40

Dose in renal impairment GFR (mL/min)

Contra-indicated in renal impairment

20–50	Avoid if possible or reduce dose and monitor plasma concentration carefully
10–20	Avoid if possible or reduce dose and monitor plasma concentration carefully
<10	Avoid if possible or reduce dose and monitor plasma concentration carefully

Dose in patients undergoing renal replacement therapies

CAPD	Dialysed in lithium intoxication. Dose as in GFR < 10 mL/min
HD	Dialysed in lithium intoxication. Dose as in GFR < 10 mL/min
CAV/VVHD	Unknown dialysability. Dose as in GFR = 10–20 mL/min

Important drug interactions

POTENTIALLY HAZARDOUS INTERACTIONS WITH OTHER DRUGS

- ACE inhibitors and AT-II antagonists: lithium excretion reduced
- NSAIDs: excretion of lithium reduced
- Antidepressants (SSRIs): increased risk of CNS effects
- Antipsychotics: increased risk of extrapyramidal side-effects and possibly neurotoxicity
- Methyldopa: neurotoxicity may occur without increased plasma lithium levels
- Diuretics: lithium excretion reduced by loop diuretics, potassium-sparing diuretics and thiazides. Lithium excretion increased by acetazolamide
- Sumatriptan: increases risk of CNS toxicity

Administration

RECONSTITUTION

–

ROUTE

- Oral

RATE OF ADMINISTRATION

–

COMMENTS

- Different preparations vary widely in bioavailability; a change in the preparation used requires the same precautions as initiation of treatment

Other information

- Doses are adjusted to achieve plasma concentrations of 0.4–1.0 mmol Li⁺/L (lower end of range for maintenance therapy and elderly patients) on samples taken 12 hours after the preceding dose
- Long-term treatment may result in permanent changes in kidney histology and impairment of renal function. High serum concentration of lithium, including episodes of acute lithium toxicity, may aggravate these changes. The minimum clinically effective dose of lithium should always be used
- Bennett suggests 25–50% of normal dose if GFR < 10 and 50–75% of normal dose if GFR between 10–50 mL/min. Closely monitor lithium plasma concentrations
- Lithium generally should not be used in patients with severe renal disease because of increased risk of toxicity
- Dialysability: serum lithium concentrations rebound within 5–8 hours post haemodialysis because of redistribution of the drug, often necessitating repeated courses of haemodialysis. Peritoneal dialysis is less effective at removing lithium and is only used if haemodialysis is not possible
- Up to one-third of patients on lithium may develop polyuria, usually due to lithium blocking the effect of ADH. This reaction is reversible on withdrawal of lithium therapy

Lomustine

Clinical use

Treatment of Hodgkin's disease and certain solid tumours

Dose in normal renal function

120–130 mg/m² every 6–8 weeks if used alone, lower dose is used in combination treatment and compromised bone marrow function

Pharmacokinetics

Molecular weight (daltons)	233.7
% Protein binding	60
% Excreted unchanged in urine	50 (as metabolites)
Volume of distribution (L/kg)	No data
Half-life – normal/ESRF (hrs)	16–48 (metabolites)

Dose in renal impairment GFR (mL/min)

45–60	75% of dose
30–45	70% of dose
<30	Not recommended

Dose in patients undergoing renal replacement therapies

CAPD	Unlikely removal. Avoid
HD	Not dialysed. Avoid
CAV/VVHD	Unlikely removal. Avoid

Important drug interactions

POTENTIALLY HAZARDOUS INTERACTIONS WITH OTHER DRUGS

• None known

Administration

RECONSTITUTION

–

ROUTE

• Oral

RATE OF ADMINISTRATION

–

COMMENTS

–

Other information

• Bone marrow toxicity is delayed
• Doses in renal failure from Kintzel et al. (1995) Cancer Treatment Reviews. 21: 33–64

Loperamide

Clinical use

Anti-diarrhoeal agent

Dose in normal renal function

4 mg stat, then 2 mg after each loose stool,
maximum 16 mg daily

Pharmacokinetics

Molecular weight (daltons)	514 (hydrochloride)
% Protein binding	80
% Excreted unchanged in urine	<10
Volume of distribution (L/kg)	–
Half-life – normal/ESRF (hrs)	7–15/–

Dose in renal impairment GFR (mL/min)

20–50	Dose as in normal renal function
10–20	Dose as in normal renal function
<10	Dose as in normal renal function

Dose in patients undergoing renal replacement therapies

CAPD	Unlikely dialysability. Dose as in normal renal function
HD	Unlikely dialysability. Dose as in normal renal function
CAV/VVHD	Unlikely dialysability. Dose as in normal renal function

Important drug interactions

POTENTIALLY HAZARDOUS INTERACTIONS WITH OTHER DRUGS

• None known

Administration

RECONSTITUTION

–

ROUTE

• Oral

RATE OF ADMINISTRATION

–

COMMENTS

–

Other information

–

Lorazepam

Clinical use

Benzodiazepine: short-term use in anxiety or insomnia; status epilepticus; peri-operative

Dose in normal renal function

Anxiety: 1–4 mg daily in divided doses;
Insomnia associated with anxiety: 1–2 mg at bedtime

Acute panic attacks: (IV/IM): 25–30 micrograms/kg repeat 6-hourly if required

Pharmacokinetics

Molecular weight (daltons)	321
% Protein binding	85
% Excreted unchanged in urine	<5
Volume of distribution (L/kg)	0.9–1.3
Half-life – normal/ESRF (hrs)	5–10/32–70

Dose in renal impairment GFR (mL/min)

20–50	Dose as in normal renal function
10–20	Dose as in normal renal function
<10	Dose as in normal renal function

Dose in patients undergoing renal replacement therapies

CAPD	Unlikely dialysability. Dose as in normal renal function
HD	Not dialysed. Dose as in normal renal function
CAV/VVHD	Unknown dialysability. Dose as in normal renal function

Important drug interactions

POTENTIALLY HAZARDOUS INTERACTIONS WITH OTHER DRUGS

• None known

Administration

RECONSTITUTION

–

ROUTE

• Oral, IV, IM, sublingual

RATE OF ADMINISTRATION

• Slow IV bolus

COMMENTS

• Onset of effect after IM injection is similar to oral administration

• IV route preferred over IM route

• Dilute 1:1 with sodium chloride 0.9% or water for injection

Other information

• Patients with impaired renal or hepatic function should be monitored frequently and have their dosage adjusted carefully according to response. Lower doses may be sufficient in these patients

• Lorazepam as intact drug is not removed by dialysis. The glucuronide metabolite is highly dialysable, but is pharmacologically inactive

• Increased CNS sensitivity in patients with renal impairment

Losartan

Clinical use

AT-II receptor antagonist, used for hypertension, treatment of type 2 diabetic nephropathy

Dose in normal renal function

25–100 mg daily

Pharmacokinetics

Molecular weight (daltons)	461
% Protein binding	>99
% Excreted unchanged in urine	4
Volume of distribution (L/kg)	34 litres
Half-life – normal/ESRF (hrs)	2 (active metabolite 6–9)/ unchanged

Dose in renal impairment GFR (mL/min)

20–50	Dose as in normal renal function
10–20	Initial dose 25 mg, adjust according to response
<10	Initial dose 25 mg, adjust according to response

Dose in patients undergoing renal replacement therapies

CAPD	Not dialysed. Initial dose 25 mg, adjust according to response
HD	Not dialysed. Initial dose 25 mg, adjust according to response
CAV/VVHD	Not dialysed. Initial dose 25 mg, adjust according to response

Important drug interactions

POTENTIALLY HAZARDOUS INTERACTIONS WITH OTHER DRUGS

- Ciclosporin: increased risk of hyperkalaemia and nephrotoxicity
- Anaesthetics: enhanced hypotensive effect
- Analgesics: antagonism of hypotensive effect and increased risk of renal impairment with NSAIDs; hyperkalaemia with ketorolac and other NSAIDs
- Diuretics: enhanced hypotensive effect; hyperkalaemia with potassium-sparing diuretics
- Lithium: reduced excretion. Possibility of enhanced lithium toxicity
- Potassium salts: increased risk of hyperkalaemia
- Tacrolimus: increased risk of hyperkalaemia and nephrotoxicity

Administration

RECONSTITUTION

–

ROUTE

- Oral

RATE OF ADMINISTRATION

–

COMMENTS

–

Other information

- Adverse reactions, especially hyperkalaemia, are more common in patients with renal impairment
- Renal failure has been reported in association with AT-II antagonists in patients with renal artery stenosis, post renal transplant, or in those with congestive heart failure
- Close monitoring of renal function during therapy is necessary in those with renal insufficiency

Mebendazole

Clinical use

Treatment of threadworm, roundworm, whipworm, and hookworm infections

Dose in normal renal function

Threadworm: 100 mg as a single dose, if re-infection occurs repeat after 2–3 weeks

Whipworm, roundworm, hookworm: 100 mg twice daily for 3 days

Echinococcosis: 40–50 mg/kg for at least 3–6 months

Pharmacokinetics

Molecular weight (daltons)	295.3
% Protein binding	90
% Excreted unchanged in urine	2
Volume of distribution (L/kg)	1–1.2
Half-life – normal/ESRF (hrs)	1.5–8

Dose in renal impairment GFR (mL/min)

20–50	Dose as in normal renal function
10–20	Dose as in normal renal function
<10	Dose as in normal renal function

Dose in patients undergoing renal replacement therapies

CAPD	Unlikely dialysability. Dose as in normal renal function
HD	Unlikely dialysability. Dose as in normal renal function
CAV/VVHD	Unlikely dialysability. Dose as in normal renal function

Important drug interactions

POTENTIALLY HAZARDOUS INTERACTIONS WITH OTHER DRUGS

• Cimetidine: possibly inhibits metabolism of mebendazole
• Phenytoin, carbamazepine: lower plasma mebendazole concentrations, only relevant when being used in high doses for echinococcosis

Administration

RECONSTITUTION

–

ROUTE

• Oral

RATE OF ADMINISTRATION

–

COMMENTS

–

Other information

• Contra-indicated in pregnancy
• Undergoes first-pass metabolism
• Poorly absorbed from the GI tract (5–10%)

Mefenamic acid

Clinical use

NSAID: mild to moderate rheumatic pain, dysmenorrhoea and menorrhagia

Dose in normal renal function

500 mg three times daily

Pharmacokinetics

Molecular weight (daltons)	241
% Protein binding	99
% Excreted unchanged in urine	<6
Volume of distribution (L/kg)	1.3
Half-life – normal/ESRF (hrs)	2–4/unchanged

Dose in renal impairment GFR (mL/min)

20–50	250–500 mg three times a day, but avoid if possible
10–20	250–500 mg three times a day, but avoid if possible
<10	250 mg three times a day, but only use if ESRD on dialysis

Dose in patients undergoing renal replacement therapies

CAPD	Unlikely removal. Dose as in GFR < 10 mL/min
HD	Not dialysed. Dose as in GFR < 10 mL/min
CAV/VVHD	Unlikely removal. Dose as in GFR = 10–20 mL/min

Important drug interactions

POTENTIALLY HAZARDOUS INTERACTIONS WITH OTHER DRUGS

- Ciclosporin: increased risk of nephrotoxicity
- ACE inhibitors and AT-II antagonists: antagonism of hypotensive effect; increased risk of renal damage and hyperkalaemia
- Antibacterials: possibly increased risk of convulsions with quinolones
- Antidiabetic agents: effects of sulphonylureas enhanced
- Antivirals: increased risk of haematological toxicity with zidovudine
- Cytotoxic agents: reduced excretion of methotrexate
- Diuretics: increased risk of nephrotoxicity, hyperkalaemia with potassium-sparing diuretics
- Lithium: excretion reduced
- Anticoagulants: effects of warfarin and acenocoumarol enhanced
- Anti-epileptic agents: effects of phenytoin enhanced
- Tacrolimus: increased risk of nephrotoxicity

Administration

RECONSTITUTION

–

ROUTE

- Oral

RATE OF ADMINISTRATION

–

COMMENTS

–

Other information

- As with other prostaglandin inhibitors, allergic glomerulonephritis has occurred occasionally. There have also been reports of acute interstitial nephritis with haematuria and proteinuria and occasionally nephrotic syndrome
- Inhibition of renal prostaglandin synthesis by NSAIDs may interfere with renal function, especially in the presence of existing renal disease. Avoid use if possible; if not, check serum creatinine 48–72 hours after starting NSAID. If raised, discontinue NSAID therapy
- Use normal doses in patients with ESRD on dialysis
- Use with caution in renal transplant recipients – can reduce intra-renal autocoid synthesis

Mefloquine

Clinical use

Malaria prophylaxis and treatment

Dose in normal renal function

Prophylaxis: 250 mg weekly

Treatment: non-immune patients 20–25 mg/kg in 2–3 divided doses; partially-immune patients 15 mg/kg in 2–3 divided doses

Pharmacokinetics

Molecular weight (daltons)	414.8
% Protein binding	98
% Excreted unchanged in urine	9 (+4% metabolites)
Volume of distribution (L/kg)	20
Half-life – normal/ESRF (hrs)	21 days

Dose in renal impairment GFR (mL/min)

20–50	Dose as in normal renal function
10–20	Dose as in normal renal function
<10	Use with caution

Dose in patients undergoing renal replacement therapies

CAPD	Not dialysed. Dose as in GFR = <10 mL/min
HD	Not dialysed. Dose as in GFR = <10 mL/min
CAV/VVHD	Not dialysed. Dose as in GFR = 10–20 mL/min

Important drug interactions

POTENTIALLY HAZARDOUS INTERACTIONS WITH OTHER DRUGS

• Anti-arrhythmics: increased risk of ventricular arrhythmias with amiodarone and quinidine (avoid concomitant use)

• Anti-epileptics: antagonism of anticonvulsant effect

• Antipsychotics: increased risk of ventricular arrhythmias, avoid concomitant use with pimozide

• Other anti-malarials: increased risk of convulsions with chloroquine and quinine; avoid concomitant use with artemether with lumefantrine

Administration

RECONSTITUTION

–

ROUTE

• Oral

RATE OF ADMINISTRATION

–

COMMENTS

–

Other information

• Start prophylaxis 1–3 weeks before arriving in malarious area. Continue for 4 weeks after leaving the malarious area

• Increased risk of convulsions in patients with epilepsy

Meloxicam

Clinical use

COX-2 inhibitor, used for the short-term treatment of osteoarthritis (OA) or long-term treatment of rheumatoid arthritis (RA) or ankylosing spondylitis

Dose in normal renal function

Oral: 7.5–15 mg

Rectal: OA – 7.5 mg daily; RA and ankylosing spondylitis – 15 mg daily

Pharmacokinetics

Molecular weight (daltons)	351.4
% Protein binding	99
% Excreted unchanged in urine	3
Volume of distribution (L/kg)	11 litres
Half-life – normal/ESRF (hrs)	20/–

Dose in renal impairment GFR (mL/min)

20–50	Dose as in normal renal function
10–20	Dose as in normal renal function, but avoid if possible
<10	7.5 mg daily, but only use if ESRD on dialysis

Dose in patients undergoing renal replacement therapies

CAPD	Not dialysed. Dose as in GFR = <10 mL/min
HD	Not dialysed. Dose as in GFR = <10 mL/min
CAV/VVHD	Not dialysed. Dose as in GFR = 10–20 mL/min

Important drug interactions

POTENTIALLY HAZARDOUS INTERACTIONS WITH OTHER DRUGS

- Ciclosporin: may enhance nephrotoxicity
- Other analgesics: avoid concomitant administration of two or more NSAIDs including aspirin (increased side-effects)
- Antibacterials: possibly increased risk of convulsions with quinolones
- Anticoagulants: anticoagulant effect of acenocoumarol and warfarin enhanced
- Antivirals: increased risk of haematological toxicity with zidovudine; plasma concentration possibly increased by ritonavir
- Lithium: decreased excretion leading to increased lithium levels
- Diuretics: risk of acute renal failure in dehydrated patients
- ACE inhibitors and AT-II antagonists: increased risk of renal damage and hyperkalaemia; antagonism of hypotensive effects
- Tacrolimus: possibly increased risk of nephrotoxicity
- Methotrexate: excretion of methotrexate reduced, increased risk of toxicity

Administration

RECONSTITUTION

–

ROUTE

- Oral, PR

RATE OF ADMINISTRATION

–

COMMENTS

–

Other information

- SPC states meloxicam is contra-indicated in non-dialysed severe renal failure
- Clinical trials have shown renal effects similar to those observed with comparator NSAIDs. Monitor patient for deterioration in renal function and fluid retention
- Inhibition of renal prostaglandin synthesis by NSAIDs may interfere with renal function, especially in the presence of existing renal disease. Avoid if possible; if not, check serum creatinine 48–72 hours after starting NSAID. If raised, discontinue NSAID therapy
- Use normal doses in patients with ESRD on dialysis
- Use with caution in renal transplant recipients – can reduce intra-renal autocoid synthesis
- Meloxicam should be used with caution in uraemic patients predisposed to GI bleeding or uraemic coagulopathies

Melphalan

Clinical use

Antineoplastic agent: myelomatosis, solid tumours and lymphomas

Dose in normal renal function

Orally: 150–200 micrograms/kg daily for 4–6 days, repeated after 4–8 weeks

IV administration: 16–200 mg/m^2 according to indication and local protocol

Pharmacokinetics

Molecular weight (daltons)	305
% Protein binding	90
% Excreted unchanged in urine	12
Volume of distribution (L/kg)	0.6–0.75
Half-life – normal/ESRF (hrs)	1.1–1.4/4–6

Dose in renal impairment GFR (mL/min)

20–50	See 'Other information'
10–20	See 'Other information'
<10	See 'Other information'

Dose in patients undergoing renal replacement therapies

CAPD	Unknown dialysability. Dose as in GFR = <10 mL/min
HD	Not dialysed. Dose as in GFR = <10 mL/min
CAV/VVHD	Unknown dialysability. Dose as in GFR = 10–20 mL/min

Important drug interactions

POTENTIALLY HAZARDOUS INTERACTIONS WITH OTHER DRUGS

• Ciclosprin: increased risk of nephrotoxicity

Administration

RECONSTITUTION

• Reconstitute with 10 mL of provided diluent
• Further dilution with 0.9% sodium chloride

ROUTE

• IV, oral

RATE OF ADMINISTRATION

• Inject slowly into a fast-running infusion solution or via an infusion bag

COMMENTS

–

Other information

• Melphalan clearance, though variable, is decreased in renal impairment

• Currently available pharmacokinetic data do not justify an absolute recommendation on dosage reduction when administering melphalan tablets to patients with renal impairment, but it may be prudent to use a reduced dosage initially until tolerance is established

• When melphalan injection is used at conventional IV dosage (8–40 mg/m^2 BSA), it is recommended that the initial dose should be reduced by 50% in patients with moderate to severe renal impairment and subsequent dosage determined by the degree of haematological suppression

• For high IV doses of melphalan (100–240 mg/m^2 BSA), the need for dose reduction depends upon the degree of renal impairment, whether autologous bone marrow stem cells are reinfused, and therapeutic need. High-dose melphalan is not recommended in patients with more severe renal impairment (EDTA clearance less than 30 mL/minute)

• It should be borne in mind that dose reduction of melphalan in renal impairment is somewhat arbitrary. At moderate doses, where melphalan is used as part of a combined regimen, dosage reductions of up to 50% may be appropriate. However, at high doses, e.g. conditioning for bone marrow transplant, there is a risk of underdosing the patient and not achieving the desired therapeutic effect, so the dose should be reduced with caution in these instances

• Adequate hydration and forced diuresis may be necessary in patients with poor renal function

• In myeloma patients with renal damage, temporary but significant increases in blood urea levels have been observed during melphalan therapy

Mercaptopurine

Clinical use

Antineoplastic agent: acute leukaemias

Dose in normal renal function

Usual dose is 2.5 mg/kg/day, but the dose and duration of administration depend on the nature and dosage of other cytotoxic agents given in conjunction with mercaptopurine

Pharmacokinetics

Molecular weight (daltons)	170
% Protein binding	20
% Excreted unchanged in urine	8–21
Volume of distribution (L/kg)	0.1–1.7
Half-life – normal/ESRF (hrs)	0.9–1.5/–

Dose in renal impairment GFR (mL/min)

20–50	Caution – reduce dose. See 'Other information'
10–20	Caution – reduce dose. See 'Other information'
<10	Caution – reduce dose. See 'Other information'

Dose in patients undergoing renal replacement therapies

CAPD	Unknown dialysability. Dose as in GFR = <10 mL/min
HD	Dialysed. Dose as in GFR = <10 mL/min
CAV/VVHD	Unknown dialysability. Dose as in GFR = 10–20 mL/min

Important drug interactions

POTENTIALLY HAZARDOUS INTERACTIONS WITH OTHER DRUGS

• Allopurinol: decreases rate of metabolism of mercaptopurine – reduce dose of mercaptopurine to a quarter of normal dose
• Antibacterials: increased risk of haematological toxicity with co-trimoxazole and trimethoprim

Administration

RECONSTITUTION

–

ROUTE

• Oral

RATE OF ADMINISTRATION

–

COMMENTS

–

Other information

• Mercaptopurine is extensively metabolised and excreted via the kidneys and the active metabolites have a longer half-life than the parent drug
• Wellcome UK recommend consideration be given to reducing the dose in patients with impaired hepatic or renal function, although no specific dosing guidelines are available
• A study on anti-cancer drug renal toxicity and elimination concluded that the dose of 6-mercaptopurine does not require modification in patients with decreased renal function (except in conjunction with allopurinol). This study also gives % excreted unchanged in urine as 21% (*Cancer Treatment Reviews.* (1995) **21**: 33–64)

Meropenem

Clinical use

Antibacterial agent

Dose in normal renal function

500 mg – 1 g every 8 hours
Higher doses used in cystic fibrosis and meningitis
– up to 2 g every 8 hours

Pharmacokinetics

Molecular weight (daltons)	437.5
% Protein binding	2
% Excreted unchanged in urine	70
Volume of distribution (L/kg)	0.35
Half-life – normal/ESRF (hrs)	1/6–8

Dose in renal impairment
GFR (mL/min)

20–50	500 mg – 1 g every 12 hours
10–20	250 mg – 1 g every 12 hours *or* 500 mg every 8 hours
<10	250 mg – 1 g every 24 hours

Dose in patients undergoing renal replacement therapies

CAPD	Dialysed. Dose as in GFR = <10 mL/min
HD	Dialysed. Dose as in GFR = <10 mL/min
CAV/VVHD	Dialysed. Dose as in GFR = 10–20 mL/min. See 'Other information'

Important drug interactions

POTENTIALLY HAZARDOUS INTERACTIONS WITH OTHER DRUGS

• None known

Administration

RECONSTITUTION

• Add 5 mL water for injection to each 250 mg of meropenem

ROUTE

• IV

RATE OF ADMINISTRATION

• Bolus: 5 minutes
• IV infusion: 15–30 minutes

COMMENTS

• Further dilute in 50–200 mL sodium chloride 0.9%, glucose 5% or glucose 10% if for infusion
• Stable for 24 hours once reconstituted

Other information

• Metabolite is inactive
• Each 1-g vial contains 3.9 mmol of sodium
• Has less potential to induce seizures than imipenem
• Thalhammer and Hörl (2000) *Clin Pharmacokinet.* **39**(4): 271–9 – haemofiltration dose, recommends 1 g three times a day in haemodiafiltration
• Other references:
  • Ververs TF *et al.* (2000) *Crit Care Med.* **28**(10): 3412–16
  • Giles LJ *et al.* (2000) *Crit Care Med.* **28**(3): 632–7
  • Valtonen M *et al.* (2000) *J Antimicrob Chemother.* **45**(5): 701–4
• Has been used IP for pseudomonas PD peritonitis at concentration of 100 mg/L

Mesalazine

Clinical use

Induction and maintenance of remission in ulcerative colitis

Dose in normal renal function

Acute attack: 1.5–4.0 g daily in divided doses

Maintenance: 750 mg – 1.5 g daily in divided doses

Pharmacokinetics

Molecular weight (daltons)	153
% Protein binding	40–50
% Excreted unchanged in urine	–
Volume of distribution (L/kg)	–
Half-life – normal/ESRF (hrs)	1.0/–

Dose in renal impairment GFR (mL/min)

20–50	Caution – use only if necessary – start with low dose and increase according to response
10–20	Caution – use only if necessary – start with low dose and monitor closely
<10	Caution – use only if necessary – start with low dose and monitor closely

Dose in patients undergoing renal replacement therapies

CAPD	Unlikely dialysability. Dose as in GFR = <10 mL/min
HD	Unlikely dialysability. Dose as in GFR = <10 mL/min
CAV/VVHD	Unknown dialysability. Dose as in GFR = 10–20 mL/min

Important drug interactions

POTENTIALLY HAZARDOUS INTERACTIONS WITH OTHER DRUGS

• None known

Administration

RECONSTITUTION

–

ROUTE

• Oral, PR

RATE OF ADMINISTRATION

–

COMMENTS

–

Other information

• Mesalazine is excreted rapidly by the kidney, mainly as its metabolite N-acetyl-5-aminosalicylic acid. Nephrotoxicity has been reported

• Mesalazine is best avoided in patients with established renal impairment, but if necessary should be used with caution, and the patient carefully monitored

Mesna

Clinical use

Prophylaxis of urothelial toxicity in patients treated with ifosfamide or cyclophosphamide

Dose in normal renal function

Dose and timing depends on cytotoxic agent and on route of administration of mesna

Pharmacokinetics

Molecular weight (daltons)	164
% Protein binding	<10
% Excreted unchanged in urine	16–32
Volume of distribution (L/kg)	0.65
Half-life – normal/ESRF (hrs)	0.25–0.5/–

Dose in renal impairment GFR (mL/min)

20–50	See 'Other information'
10–20	See 'Other information'
<10	See 'Other information'

Dose in patients undergoing renal replacement therapies

CAPD	Unknown dialysability. Dose as in GFR = <10 mL/min
HD	Probably dialysed. Dose as in GFR = <10 mL/min
CAV/VVHD	Unknown dialysability. Dose as in GFR = 10–20 mL/min

Important drug interactions

POTENTIALLY HAZARDOUS INTERACTIONS WITH OTHER DRUGS

• None known

Administration

RECONSTITUTION

–

ROUTE

• Oral, IV bolus, IV infusion

RATE OF ADMINISTRATION

• IV infusion: over 15–30 minutes

COMMENTS

• Compatible with sodium chloride 0.9%
• Mesna injection can be administered orally in orange juice or cola to improve palatability

Other information

• Urinary output should be maintained at 100 mL/hour (as required for oxazaphosphorine treatment)
• The dose of mesna is dependent on the dose of oxazaphosphorine, e.g. reduce dose of cyclophosphamide to 50% normal dose if GFR < 10 mL/min, hence dose of mesna will consequently be reduced
• From what is known about the pharmacokinetics and mechanism of action of mesna, its availability in the urinary tract depends on renal function
• In the case of complete anuric patients (extremely rare) neither cyclophosphamide nor its metabolites should appear in the urinary tract: the use of mesna concomitantly may therefore be unnecessary in anuric patients. If there is any risk of cyclophosphamide or its metabolites entering the urinary tract, mesna should probably be given to prevent urothelial toxicity
• Limited kinetic information would suggest mesna would be eliminated by haemodialysis

Metformin

Clinical use

Non-insulin-dependent diabetes mellitus

Dose in normal renal function

500 mg three times a day

Maximum dose: 2–3 g daily in divided doses

Pharmacokinetics

Molecular weight (daltons)	165.6
% Protein binding	Negligible
% Excreted unchanged in urine	100
Volume of distribution (L/kg)	63–276 litres
Half-life – normal/ESRF (hrs)	2–6/prolonged

Dose in renal impairment GFR (mL/min)

40–50	25–50% of dose
10–40	Avoid
<10	Avoid

Dose in patients undergoing renal replacement therapies

CAPD	Unknown dialysability. Avoid
HD	Dialysed. Avoid
CAV/VVHD	Probably dialysed. Avoid

Important drug interactions

POTENTIALLY HAZARDOUS INTERACTIONS WITH OTHER DRUGS

• Cimetidine: inhibits renal excretion of metformin
• Alcohol: increased risk of lactic acidosis

Administration

RECONSTITUTION

–

ROUTE

• Oral

RATE OF ADMINISTRATION

–

COMMENTS

–

Other information

• Lactic acidosis is a rare but serious metabolic complication that can occur due to metformin accumulation. Reported cases have occurred primarily in diabetic patients with significant renal impairment

• As metformin is renally excreted serum creatinine levels should be determined before initiating treatment and regularly thereafter:

  • at least annually in patients with normal renal function

  • at least 2–4 times a year in patients with serum creatinine levels at the upper limit of normal and in elderly subjects

• Special caution should be exercised in the elderly in situations where renal function may become impaired, e.g. initiating therapy with antihypertensives, diuretics or NSAIDs

Methadone hydrochloride

Clinical use

Treatment of opioid drug addiction; analgesic for moderate to severe pain

Dose in normal renal function

Opioid addiction: 10–20 mg per day increasing by 10–20 mg per day until there are no signs of withdrawal or intoxication. Reduce gradually

Analgesia: 5–10 mg every 6–8 hours

Pharmacokinetics

Molecular weight (daltons)	346
% Protein binding	60–90
% Excreted unchanged in urine	33
Volume of distribution (L/kg)	3–6
Half-life – normal/ESRF (hrs)	13–58/–

Dose in renal impairment GFR (mL/min)

20–50	Dose as in normal renal function
10–20	Dose as in normal renal function
<10	50% of normal dose, and titrate according to response

Dose in patients undergoing renal replacement therapies

CAPD	Not dialysed. Dose as in GFR < 10 mL/min
HD	Not dialysed. Dose as in GFR < 10 mL/min
CAV/VVHD	Unknown dialysability. Dose as in normal renal function

Important drug interactions

POTENTIALLY HAZARDOUS INTERACTIONS WITH OTHER DRUGS

- MAOIs: possible CNS excitation or depression
- Antivirals: methadone possibly increases plasma concentration of zidovudine. Methadone levels possibly reduced by ritonavir, abacavir and nevirapine
- Dopaminergics: hyperpyrexia and CNS toxicity reported with selegiline and opioids

Administration

RECONSTITUTION

–

ROUTE

- IM, SC, oral

RATE OF ADMINISTRATION

–

COMMENTS

- Methadone is probably not suitable to be used as an analgesic for patients with severe renal impairment

Other information

- Overdosage with methadone can be reversed using naloxone

Methotrexate

Clinical use

Antineoplastic agent: neoplastic disease, severe uncontrolled psoriasis, severe rheumatoid arthritis

Dose in normal renal function

Rheumatoid arthritis: 5–10 mg per week

Psoriasis: 10–25 mg orally once weekly, adjusted to response

Neoplastic disease: dose by weight or BSA according to specific indication

Pharmacokinetics

Molecular weight (daltons)	454
% Protein binding	45–60
% Excreted unchanged in urine	80–90
Volume of distribution (L/kg)	0.76–1.0
Half-life – normal/ESRF (hrs)	8–12/increased

Dose in renal impairment GFR (mL/min)

20–50	50–100% of normal dose
10–20	50% of normal dose
<10	Contra-indicated

Dose in patients undergoing renal replacement therapies

CAPD	Not dialysed. Contra-indicated
HD	Not dialysed. Haemodialysis clearance is 38–40 mL/minute. Contra-indicated
CAV/VVHD	Unknown dialysability. Dose as in GFR = 10–20 mL/min

Important drug interactions

POTENTIALLY HAZARDOUS INTERACTIONS WITH OTHER DRUGS

- Ciclosporin: methotrexate may inhibit the clearance of ciclosporin or its metabolites. Ciclosporin may inhibit methotrexate elimination
- NSAIDs: increased risk of toxicity
- Antibacterials: antifolate effect increased with co-trimoxazole and trimethoprim. Penicillin reduces excretion of methotrexate – increased risk of toxicity
- Acitretin: plasma concentration of methotrexate increased
- Anti-malarials: antifolate effect enhanced by pyrimethamine
- Corticosteroids: increased risk of haematological toxicity
- Probenecid: excretion of methotrexate reduced

Administration

RECONSTITUTION

- Methotrexate compatible with glucose 5%, sodium chloride 0.9%, compound sodium lactate, or Ringer's solution

ROUTE

- Oral, IM, IV (bolus injection or infusion), intrathecal, intra-arterial, intraventricular

RATE OF ADMINISTRATION

- Slow IV injection

COMMENTS

- High-dose methotrexate may cause precipitation of methotrexate or its metabolites in renal tubules. A high fluid throughput and alkalinisation of urine, using sodium bicarbonate if necessary, is recommended

Other information

- Calcium folinate (calcium leucovorin) is a potent agent for neutralising the immediate toxic effects of methotrexate on the haematopoietic system
- Calcium folinate rescue may begin 24/32/36 hours post start of methotrexate therapy, according to local protocol. Doses of up to 120 mg may be given over 12–24 hours by IM or IV injection or infusion, followed by 12–15 mg IM, or 15 mg orally every 6 hours for the next 48 hours
- Renal function should be closely monitored throughout treatment
- An approximate correction for renal function may be made by reducing the dose in proportion to the reduction in CL_{CR} based on a normal CL_{CR} of 60 mL/minute/m^2

Methyldopa

Clinical use

Hypertension

Dose in normal renal function

250–500 mg 2–3 times a day. Maximum daily dose: 3 g

Pharmacokinetics

Molecular weight (daltons)	238 (hydrate)
% Protein binding	10–20
% Excreted unchanged in urine	25–40
Volume of distribution (L/kg)	0.5
Half-life – normal/ESRF (hrs)	1.5–6/6–16

Dose in renal impairment GFR (mL/min)

20–50	250–500 mg three times a day
10–20	250–500 mg two to three times a day
<10	250–500 mg once or twice a day

Dose in patients undergoing renal replacement therapies

CAPD	Dialysed. Dose as in GFR < 10 mL/min
HD	Dialysed. Dose as in GFR < 10 mL/min
CAV/VVHD	Probably dialysed. Dose as in GFR = 10–20 mL/min

Important drug interactions

POTENTIALLY HAZARDOUS INTERACTIONS WITH OTHER DRUGS

• Anaesthetics: enhanced hypotensive effect
• Lithium: neurotoxicity (without increased plasma-lithium concentrations)
• Salbutamol: acute hypotension reported with salbutamol infusions

Administration

RECONSTITUTION

• Add dose to 100 mL glucose 5%

ROUTE

• Oral, IV peripherally

RATE OF ADMINISTRATION

• 30 minutes

COMMENTS

–

Other information

• Active metabolites with long half-life
• Interferes with serum creatinine measurement
• Orthostatic hypotension more common in renally impaired patients

Methylprednisolone

Clinical use

Corticosteroid. Suppression of inflammatory and allergic disorders. Immunosuppressant. Rheumatic disease

Dose in normal renal function

Oral: 2–40 mg daily

IM/IV: 10–500 mg

Graft rejection: IM up to 1 g daily for up to 3 days

Pharmacokinetics

Molecular weight (daltons)	375
% Protein binding	50–77
% Excreted unchanged in urine	2.6–7.2
Volume of distribution (L/kg)	1.0–1.5
Half-life – normal/ESRF (hrs)	1.9–6.0/ unchanged

Dose in renal impairment GFR (mL/min)

20–50	Dose as in normal renal function
10–20	Dose as in normal renal function
<10	Dose as in normal renal function

Dose in patients undergoing renal replacement therapies

CAPD	Dialysed. Dose as in normal renal function
HD	Dialysed. Dose as in normal renal function, after haemodialysis
CAV/VVHD	Dialysed. Dose as in normal renal function

Important drug interactions

POTENTIALLY HAZARDOUS INTERACTIONS WITH OTHER DRUGS

- Ciclosprin: levels of ciclosporin increased
- Rifampicin accelerates metabolism
- Anti-epileptics: carbamazepine, phenobarbital, phenytoin and primidone accelerate metabolism
- Antifungals: increased risk of hypokalaemia with amphotericin. Ketoconazole inhibits metabolism

Administration

RECONSTITUTION

- Use solvent supplied (Solu-Medrone) or see manufacturer's recommendations

ROUTE

- Oral, IM, IV peripherally or centrally

RATE OF ADMINISTRATION

- 30 minutes

COMMENTS

- NB: Rapid bolus injection may be associated with arrhythmias or cardiovascular collapse

Other information

- A single dose of 1 g is often given at transplantation
- Three 1-g doses at 24-hour intervals are often used as first line for reversal of acute rejection episodes. (Some units use 300–500 mg daily for 3 days.)
- Anecdotally possesses less mineralocorticoid activity than equipotent doses of prednisolone

Metoclopramide

Clinical use

Nausea and vomiting

Dose in normal renal function

10 mg three times daily. The use of
metoclopramide in patients under 20 years should
be restricted

Pharmacokinetics

Molecular weight (daltons)	354 (hydrochloride)
% Protein binding	40
% Excreted unchanged in urine	10–22
Volume of distribution (L/kg)	2–3.4
Half-life – normal/ESRF (hrs)	2.5–5.4/14–15

Dose in renal impairment GFR (mL/min)

20–50	Dose as in normal renal function
10–20	75% – 100% of normal dose
<10	50% – 100% of normal dose

Dose in patients undergoing renal replacement therapies

CAPD	Not dialysed. Dose as in GFR < 10 mL/min
HD	Dialysed. Dose as in GFR < 10 mL/min
CAV/VVHD	Possibly dialysed. Dose as in GFR = 10–20 mL/min

Important drug interactions

POTENTIALLY HAZARDOUS INTERACTIONS WITH OTHER DRUGS

• Ciclosporin: increased ciclosporin blood levels

Administration

RECONSTITUTION

–

ROUTE

• Oral or IV/IM

RATE OF ADMINISTRATION

• 1–2 minutes

COMMENTS

–

Other information

• Increased risk of extrapyramidal reactions in severe renal impairment

Metolazone

Clinical use

Hypertension. Oedema. Acts synergistically with loop diuretics

Dose in normal renal function

Oedema: 5–10 mg increased to 20 mg daily. Maximum 80 mg daily

Hypertension: 5 mg initially, maintenance – 5 mg on alternate days

Pharmacokinetics

Molecular weight (daltons)	366
% Protein binding	95
% Excreted unchanged in urine	70
Volume of distribution (L/kg)	1.6
Half-life – normal/ESRF (hrs)	4–20/–

Dose in renal impairment GFR (mL/min)

20–50	Dose as in normal renal function
10–20	Dose as in normal renal function
<10	Dose as in normal renal function

Dose in patients undergoing renal replacement therapies

CAPD	Unlikely dialysability. Dose as in normal renal function
HD	Not dialysed. Dose as in normal renal function
CAV/VVHD	Probably not dialysed. Dose as in normal renal function

Important drug interactions

POTENTIALLY HAZARDOUS INTERACTIONS WITH OTHER DRUGS

- Ciclosporin: impaired renal function
- Anti-arrhythmics: hypokalaemia leads to increased cardiac toxicity
- Antipsychotics: hypokalaemia increases risk of ventricular arrhythmias with pimozide and thioridazine – avoid concomitant use
- Lithium excretion reduced
- Antihypertensives: enhanced hypotensive effect
- Antihistamines: hypokalaemia increases risk of ventricular arrhythmias with terfenadine
- Cardiac glycosides: increased toxicity if hypokalaemia occurs
- NSAIDs: increased risk of nephrotoxicity

Administration

RECONSTITUTION

–

ROUTE

- Oral

RATE OF ADMINISTRATION

–

COMMENTS

–

Other information

- May result in profound diuresis. Monitor patient's fluid balance carefully
- Monitor for hypokalaemia
- In patients with CL_{CR} less than 50 mL/minute there is no clinical evidence of accumulation

Metoprolol

Clinical use

Beta-adrenoceptor blocker: hypertension, angina, cardiac arrhythmias, migraine prophylaxis

Dose in normal renal function

Oral: 50–100 mg 2–3 times daily
IV: 5–15 mg
Migraine: 100–200 mg orally daily in divided doses

Pharmacokinetics

Molecular weight (daltons)	685 (tartrate)
% Protein binding	8–12
% Excreted unchanged in urine	5
Volume of distribution (L/kg)	5.5
Half-life – normal/ESRF (hrs)	3.5/2.5–4.5

Dose in renal impairment GFR (mL/min)

20–50	Dose as in normal renal function
10–20	Start with small doses/Normal interval
<10	Start with small doses/Normal interval

Dose in patients undergoing renal replacement therapies

CAPD	Not dialysed. Start with small doses
HD	Dialysed. Start with small doses
CAV/VVHD	Probably dialysed. Start with small doses and titrate in accordance with response

Important drug interactions

POTENTIALLY HAZARDOUS INTERACTIONS WITH OTHER DRUGS

- Anaesthetics: enhanced hypotensive effect
- Anti-arrhythmics: increased risk of myocardial depression and bradycardia. Amiodarone increases risk of bradycardia and AV block
- Antihypertensives: enhanced effect
- Calcium-channel blockers: increased risk of bradycardia and AV block with diltiazem. Care if used with nifedipine. Asystole, severe hypotension and heart failure with verapamil
- Moxisylyte: possibly severe postural hypotension
- Sympathomimetics: severe hypertension with adrenaline and noradrenaline. Severe hypertension also possible with sympathomimetics in anorectics and cough and cold remedies

Administration

RECONSTITUTION

–

ROUTE

- Oral or IV

RATE OF ADMINISTRATION

- For bolus injection 1–2 mg/minute or by continuous infusion via CRIP

COMMENTS

- A total IV dose of 10–15 mg is usually sufficient

Other information

- Can cause hypoglycaemia in dialysis patients
- Almost all the drug is excreted as inactive metabolites. Accumulation of the metabolites will occur in renal failure, but does not seem to cause any side-effects

Metronidazole

Clinical use

Antibiotic: anaerobic and protozoal infections

Dose in normal renal function

Oral: 200–400 mg every 8–12 hours

IV: 500 mg every 8 hours

PR: 1 g every 8–12 hours

Pharmacokinetics

Molecular weight (daltons)	171
% Protein binding	20
% Excreted unchanged in urine	20
Volume of distribution (L/kg)	0.76–1.02
Half-life – normal/ESRF (hrs)	6–14/7–21

Dose in renal impairment GFR (mL/min)

20–50	Dose as in normal renal function
10–20	Dose as in normal renal function
<10	Normal dose every 12 hours

Dose in patients undergoing renal replacement therapies

CAPD	Not dialysed. Dose as in GFR < 10 mL/min
HD	Dialysed. Dose as in normal renal function
CAV/VVHD	Unknown dialysability. Dose as in normal renal function

Important drug interactions

POTENTIALLY HAZARDOUS INTERACTIONS WITH OTHER DRUGS

- Ciclosporin: raised blood level of ciclosporin
- Effects of warfarin and acenocoumarol enhanced
- Anti-epileptics: metabolism of phenytoin inhibited. Phenobarbital accelerates metabolism of metronidazole
- Alcohol: disulfiram-like reaction

Administration

RECONSTITUTION

–

ROUTE

- IV, oral, PR

RATE OF ADMINISTRATION

- IV: 5 mL/minute, i.e. 500 mg over 20 minutes

COMMENTS

–

Other information

- Active metabolites have long half-life in renal impairment
- Increased incidence of GI tract reactions and vestibular toxicity in renal failure
- Drug-induced lupus is a rare adverse drug reaction
- Rectally: dose frequency reduced to 12 hours after 3 days
- 500 mg/100 mL infusion provides 14 mmol sodium

Mexiletine hydrochloride

Clinical use

Ventricular arrhythmias, especially after MI

Dose in normal renal function

Oral: 400 mg loading dose followed by
200–250 mg 3–4 times daily commencing 2 hours
after the loading dose

IV injection: 100–250 mg with ECG monitoring
followed by infusion of 250 mg as a 0.1% solution
over I hour, then 125 mg/hour for 2 hours, then
500 micrograms/minute thereafter

Pharmacokinetics

Molecular weight (daltons)	216
% Protein binding	50–70
% Excreted unchanged in urine	10
Volume of distribution (L/kg)	5.5–6.6
Half-life – normal/ESRF (hrs)	8–13/16

Dose in renal impairment GFR (mL/min)

20–50	Dose as in normal renal function
10–20	Dose as in normal renal function
<10	50% of normal dose and titrate according to response

Dose in patients undergoing renal replacement therapies

CAPD	Not dialysed. Dose as in GFR < 10 mL/min
HD	Not dialysed. Dose as in GFR < 10 mL/min
CAV/VVHD	Not dialysed. Dose as in normal renal function

Important drug interactions

POTENTIALLY HAZARDOUS INTERACTIONS WITH
OTHER DRUGS

- Anti-arrhythmics: increased myocardial
  depression with any combination of anti-
  arrhythmics
- Analgesics: opioids delay absorption
- Antihistamines: increased risk of ventricular
  arrhythmias with mizolastine and terfenadine –
  avoid concomitant use
- Antivirals: possibly increased risk of arrhythmias
  with ritonavir

Administration

RECONSTITUTION

- Add 250–500 mg mexiletine to 500 mL of
  infusion solution (depends on whether for
  loading of maintenance dose)

ROUTE

- IV infusion, oral

RATE OF ADMINISTRATION

- Variable

COMMENTS

- Mexiletine should never be injected in bolus
  form – loading dose IV injection of 25 mg/min

Other information

- Mexiletine has a narrow therapeutic index. Its
  therapeutic effect has been correlated with
  plasma concentrations of 0.5–2 micrograms
  per mL
- Mexiletine is metabolised in the liver and is
  excreted in the urine, mainly in the form of
  metabolites
- Rate of elimination increased with acidic urine
- Injection can be given orally, however due to
  local anaesthetic effect, care with hot foods

Miconazole

Clinical use

Antifungal agent

Dose in normal renal function

Oral gel: 5–10 mL in mouth, after food,
four times daily

Pharmacokinetics

Molecular weight (daltons)	416
% Protein binding	90
% Excreted unchanged in urine	1
Volume of distribution (L/kg)	20
Half-life – normal/ESRF (hrs)	20–24/unchanged

Dose in renal impairment
GFR (mL/min)

20–50	Dose as in normal renal function
10–20	Dose as in normal renal function
<10	Dose as in normal renal function

Dose in patients undergoing renal replacement therapies

CAPD	Not dialysed. Dose as in normal renal function
HD	Not dialysed. Dose as in normal renal function
CAV/VVHD	Unlikely to be significantly dialysed. Dose as in normal renal function

Important drug interactions

POTENTIALLY HAZARDOUS INTERACTIONS WITH OTHER DRUGS

- Ciclosporin: possibly increased plasma ciclosporin concentrations
- Anti-arrhythmics: plasma concentration of quinidine increased
- Anticoagulants: effect of acenocoumarol and warfarin enhanced
- Antidepressants: avoid concomitant use with reboxetine
- Anti-epileptics: effect of phenytoin enhanced
- Terfenadine: avoid concomitant use
- Antidiabetics: plasma concentrations of sulphonylureas increased
- Sirolimus: plasma concentration increased by miconazole
- Tacrolimus: possibly increased tacrolimus concentration

Administration

RECONSTITUTION

–

ROUTE

- Oral gel, topical

RATE OF ADMINISTRATION

–

COMMENTS

- Oral gel absorbed

Other information

- Miconazole is metabolised in the liver to inactive metabolites, 10–20% of an oral dose is excreted in the urine as metabolites. About 50% of an oral dose may be excreted mainly unchanged in the faeces
- There is little absorption through skin or mucous membranes when miconazole nitrate is applied topically

Midazolam

Clinical use

Benzodiazepine: sedation with amnesia, and in conjunction with local anaesthesia; premedication, induction

Dose in normal renal function

Sedation: IV injection over 30 seconds, 2 mg followed after 2 minutes by increments of 0.5–1 mg if sedation not adequate; usual range 2.5–7.5 mg
See data sheet for dosing guidelines in other indications

Pharmacokinetics

Molecular weight (daltons)	362
% Protein binding	93–96
% Excreted unchanged in urine	<1
Volume of distribution (L/kg)	1.0–6.6
Half-life – normal/ESRF (hrs)	1.2–12.3/ unchanged

Dose in renal impairment GFR (mL/min)

20–50	Dose as in normal renal function
10–20	Dose as in normal renal function
<10	50% of normal dose

Dose in patients undergoing renal replacement therapies

CAPD	Unlikely dialysability. Dose as in GFR < 10 mL/min
HD	Not dialysed. Dose as in GFR < 10 mL/min
CAV/VVHD	Unknown dialysability. Dose as in normal renal function

Important drug interactions

POTENTIALLY HAZARDOUS INTERACTIONS WITH OTHER DRUGS

• Ciclosporin: in vitro studies suggested that ciclosporin could inhibit the metabolism of midazolam. However, blood ciclosporin concentrations in patients given ciclosporin to prevent graft rejection were considered too low to result in an interaction

• Antivirals: efavirenz, nelfinavir, saquinavir, ritonavir, amprenavir and indinavir increase risk of prolonged sedation with midazolam

• Antibacterials: erythromycin, clarithromycin and quinupristin/dalfopristin increase plasma midazolam concentration with profound sedation

• Antifungals: itraconazole, ketoconazole and possibly fluconazole increase plasma concentration of midazolam (prolonged sedative effect)

Administration

RECONSTITUTION

• Compatible with glucose 5%, sodium chloride 0.9%, glucose 4% with sodium chloride 0.18%

ROUTE

• IV, IM

RATE OF ADMINISTRATION

• 1–10 mL/hour according to response

COMMENTS

–

Other information

• Protein binding of midazolam is decreased in ESRD, hence more unbound drug is available to produce CNS effects, hence a decrease in dose is recommended

• CSM has received reports of respiratory depression, sometimes associated with severe hypotension, following intravenous administration

• Caution with use for sedation in severe renal impairment especially when used with opiates and/or neuromuscular blocking agents – monitor sedation and titrate to response

• Increased CNS sensitivity in patients with renal impairment

• One study reports midazolam as having a sieving coefficient = 0.06 and unlikely to be removed by haemofiltration

Midodrine (unlicensed product)

Clinical use

Treatment of orthostatic hypotension, including dialysis related hypotension, urinary incontinence

Dose in normal renal function

Hypotension: 2.5 mg twice daily up to 10 mg three times a day

Urinary incontinence: 2.5–5 mg twice to three times a day

Pharmacokinetics

Molecular weight (daltons)	290.7
% Protein binding	Negligible
% Excreted unchanged in urine	Negligible
Volume of distribution (L/kg)	No data
Half-life – normal/ESRF (hrs)	25 minutes/increased (3.5 hours for active metabolite/9)

Dose in renal impairment GFR (mL/min)

20–50	Dose as in normal renal function
10–20	Dose as in normal renal function. Start with a lower dose and titrate according to response
<10	Dose as in normal renal function. Start with a lower dose and titrate according to response

Dose in patients undergoing renal replacement therapies

CAPD	Dialysed. Dose as in GFR < 10 mL/min
HD	Dialysed. Initial dose, 2.5 if <70 kg, 5 mg if >70 kg. See 'Other information'
CAV/VVHD	Dialysed. Dose as in GFR = 10–20 mL/min

Important drug interactions

POTENTIALLY HAZARDOUS INTERACTIONS WITH OTHER DRUGS

- Risk of arrhythmias if given with volatile anaesthetics
- Risk of arrhythmias and hypertension if given with tricyclic antidepressants
- Risk of severe hypertension if given with beta-blockers

Administration

RECONSTITUTION

–

ROUTE

- Oral

RATE OF ADMINISTRATION

–

COMMENTS

–

Other information

- Metabolised to an active metabolite (desglymidodrine)
- After dialysis only 15% of drug remaining, so effectively removed by dialysis
- Hypertension post dialysis is also not a problem because it is dialysed out
- Peak levels occur 90 minutes after administration so give 30 minutes before dialysis. Avoid in patients with active coronary ischaemia
- 93% bioavailability
- For haemodialysis patients start at a low dose and increase to a maximum of 30 mg, a second dose can be given at midway of dialysis (maximum dose 10 mg)

Minoxidil

Clinical use

Severe hypertension, in addition to a diuretic and a beta-blocker

Dose in normal renal function

Initially 5 mg (elderly 2.5 mg) daily in 1–2 doses increased by 5–10 mg every three or more days; maximum 50 mg daily

Pharmacokinetics

Molecular weight (daltons)	209
% Protein binding	0
% Excreted unchanged in urine	15–20
Volume of distribution (L/kg)	2–3
Half-life – normal/ESRF (hrs)	2.8–4.2/8.9

Dose in renal impairment GFR (mL/min)

<50   Start with small doses and titrate according to response. See 'Other information'

Dose in patients undergoing renal replacement therapies

CAPD	Dialysed. Dose as in GFR < 50 mL/min
HD	Dialysed. Dose as in GFR < 50 mL/min
CAV/VVHD	Unknown dialysability. Dose as in GFR < 50 mL/min

Important drug interactions

POTENTIALLY HAZARDOUS INTERACTIONS WITH OTHER DRUGS

• Anaesthetics: enhanced hypotensive effect

Administration

RECONSTITUTION

–

ROUTE

• Oral

RATE OF ADMINISTRATION

–

COMMENTS

–

Other information

• A study of the pharmacokinetics of minoxidil in patients with varying degrees of renal impairment found that the non-renal clearance was also impaired as renal function worsened. Substantial accumulation of minoxidil might occur in these patients during multiple-dose therapy. It is advised that minoxidil therapy be initiated with smaller doses or a longer dose interval in patients with significant renal impairment

• Minoxidil is a peripheral vasodilator and should be given in conjunction with a diuretic to control salt and water retention and a beta-blocker to control reflex tachycardia. Patients on dialysis do not need to be given minoxidil in conjunction with a diuretic

• Following topical application between 0.3% and 4.5% of the total applied dose of minoxidil is absorbed from intact scalp

Mirtazapine

Clinical use

Antidepressant

Dose in normal renal function

15–45 mg daily, once or in two divided doses

Pharmacokinetics

Molecular weight (daltons)	265.4
% Protein binding	85
% Excreted unchanged in urine	75
Volume of distribution (L/kg)	107 ± 42 litres (339 ± 125 litres at steady state)
Half-life – normal/ESRF (hrs)	20–40/increased

Dose in renal impairment GFR (mL/min)

20–50	Dose as in normal renal function
10–20	Dose as in normal renal function
<10	Start at low dose and monitor closely

Dose in patients undergoing renal replacement therapies

CAPD	Unlikely dialysability. Dose as in GFR = <10 mL/min
HD	Unlikely dialysability. Dose as in GFR = <10 mL/min
CAV/VVHD	Unlikely dialysability. Dose as in GFR = 10–20 mL/min

Important drug interactions

POTENTIALLY HAZARDOUS INTERACTIONS WITH OTHER DRUGS

- Other antidepressants: CNS excitation and hypertension with MAOIs, plasma concentration possibly increased with SSRIs, manufacturer of reboxetine advises use with caution
- Anti-malarials: manufacturer advises avoid concomitant use with artemether with lumefantrine
- Sibutramine: increased risk of CNS toxicity – avoid concomitant use

Administration

RECONSTITUTION

–

ROUTE

- Oral

RATE OF ADMINISTRATION

–

COMMENTS

–

Other information

–

Misoprostol

Clinical use

Benign gastric and duodenal ulceration and NSAID-associated ulceration. Prophylaxis of NSAID-induced ulceration

Dose in normal renal function

Treatment: 800 micrograms daily in 2–4 divided doses

Prophylaxis: 200–800 micrograms daily in divided doses

Pharmacokinetics

Molecular weight (daltons)	382.5
% Protein binding	85 (as misoprostol acid)
% Excreted unchanged in urine	<1
Volume of distribution (L/kg)	858 litres
Half-life – normal/ESRF (hrs)	0.5/– (as misoprostol acid)

Dose in renal impairment GFR (mL/min)

20–50	Dose as in normal renal function
10–20	Dose as in normal renal function
<10	Dose as in normal renal function

Dose in patients undergoing renal replacement therapies

CAPD	Unlikely dialysability. Dose as in normal renal function
HD	Unlikely dialysability. Dose as in normal renal function
CAV/VVHD	Unknown dialysability. Dose as in normal renal function

Important drug interactions

POTENTIALLY HAZARDOUS INTERACTIONS WITH OTHER DRUGS

• None known

Administration

RECONSTITUTION

–

ROUTE

• Oral

RATE OF ADMINISTRATION

–

COMMENTS

–

Other information

• Plasma concentrations of misoprostol are generally undetectable due to its rapid metabolic conversion to misoprostol acid

• Although there is an approximate doubling of half-life, C_{max} and AUC in patients with varying degrees of renal impairment, dosing adjustment is not usually necessary. If renal patients are unable to tolerate it, then the dose can be reduced

Mitomycin C

Clinical use

Antitumour antibiotic used in a range of neoplastic conditions

Dose in normal renal function

IV: 10–20 mg/m^2 or 0.06–0.15 mg/kg given every 6–8 weeks depending on concurrent therapy and bone marrow recovery

For instillation into bladder: 20–40 mg potency

Pharmacokinetics

Molecular weight (daltons)	334
% Protein binding	–
% Excreted unchanged in urine	10
Volume of distribution (L/kg)	0.5
Half-life – normal/ESRF (hrs)	0.5–1/–

Dose in renal impairment GFR (mL/min)

20–50	Dose as in normal renal function
10–20	Dose as in normal renal function
<10	75% of normal dose

Dose in patients undergoing renal replacement therapies

CAPD	Unknown dialysability. Dose as in GFR < 10 mL/min
HD	Unknown dialysability. Dose as in GFR < 10 mL/min
CAV/VVHD	Unknown dialysability. Dose as in normal renal function

Important drug interactions

POTENTIALLY HAZARDOUS INTERACTIONS WITH OTHER DRUGS

• None known

Administration

RECONSTITUTION

• Reconstitute with water for injection or sodium chloride 0.9%; 5 mL for the 2-mg vial, at least 10 mL for the 10-mg vial and at least 20 mL for the 20-mg vial

ROUTE

• IV, intra-arterial, bladder instillation

RATE OF ADMINISTRATION

• Bolus injection over 3–5 mins (1 mL/min)
• Infusion over 60 minutes

COMMENTS

–

Other information

• A syndrome of thrombotic microangiopathy resembling the haemolytic-uraemic syndrome has been seen in patients receiving mitomycin, either alone or, more frequently, combined with other agents. Symptoms of haemolysis and renal failure may be accompanied by ATN and cardiovascular problems, pulmonary oedema and neurological symptoms

• The percentage dose excreted in the urine increases with increasing dose

• The principal toxicity of mitomycin C is bone marrow suppression. The nadir is usually around 4 weeks after treatment and toxicity is cumulative, with increasing risk after each course of treatment

Mivacurium

Clinical use

Non-depolarising muscle relaxant of short duration

Dose in normal renal function

IV injection: 70–250 micrograms/kg; maintenance 100 micrograms/kg every 15 minutes

IV infusion: maintenance of block 8–10 micrograms/kg/minute adjusted to maintenance dose of 6–7 micrograms/kg/minute according to response

Pharmacokinetics

Molecular weight (daltons)	940
% Protein binding	–
% Excreted unchanged in urine	<7
Volume of distribution (L/kg)	0.1–0.3
Half-life – normal/ESRF (hrs)	0.03–0.08/–

Dose in renal impairment GFR (mL/min)

20–50	Adjust to response. Slower infusion rate may be required
10–20	Adjust to response. Slower infusion rate may be required
<10	Reduce dose. See 'Other information'

Dose in patients undergoing renal replacement therapies

CAPD	Unknown dialysability. Adjust infusion to response
HD	Unknown dialysability. Adjust infusion to response
CAV/VVHD	Unknown dialysability. Adjust infusion to response

Important drug interactions

POTENTIALLY HAZARDOUS INTERACTIONS WITH OTHER DRUGS

• Anti-arrhythmics: procainamide and quinidine enhance muscle relaxant effect

• Antibacterials: effect enhanced by aminoglycosides, clindamycin, colistin and piperacillin

• Botulinum toxin: neuromuscular blockade enhanced, risk of toxicity

Administration

RECONSTITUTION

• Compatible with sodium chloride 0.9%; glucose 5%, sodium chloride 0.18% and glucose 4%; compound sodium lactate

• Dilute to 500 micrograms/mL

ROUTE

• IV bolus, IV infusion

RATE OF ADMINISTRATION

• IV bolus: doses of up to 0.15 mg/kg may be administered over 5–15 seconds. Higher doses should be administered over 30 seconds

COMMENTS

• Compatible with fentanyl, alfentanil and midazolam

Other information

• Spontaneous recovery is complete in approximately 15 minutes and is independent of dose administered

• In patients with ESRD the clinically effective duration of block produced by 0.15 mg/kg is approximately 1.5 times longer than in patients with normal renal function. Subsequently, dosage should be adjusted according to individual clinical response

• The results from a study which compared 20 anephric patients with 20 healthy patients also highlight the need for reduced dosages of Mivacron in patients with renal failure; patients with renal failure had a slightly shorter time to maximum depression of T1/T0, a slower recovery of T1/T0 to 5% (15.3 vs 9.8 min), required a slower infusion rate (6.3 vs 10.4 micrograms/kg/min) and experienced slower spontaneous recovery (12.2 vs 7.7 min). The drug company have no specific guidelines as to the extent of dose reduction required

Mizolastine

Clinical use

Antihistamine, used for symptomatic relief of allergy, e.g. hayfever, urticaria

Dose in normal renal function

10 mg daily

Pharmacokinetics

Molecular weight (daltons)	432.5
% Protein binding	98.4
% Excreted unchanged in urine	<0.5
Volume of distribution (L/kg)	1.4
Half-life – normal/ESRF (hrs)	13/–

Dose in renal impairment GFR (mL/min)

20–50	Dose as in normal renal function
10–20	Dose as in normal renal function
<10	Dose as in normal renal function

Dose in patients undergoing renal replacement therapies

CAPD	Not dialysed. Dose as in normal renal function
HD	Not dialysed. Dose as in normal renal function
CAV/VVHD	Not dialysed. Dose as in normal renal function

Important drug interactions

POTENTIALLY HAZARDOUS INTERACTIONS WITH OTHER DRUGS

- Ciclosporin: use with caution due to inhibition of ciclosporin metabolism
- Anti-arrhythmics: increased risk of ventricular arrhythmias (avoid concomitant use with amiodarone, quinidine, disopyramide, flecainide, mexiletine, procainamide, propafenone)
- Imidazole antifungals: metabolism of mizolastine inhibited, avoid concomitant use
- Macrolide antibiotics: metabolism of mizolastine inhibited, avoid concomitant use
- Sotalol: increased risk of ventricular arrhythmias (avoid concomitant use)
- Avoid concomitant treatment with any drug that could prolong QT interval
- Caution with drugs that inhibit CYP 450 enzymes (may elevate mizolastine levels)

Administration

RECONSTITUTION

–

ROUTE

- Oral

RATE OF ADMINISTRATION

–

COMMENTS

–

Other information

- Contra-indicated in patients with electrolyte imbalances, particularly hypokalaemia

Modafinil

Clinical use

Narcolepsy, excessive daytime drowsiness associated with obstructive sleep apnoea or hypopnoea syndrome

Dose in normal renal function

200–400 mg daily, once or in two divided doses

Pharmacokinetics

Molecular weight (daltons)	273.4
% Protein binding	62
% Excreted unchanged in urine	<10
Volume of distribution (L/kg)	0.9
Half-life – normal/ESRF (hrs)	10–12 hours

Dose in renal impairment GFR (mL/min)

20–50	Dose as in normal renal function
10–20	Dose as in normal renal function
<10	Reduce dose by 50%

Dose in patients undergoing renal replacement therapies

CAPD	Unknown dialysability. Dose as in GFR = <10 mL/min
HD	Unknown dialysability. Dose as in GFR = <10 mL/min
CAV/VVHD	Unknown dialysability. Dose as in GFR = 10–20 mL/min

Important drug interactions

POTENTIALLY HAZARDOUS INTERACTIONS WITH OTHER DRUGS

• Oral contraceptives: metabolism accelerated, reduced contraceptive effect

Administration

RECONSTITUTION

–

ROUTE

• Oral

RATE OF ADMINISTRATION

–

COMMENTS

–

Other information

• Major metabolite is not pharmacologically active
• Recommended that modafinil not be used in patients with left ventricular hypertrophy or ischaemic ECG changes

Moexipril hydrochloride

Clinical use

ACE inhibitor used for hypertension

Dose in normal renal function

3.75–30 mg daily (depending on age or other antihypertensive therapy)

Pharmacokinetics

Molecular weight (daltons)	535
% Protein binding	Moderate
% Excreted unchanged in urine	50
Volume of distribution (L/kg)	183 litres
Half-life – normal/ESRF (hrs)	12 (of active metabolite)

Dose in renal impairment GFR (mL/min)

20–40	Initial dose: 3.75 mg daily
10–20	Initial dose: 3.75 mg daily, adjust according to response
<10	Initial dose: 3.75 mg daily, adjust according to response

Dose in patients undergoing renal replacement therapies

CAPD	Unknown dialysability. Dose as in GFR = <10 mL/min
HD	Unknown dialysability. Dose as in GFR = <10 mL/min
CAV/VVHD	Unknown dialysability. Dose as in GFR = 0–20 mL/min

Important drug interactions

POTENTIALLY HAZARDOUS INTERACTIONS WITH OTHER DRUGS

- Ciclosporin: increased risk of hyperkalaemia and nephrotoxicity
- Anaesthetics: enhanced hypotensive effect
- Analgesics: antagonism of hypotensive effect and increased risk of renal impairment with NSAIDs; hyperkalaemia with ketorolac and other NSAIDs
- Diuretics: enhanced hypotensive effect; hyperkalaemia with potassium-sparing diuretics
- Lithium: reduced excretion, possibility of enhanced lithium toxicity
- Potassium salts: increased risk of hyperkalaemia
- Tacrolimus: increased risk of hyperkalaemia and nephrotoxicity

Administration

RECONSTITUTION

–

ROUTE

- Oral

RATE OF ADMINISTRATION

–

COMMENTS

–

Other information

- Moexipril is a pro-drug converted to its active metabolite moexiprilat
- Close monitoring of renal function during therapy is necessary in those with renal insufficiency
- Renal failure has been reported in association with ACE inhibitors and has been mainly in patients with severe congestive heart failure, renal artery stenosis, or post renal transplant
- A high incidence of anaphylactoid reactions has been reported in patients dialysed with high-flux polyacrylonitrile membranes and treated concomitantly with an ACE inhibitor. This combination should therefore be avoided
- Hyperkalaemia and other side-effects are more common in patients with impaired renal function

Molgramostim

Clinical use

Recombinant human granulocyte-macrophage colony-stimulating factor, for treatment and prophylaxis of neutropenia in patients receiving myelosuppressive chemotherapy

Dose in normal renal function

SC: 5–10 micrograms/kg/day for 7–10 days after chemotherapy

IV: 10 micrograms/kg/day for a maximum of 30 days post bone marrow transplant

Both to commence the day after the last dose of chemotherapy is given or the bone marrow is transplanted

Pharmacokinetics

Molecular weight (daltons)	14478.275
% Protein binding	–
% Excreted unchanged in urine	<0.2
Volume of distribution (L/kg)	–
Half-life – normal/ESRF (hrs)	(SC) 2–3 (IV) 0.5–2.0/unchanged

Dose in renal impairment GFR (mL/min)

20–50	Dose as in normal renal function
10–20	Dose as in normal renal function
<10	Dose as in normal renal function

Dose in patients undergoing renal replacement therapies

CAPD	Not dialysed. Dose as in normal renal function
HD	Not dialysed. Dose as in normal renal function
CAV/VVHD	Not dialysed. Dose as in normal renal function

Important drug interactions

POTENTIALLY HAZARDOUS INTERACTIONS WITH OTHER DRUGS

• None

Administration

RECONSTITUTION

• Add 1.0 mL water for injection

ROUTE

• IV: in sodium chloride 0.9% or glucose 5% at a concentration not <7 micrograms/mL
• SC: bolus

RATE OF ADMINISTRATION

–

COMMENTS

–

Other information

• In a series of nine patients given prolonged treatment with molgramostim, four developed hypoalbuminaemia that was symptomatic in two of the patients
• Use with caution in patients with fluid retention or heart failure, as fluid retention may be aggravated
• Treatment has been associated with heart failure, capillary leak syndrome, hypotension, cardiac arrhythmias, intracranial hypertension and fever
• Renal insufficiency occurred in 3% of bone marrow transplant patients receiving molgramostim 60–125 micrograms/m^2/day

Montelukast

Clinical use

Add-on therapy for asthma

Dose in normal renal function

10 mg at night

Pharmacokinetics

Molecular weight (daltons)	608.2
% Protein binding	>99
% Excreted unchanged in urine	<0.2
Volume of distribution (L/kg)	8–11 litres
Half-life – normal/ESRF (hrs)	2.7–5.5

Dose in renal impairment GFR (mL/min)

20–50	Dose as in normal renal function
10–20	Dose as in normal renal function
<10	Dose as in normal renal function

Dose in patients undergoing renal replacement therapies

CAPD	Not dialysed. Dose as in normal renal function
HD	Not dialysed. Dose as in normal renal function
CAV/VVHD	Not dialysed. Dose as in normal renal function

Important drug interactions

POTENTIALLY HAZARDOUS INTERACTIONS WITH OTHER DRUGS

• None known

Administration

RECONSTITUTION

–

ROUTE

• Oral

RATE OF ADMINISTRATION

–

COMMENTS

–

Other information

• Metabolites have minimal therapeutic activity

Morphine

Clinical use

Opiate analgesic

Dose in normal renal function

5–20 mg every 4 hours (higher in very severe pain or terminal illness)

Pharmacokinetics

Molecular weight (daltons)	759 (sulphate)
% Protein binding	20–30
% Excreted unchanged in urine	10
Volume of distribution (L/kg)	3.5
Half-life – normal/ESRF (hrs)	1–4/unchanged

Dose in renal impairment GFR (mL/min)

20–50	75% of normal
10–20	Use small doses, e.g. 2.5–5 mg
<10	Use small doses, e.g. 1.25–2.5 mg

Dose in patients undergoing renal replacement therapies

CAPD	Probably not dialysed. Dose as in GFR < 10 mL/min
HD	Dialysed, active metabolite removed significantly. Dose as in GFR < 10 mL/min
CAV/VVHD	Dialysed. Dose as in GFR = 10–20 mL/min

Important drug interactions

POTENTIALLY HAZARDOUS INTERACTIONS WITH OTHER DRUGS

- Beta-blockers: possibly increased plasma concentration of esmolol
- MAOIs: avoid concomitant use. CNS excitation or depression (hypertension or hypotension)
- Selegiline: hyperpyrexia and CNS toxicity reported

Administration

RECONSTITUTION

–

ROUTE

- Oral, SC, IM or IV

RATE OF ADMINISTRATION

- IV 2 mg/minute (titrate according to response)

COMMENTS

–

Other information

- Extreme caution with all opiates in patients with impaired renal function
- Potential accumulation of morphine 6-glucuronide (an active, renally excreted metabolite – more potent than morphine). The half-life of morphine 6-glucuronide is increased from 3–5 hours in normal renal function to about 50 hours in ESRD
- **ENSURE NALOXONE READILY AVAILABLE**
- Some units avoid slow-release oral preparations as any side-effects may be prolonged

Movicol

Clinical use

Laxative

Dose in normal renal function

1–3 sachets daily in divided doses in
125 mL of water

Maintenance: 1–2 sachets daily

Pharmacokinetics

Molecular weight (daltons)	3350
% Protein binding	Not absorbed
% Excreted unchanged in urine	Not absorbed
Volume of distribution (L/kg)	Not absorbed
Half-life – normal/ESRF (hrs)	Not absorbed

Dose in renal impairment GFR (mL/min)

20–50	Dose as in normal renal function
10–20	Dose as in normal renal function
<10	Dose as in normal renal function

Dose in patients undergoing renal replacement therapies

CAPD	Dose as in normal renal function
HD	Dose as in normal renal function
CAV/VVHD	Dose as in normal renal function

Important drug interactions

POTENTIALLY HAZARDOUS INTERACTIONS WITH OTHER DRUGS

• None known

Administration

RECONSTITUTION

–

ROUTE

• Oral

RATE OF ADMINISTRATION

–

COMMENTS

–

Other information

• Movicol contains polyethylene glycol, sodium chloride, sodium bicarbonate and potassium chloride

• The electrolyte content of a sachet when made up with 125 mL water is:

sodium 65 mmol/L

chloride 53 mmo/L

potassium 5.4 mmol/L

bicarbonate 17 mmol/L

• Sachets are formulated to ensure that there is virtually no net gain or loss of sodium, potassium or water

• active ingredient is the osmotic laxative polyethylene glycol

Moxonidine

Clinical use

Antihypertensive agent (centrally acting agonist at imidazoline I_1 receptor and alpha$_2$ adrenoceptors)

Dose in normal renal function

200–600 micrograms daily

(Doses >400 micrograms should be in two divided doses)

Pharmacokinetics

Molecular weight (daltons)	241.7
% Protein binding	7
% Excreted unchanged in urine	50–75
Volume of distribution (L/kg)	1.8
Half-life – normal/ESRF (hrs)	2–3/6.9 ± 3.7

Dose in renal impairment GFR (mL/min)

30–60	200 micrograms twice daily
10–30	Use with caution. See 'Other information'
<10	Use with caution. See 'Other information'

Dose in patients undergoing renal replacement therapies

CAPD	Probably dialysed. Dose as in GFR = <10 mL/min
HD	Probably dialysed. Dose as in GFR = <10 mL/min
CAV/VVHD	Probably dialysed. Dose as in GFR = 10–20 mL/min

Important drug interactions

POTENTIALLY HAZARDOUS INTERACTIONS WITH OTHER DRUGS

• None known

Administration

RECONSTITUTION

–

ROUTE

• Oral

RATE OF ADMINISTRATION

–

COMMENTS

–

Other information

• In moderately impaired renal function (GFR = 30–60 mL/min) AUC is increased by 85% and clearance decreased by 52% therefore monitor patient closely

• Anecdotal evidence suggests that moxonidine can be used safely at standard doses in patients with all degrees of renal impairment

• One paper suggests that moxonidine can be used in patients at a dose of 300 micrograms daily in severe renal failure. (Kirch et al. (1988) The influence of renal function on clinical pharmacokinetics of moxonidine. Clinical Pharmacokinetics. 15: 245–53)

Muromonab CD3 (OKT3) (unlicensed drug)

Clinical use

Steroid-resistant acute transplant rejection, prophylaxis of rejection in sensitised patients

Dose in normal renal function

5 mg daily for 5–14 days (10 days most common)

Pharmacokinetics

Molecular weight (daltons)	50,000 (heavy chain) + 25,000 (light chain)
% Protein binding	–
% Excreted unchanged in urine	–
Volume of distribution (L/kg)	0.093
Half-life – normal/ESRF (hrs)	18–36/–

Dose in renal impairment GFR (mL/min)

20–50	Dose as in normal renal function
10–20	Dose as in normal renal function
<10	Dose as in normal renal function

Dose in patients undergoing renal replacement therapies

CAPD	Unlikely to be dialysed. Dose as in normal renal function
HD	Not dialysed. Dose as in normal renal function
CAV/VVHD	Unknown dialysability. Dose as in normal renal function

Important drug interactions

POTENTIALLY HAZARDOUS INTERACTIONS WITH OTHER DRUGS

- Ciclosporin: increases ciclosporin plasma levels
- Indometacin: may increase risk of encephalopathy
- Volatile anaesthetics/drugs that decrease cardiac contractility: increase risk of developing cardiovascular problems

Administration

RECONSTITUTION

–

ROUTE

- IV peripherally

RATE OF ADMINISTRATION

- FAST over less than 1 minute

COMMENTS

- * Doctor administration recommended

Other information

- * Ensure patient is not fluid overloaded prior to administration
- Possible future scope for dose titration according to CD3 or absolute T-cell count
- Reduce or stop other immunosuppressant therapy during treatment and resume 3 days prior to cessation of OKT3
- IV methylprednisolone sodium succinate 8 mg/kg given 1–4 hours prior to the first dose of OKT3 is strongly recommended to decrease the incidence and severity of reactions to the first dose. Paracetamol and antihistamine given concomitantly with OKT3 may also help to reduce some early reactions
- Side-effects pronounced. **WARN PATIENT**

Mycophenolate mofetil

Clinical use

Prophylaxis against acute transplant rejection

Dose in normal renal function

1.0–1.5 g twice a day

Pharmacokinetics

Molecular weight (daltons)	320
% Protein binding	97
% Excreted unchanged in urine	<1
Volume of distribution (L/kg)	3.6–4.0
Half-life – normal/ESRF (hrs)	11–18/–

Dose in renal impairment GFR (mL/min)

20–50	Dose as in normal renal function
10–20	1.0 g twice a day
<10	1.0 g twice a day

Dose in patients undergoing renal replacement therapies

CAPD	Not dialysed. Dose as in GFR < 10 mL/min
HD	Not dialysed. Dose as in GFR < 10 mL/min
CAV/VVHD	Not dialysed. Dose as in normal renal function

Important drug interactions

POTENTIALLY HAZARDOUS INTERACTIONS WITH OTHER DRUGS

- Antivirals: higher plasma concentrations of both MMF and aciclovir when the two are prescribed concomitantly
- Antacids: absorption of MMF decreased in presence of magnesium and aluminium salts
- Colestyramine: 40% reduction in oral bioavailability of MMF
- Ciclosporin: some studies show that ciclosporin decreases plasma MPA AUC levels – no dose change required

Administration

RECONSTITUTION

- Add 7 mL of glucose 5% per vial

ROUTE

- Oral, IV

RATE OF ADMINISTRATION

- IV: over 2 hours

COMMENTS

- Dilute reconstituted solution further with glucose 5% to achieve a concentration of 6 mg/ml. Store between 15–30°C

Other information

- Mycophenolate mofetil (MMF) rapidly undergoes complete presystemic absorption to mycophenolic acid (MPA) which in turn is metabolised to MPA glucuronide. This undergoes extensive enterohepatic recirculation, hence a secondary increase in MPA plasma levels is seen 6–12 hours post dose
- If neutrophil count drops below 1.3 x $10^3/\mu$L, consider suspending MMF therapy
- No dosage reduction is required in the event of a transplant rejection episode

Nabumetone

Clinical use

NSAID: osteoarthritis and rheumatoid arthritis

Dose in normal renal function

1 g at night, in severe conditions 0.5–1 g in the morning as well; elderly 0.5–1 g daily

Pharmacokinetics

Molecular weight (daltons)	228
% Protein binding	>99
% Excreted unchanged in urine	<1
Volume of distribution (L/kg)	0.11
Half-life – normal/ESRF (hrs)	24/unchanged

Dose in renal impairment
GFR (mL/min)

20–50	Dose as in normal renal function, but avoid if possible
10–20	0.5–1 g daily, but avoid if possible
<10	0.5–1 g daily, but avoid if possible

Dose in patients undergoing renal replacement therapies

CAPD	Not dialysed. Dose as in GFR < 10 mL/min
HD	Not dialysed. Dose as in GFR < 10 mL/min
CAV/VVHD	Not dialysed. Dose as in GFR = 10–20 mL/min

Important drug interactions

POTENTIALLY HAZARDOUS INTERACTIONS WITH OTHER DRUGS

• Ciclosporin: increased risk of nephrotoxicity
• ACE inhibitors and AT-II antagonists: antagonism of hypotensive effect. Possible increased risk of renal damage and hyperkalaemia
• Antibacterials: possibly increased risk of convulsions with quinolones
• Anticoagulants: anticoagulant effect of warfarin and acenocoumarol possibly increased
• Antivirals: increased risk of haematological toxicity with zidovudine
• Diuretics: increased risk of nephrotoxicity, hyperkalaemia with potassium-sparing diuretics
• Lithium: excretion of lithium reduced
• Methotrexate: excretion of methotrexate possibly reduced, increased risk of toxicity
• Sulphonylureas: effect of sulphonylurea possibly enhanced
• Phenytoin: effect of phenytoin possibly enhanced
• Tacrolimus: increased risk of nephrotoxicity

Administration

RECONSTITUTION

–

ROUTE

• Oral

RATE OF ADMINISTRATION

–

COMMENTS

–

Other information

• Nabumetone is absorbed from the GI tract and rapidly metabolised in the liver to the principal active metabolite 6-methoxy-2-naphthylacetic acid (6-MNA). The metabolite is a potent inhibitor of prostaglandin synthesis. Excretion of the metabolite is predominantly in the urine. The data sheet recommends a dose reduction for CL_{CR} <30 mL/minute, however, another article concluded that dosage adjustments may not be necessary with decreased renal function. The authors found an increase in the elimination half-life of 6-MNA. However, they stated that the increased half-life in patients with renal failure is offset by changes in the apparent Vd that prevent the accumulation of 6-MNA. (Brier ME et al. (1995) Clinical Pharmacology and Therapeutics. 57(6): 622–7)
• Inhibition of renal prostaglandin synthesis by NSAIDs may interfere with renal function, especially in the presence of existing renal disease. Avoid if possible; if not, check serum creatinine 48–72 hours after starting NSAID. If increased, discontinue NSAID therapy
• Use normal doses in patients with ESRD on dialysis
• Use with caution in renal transplant recipients – can reduce intra-renal autocoid synthesis

Nadolol

Clinical use

Beta-adrenoceptor blocker: management of angina pectoris, hypertension, arrhythmias, migraine, thyrotoxicosis

Dose in normal renal function

40–240 mg per day

Pharmacokinetics

Molecular weight (daltons)	309
% Protein binding	30
% Excreted unchanged in urine	90
Volume of distribution (L/kg)	1.9
Half-life – normal/ESRF (hrs)	19/45

Dose in renal impairment GFR (mL/min)

>50	Dose as in normal renal function
31–50	Normal dose every 24–36 hours
10–30	50% of dose every 24–48 hours
<10	25% of dose every 40–60 hours

Dose in patients undergoing renal replacement therapies

CAPD	Dialysed. Dose as in GFR < 10 mL/min
HD	Dialysed. Dose as in GFR < 10 mL/min
CAV/VVHD	Dialysed. Dose as in GFR = 10–30 mL/min

Important drug interactions

POTENTIALLY HAZARDOUS INTERACTIONS WITH OTHER DRUGS

- Anaesthetics: enhanced hypotensive effect
- Anti-arrhythmics: increased risk of myocardial depression and bradycardia
- Antihypertensives: enhanced hypotensive effect
- Calcium-channel blockers: increased risk of bradycardia and AV block with diltiazem; severe hypotension and heart failure occasionally with nifedipine; asystole, severe hypotension and heart failure with verapamil
- Moxisylyte: possibly severe postural hypotension
- Sympathomimetics: severe hypertension

Administration

RECONSTITUTION

–

ROUTE

- Oral

RATE OF ADMINISTRATION

–

COMMENTS

–

Other information

- Data sheet guidelines for increasing dosing interval for patients with renal impairment may be impractical with respect to patient compliance
- Unlike most other beta-blockers, nadolol is not metabolised and is excreted unchanged mainly by the kidneys

Naloxone

Clinical use

Reversal of opioid-induced respiratory depression

Dose in normal renal function

See 'Other information'

Pharmacokinetics

Molecular weight (daltons)	364 (hydrochloride)
% Protein binding	54
% Excreted unchanged in urine	<5
Volume of distribution (L/kg)	2–3
Half-life – normal/ESRF (hrs)	1–1.5/unchanged

Dose in renal impairment GFR (mL/min)

20–50	Dose as in normal renal function
10–20	Dose as in normal renal function
<10	Dose as in normal renal function

Dose in patients undergoing renal replacement therapies

CAPD	Unknown dialysability. Dose as in normal renal function
HD	Unknown dialysability. Dose as in normal renal function
CAV/VVHD	Unknown dialysability. Dose as in normal renal function

Important drug interactions

POTENTIALLY HAZARDOUS INTERACTIONS WITH OTHER DRUGS

• None known

Administration

RECONSTITUTION

–

ROUTE

• IV, IM or SC. (IV more rapid response)

RATE OF ADMINISTRATION

• Rapid if bolus injection

COMMENTS

–

Other information

• IV post-operative use: give 1.5–3 micrograms/kg. If response inadequate, increments of 100 micrograms every 2 minutes. Further dose by IM injection if needed or

• Dilute 400 micrograms in 100 mL sodium chloride 0.9% or glucose 5% (4 micrograms/mL) and give by continuous infusion. Titrate dose according to response

• Opioid overdosage: an initial dose of 400–2000 micrograms IV. If the desired degree of counter action and improvement in respiratory function is not obtained, it may be repeated at 2–3-minute intervals or give as an infusion. (If no response after 10 mg then question the diagnosis of opioid-induced toxicity.)

Naproxen

Clinical use

NSAID: rheumatic disease (including juvenile arthritis) and other musculoskeletal disorders; dysmenorrhoea; acute gout

Dose in normal renal function

500–1250 mg daily in 2–3 divided doses

Pharmacokinetics

Molecular weight (daltons)	230
% Protein binding	99
% Excreted unchanged in urine	<1
Volume of distribution (L/kg)	0.14–0.18
Half-life – normal/ESRF (hrs)	12–15/unchanged

Dose in renal impairment GFR (mL/min)

20–50	Dose as in normal renal function, but avoid if possible
10–20	Dose as in normal renal function, but avoid if possible
<10	Dose as in normal renal function, but only use if ESRD on dialysis

Dose in patients undergoing renal replacement therapies

CAPD	Slightly dialysed. Dose as in GFR < 10 mL/min
HD	Not dialysed. Dose as in GFR < 10 mL/min
CAV/VVHD	Slightly dialysed. Dose as in GFR = 10–20 mL/min

Important drug interactions

POTENTIALLY HAZARDOUS INTERACTIONS WITH OTHER DRUGS

- Ciclosporin: increased risk of nephrotoxicity
- Antibacterials: possibly increased risk of convulsions with quinolones
- Antivirals: increased risk of haematological toxicity with zidovudine
- Lithium: excretion reduced
- Cytotoxic agents: reduced excretion of methotrexate
- Diuretics: increased risk of nephrotoxicity, hyperkalaemia with potassium-sparing diuretics
- Anticoagulants: effects of warfarin and acenocoumarol enhanced
- Antidiabetic agents: effects of sulphonylureas enhanced
- Anti-epileptic agents: effects of phenytoin enhanced
- ACE inhibitors and AT-II antagonists: antagonism of hypotensive effect; increased risk of renal damage and hyperkalaemia
- Tacrolimus: increased risk of nephrotoxicity

Administration

RECONSTITUTION

–

ROUTE

- Oral, PR

RATE OF ADMINISTRATION

–

COMMENTS

- E/C preps: swallow whole, do not chew. Do not take at same time as indigestion remedies or phosphate binders

Other information

- Naproxen is associated with an intermediate risk of side-effects
- Naproxen is eliminated to a large extent (95%) as metabolites by urinary excretion via glomerular filtration. The remainder is excreted via the faeces
- Inhibition of renal prostaglandin synthesis by NSAIDs may interfere with renal function, especially in the presence of existing renal disease. Avoid if possible; if not, check serum creatinine 48–72 hours after starting NSAID. If raised, discontinue NSAID therapy
- Use normal doses in patients with ESRD on dialysis
- Use with caution in renal transplant recipients – can reduce intra-renal autocoid synthesis

Naratriptan hydrochloride

Clinical use

Acute treatment of migraine. ($5HT_1$-receptor agonist)

Dose in normal renal function

2.5 mg
Dose may be repeated after 4 hours – maximum 5 mg/24 hours

Pharmacokinetics

Molecular weight (daltons)	371.9
% Protein binding	29
% Excreted unchanged in urine	50
Volume of distribution (L/kg)	170 litres
Half-life – normal/ESRF (hrs)	6/10.45

Dose in renal impairment GFR (mL/min)

20–50	Maximum 2.5 mg daily
15–20	Maximum 2.5 mg daily
<15	Use with caution – maximum 2.5 mg daily

Dose in patients undergoing renal replacement therapies

CAPD	No data. Dose as for GFR = <15 mL/min
HD	No data. Dose as for GFR = <15 mL/min
CAV/VVHD	No data. Dose as for GFR = 15–20 mL/min

Important drug interactions

POTENTIALLY HAZARDOUS INTERACTIONS WITH OTHER DRUGS

• Ergotamine and related compounds (including methysergide): increased risk of vasospasm

Administration

RECONSTITUTION

–

ROUTE

• Oral

RATE OF ADMINISTRATION

–

COMMENTS

–

Other information

• Do not take second dose at 4 hours during an attack if the first dose was ineffectual
• Naratriptan is excreted by glomerular filtration and active secretion into the renal tubules
• Inactive metabolites are renally excreted
• Studies in patients with impaired renal function (GFR 18–115 mL/min) showed an 80% increase in half-life and a 50% decrease in clearance compared with matched individuals with normal renal function

Nebivolol

Clinical use

Beta$_1$-adrenoceptor blocker, used for essential hypertension

Dose in normal renal function

2.5–5 mg daily

Pharmacokinetics

Molecular weight (daltons)	441.9
% Protein binding	98
% Excreted unchanged in urine	<0.5
Volume of distribution (L/kg)	11.2
Half-life – normal/ESRF (hrs)	10 (32–34 in poor hydroxylators)

Dose in renal impairment GFR (mL/min)

20–50	Initial dose 2.5 mg, adjust according to response
10–20	Initial dose 2.5 mg, adjust according to response
<10	Initial dose 2.5 mg, adjust according to response

Dose in patients undergoing renal replacement therapies

CAPD	Not dialysed. Dose as for GFR = <10 mL/min
HD	Not dialysed. Dose as for GFR = <10 mL/min
CAV/VVHD	Not dialysed. Dose as for GFR = 10–20 mL/min

Important drug interactions

POTENTIALLY HAZARDOUS INTERACTIONS WITH OTHER DRUGS

• Anaesthetics: enhanced hypotensive effect
• Analgesics: NSAIDs antagonise hypotensive effects
• Anti-arrhythmics: increased risk of myocardial depression and bradycardia; with amiodarone increased risk of bradycardia and AV block
• Calcium-channel blockers: increased risk of bradycardia and AV block with diltiazem; severe hypotension and heart failure occasionally with nifedipine and possibly other dihydropyridines; asystole, severe hypotension and heart failure with verapamil (avoid concomitant verapamil use)
• Antidepressants: enhanced hypotensive effect with MAOIs
• Antihypertensives: enhanced hypotensive effect; increased risk of withdrawal hypertension with clonidine; increased risk of first-dose hypotensive effect with post-synaptic alpha-blockers
• Moxisylyte: possible severe postural hypotension
• Sympathomimetics: severe hypertension with adrenaline and noradrenaline and possibly dobutamine

Administration

RECONSTITUTION
–

ROUTE
• Oral

RATE OF ADMINISTRATION
–

COMMENTS
–

Other information

• 38% of the dose is excreted in the urine as active metabolites
• In a trial of 10 patients with renal artery stenosis given nebivolol 5 mg OD, plasma renin activity significantly decreased, although serum aldosterone levels did not change to any great extent. In addition, there was no change in effective renal plasma flow, GFR, renal blood flow or renal vascular resistance. Renal function remained well preserved

Nefopam hydrochloride

Clinical use

Analgesic – for moderate pain

Dose in normal renal function

Oral: 30–90 mg three times a day

IM: 20 mg 6-hourly

Pharmacokinetics

Molecular weight (daltons)	289.8
% Protein binding	73
% Excreted unchanged in urine	<5
Volume of distribution (L/kg)	–
Half-life – normal/ESRF (hrs)	4/–

Dose in renal impairment GFR (mL/min)

20–50	Dose as in normal renal function
10–20	Dose as in normal renal function
<10	Dose as in normal renal function. See 'Other information'

Dose in patients undergoing renal replacement therapies

CAPD	Unknown dialysability. Dose as in GFR = <10 mL/min
HD	Unlikely dialysability. Dose as in GFR = <10 mL/min
CAV/VVHD	Unknown dialysability. Dose as in GFR = 10–20 mL/min

Important drug interactions

POTENTIALLY HAZARDOUS INTERACTIONS WITH OTHER DRUGS

• Antidepressants: avoid MAOIs. Tricyclics possibly increase risk of side-effects

Administration

RECONSTITUTION

–

ROUTE

• Oral, IM

RATE OF ADMINISTRATION

–

COMMENTS

–

Other information

• Avoid repeated or chronic administration in ESRD and dialysis patients

• In the elderly a dose of 30 mg 8-hourly is recommended due to reduced metabolism and increased susceptibility to side-effects. Renal patients may also have reduced metabolism and excretion and may also have the same problems so always start with the lower dose

• Active metabolites excreted in the urine

Nelfinavir

Clinical use

Protease inhibitor for the treatment of HIV infection in combination with other antiretroviral drugs

Dose in normal renal function

750 mg three times a day, or
1.25 g twice a day

Pharmacokinetics

Molecular weight (daltons)	663.9
% Protein binding	>98
% Excreted unchanged in urine	1–2
Volume of distribution (L/kg)	2–7
Half-life – normal/ESRF (hrs)	1.8–5

Dose in renal impairment GFR (mL/min)

20–50	Dose as in normal renal function
10–20	Dose as in normal renal function
<10	Dose as in normal renal function. See 'Other information'

Dose in patients undergoing renal replacement therapies

CAPD	Unlikely dialysability. Dose as in GFR = <10 mL/min
HD	Unlikely dialysability. Dose as in GFR = <10 mL/min
CAV/VVHD	Unlikely dialysability. Dose as in GFR = 10–20 mL/min

Important drug interactions

POTENTIALLY HAZARDOUS INTERACTIONS WITH OTHER DRUGS

- Anti-arrhythmics: increased risk of arrhythmias with amiodarone and quinidine (avoid concomitant use)
- Antibacterials: rifampicin decreases plasma concentration of nelfinavir (avoid concomitant use); nelfinavir increases plasma concentration of rifabutin (halve rifabutin dose)
- Antidepressants: plasma concentration reduced by St John's Wort (avoid concomitant use)
- Anti-epileptics: carbamazepine and phenytoin possibly reduce plasma concentration of nelfinavir
- Antihistamines: increased risk of arrhythmias with terfenadine (avoid concomitant use)
- Antimuscarinics: avoid concomitant use with tolterodine
- Antipsychotics: possibly increased risk of arrhythmias with pimozide (avoid concomitant use); possible increase in plasma concentration of thioridazine
- Ergotamine: increased risk of ergotism (avoid concomitant use)
- Phenobarbital: possibly reduces nelfinavir plasma concentration
- Lipid-regulating drugs: increased risk of myopathy with simvastatin and possibly atorvastatin (avoid concomitant use)
- Midazolam: prolonged sedation (avoid concomitant use)
- Oestrogens and progestogens: possibly reduced efficacy of oral contraceptives
- 5HT$_1$ agonists: plasma concentration of eletriptan increased (avoid concomitant use)

Administration

RECONSTITUTION
–

ROUTE

- Oral

RATE OF ADMINISTRATION
–

COMMENTS
–

Other information

- There are no data available on the use of nelfinavir in renal failure but any dose adjustment is unlikely due to nelfinavir being predominantly metabolised and excreted via the liver. Use with caution

Neostigmine

Clinical use

Myasthenia gravis, antagonist to non-depolarising neuromuscular blockade; paralytic ileus; post-operative urinary retention

Dose in normal renal function

In myasthenia gravis: neostigmine bromide 15–30 mg at suitable intervals throughout day – total daily dose 75–300 mg; neostigmine metilsulfate, IM, SC, 1–2.5 mg – usual total daily dose 5–20 mg

Pharmacokinetics

Molecular weight (daltons)	223
% Protein binding	0–25
% Excreted unchanged in urine	67
Volume of distribution (L/kg)	0.5–1.0
Half-life – normal/ESRF (hrs)	1.3/3.0

Dose in renal impairment GFR (mL/min)

20–50	50–100% of normal dose
10–20	50% of normal dose
<10	25% of normal dose

Dose in patients undergoing renal replacement therapies

CAPD	Unknown dialysability. Dose as in GFR < 10 mL/min
HD	Unknown dialysability. Dose as in GFR < 10 mL/min
CAV/VVHD	Unknown dialysability. Dose as in GFR = 10–20 mL/min

Important drug interactions

POTENTIALLY HAZARDOUS INTERACTIONS WITH OTHER DRUGS

• Aminoglycosides, clindamycin and colistin antagonise effects of neostigmine

Administration

RECONSTITUTION

–

ROUTE

• Neostigmine bromide: oral
• Neostigmine metilsulfate: SC, IM, IV

RATE OF ADMINISTRATION

• IV: very slowly

COMMENTS

–

Other information

• Neostigmine 0.5 mg IV = 1–1.5 mg IM or SC = 15 mg orally
• When used for reversal of non-depolarising neuromuscular blockade, atropine (0.6–1.2 mg IV) or glycopyrronium should be given before or with neostigmine in order to prevent bradycardia, excessive salivation and other muscarinic actions of neostigmine
• The physicochemical nature of neostigmine may tend to encourage its removal by various renal replacement therapies

Netilmicin

Clinical use

Antibacterial agent

Dose in normal renal function

IM, IV: 4–7.5 mg/kg daily, as a single daily dose or in divided doses every 8 or 12 hours

Pharmacokinetics

Molecular weight (daltons)	1442
% Protein binding	<5
% Excreted unchanged in urine	95
Volume of distribution (L/kg)	0.16–0.3
Half-life – normal/ESRF (hrs)	1–3/35–72

Dose in renal impairment GFR (mL/min)

20–50	25–55% of normal dose daily. Monitor levels
10–20	15–20% of normal dose daily. Monitor levels
<10	10% of normal dose daily. Monitor levels

Dose in patients undergoing renal replacement therapies

CAPD	Dialysed. IV: 2 mg/kg on alternate days IP: 7.5–10 mg/L per exchange. Monitor levels
HD	Dialysed. Administer 2 mg/kg at the end of each dialysis session. Monitor levels
CAV/VVHD	Dialysed. Dose as in GFR = 10–20 mL/min. Monitor netilmicin levels

Important drug interactions

POTENTIALLY HAZARDOUS INTERACTIONS WITH OTHER DRUGS

- Ciclosporin: increased risk of nephrotoxicity
- Botulinum toxin: neuromuscular block enhanced
- Cisplatin: increased risk of nephrotoxicity and ototoxicity
- Loop diuretics: increased risk of ototoxicity
- Muscle relaxants: effects of non-depolarising muscle relaxants enhanced
- Parasympathomimetics: antagonised by aminoglycosides

Administration

RECONSTITUTION

- 50–200 mL of sterile water for injection, sodium chloride 0.9%, glucose 5% or 10%

ROUTE

- IM, IP, IV bolus or infusion

RATE OF ADMINISTRATION

- IV bolus: administer over 3–5 minutes
- IV infusion: administer over 0.5–2 hours

COMMENTS

- IM and IV dose are identical. Calculate on mg/kg lean body weight, or actual weight, whichever is lower

Other information

- Netilmicin serum concentrations should be monitored and used for basis of dosage adjustment, otherwise follow guidelines in data sheet according to serum creatinine/creatinine clearance
- Once-daily administration of netilmicin may lead to transient peak concentrations of 20–30 micrograms/mL. Other dosage regimens will result in peak levels not exceeding 12 micrograms/mL. Prolonged levels above 16 micrograms/mL should be avoided. If trough levels are monitored they will usually be 3 micrograms/mL or less with the recommended dosage. Increasing trough concentrations above 4 micrograms/mL should be avoided
- Removed by PD if given IV/IM

Nevirapine

Clinical use

Non-nucleoside reverse transcriptase inhibitor for the treatment of progressive or advanced HIV infection, in combination with at least two other antivirals

Dose in normal renal function

200 mg daily increasing to twice daily after 14 days if tolerated

Pharmacokinetics

Molecular weight (daltons)	266.3
% Protein binding	60
% Excreted unchanged in urine	<3
Volume of distribution (L/kg)	1.2–1.4
Half-life – normal/ESRF (hrs)	40–45 (single dose) 25–30 (multiple dosing)

Dose in renal impairment GFR (mL/min)

20–50	Dose as in normal renal function
10–20	Dose as in normal renal function
<10	Dose as in normal renal function. See 'Other information'

Dose in patients undergoing renal replacement therapies

CAPD	Unknown dialysability. Dose as in GFR = <10 mL/min
HD	Likely to be dialysed. Dose as in GFR = <10 mL/min
CAV/VVHD	Unknown dialysability. Dose as in GFR = 10–20 mL/min

Important drug interactions

POTENTIALLY HAZARDOUS INTERACTIONS WITH OTHER DRUGS

- Antibacterials: plasma concentrations decreased by rifampicin (avoid concomitant use)
- Antidepressants: plasma concentration reduced by St John's Wort (avoid concomitant use)
- Antifungals: plasma concentration of ketoconazole reduced (avoid concomitant use)
- Other antivirals: plasma concentration of saquinavir reduced (avoid concomitant use). Plasma concentration of indinavir and possibly amprenavir, lopinavir and efavirenz reduced by nevirapine
- Oestrogens and progestogens: accelerated metabolism of oral contraceptives and other hormonal contraceptives, reduced contraceptive effect

Administration

RECONSTITUTION

–

ROUTE

- Oral

RATE OF ADMINISTRATION

–

COMMENTS

–

Other information

- There is little data available on the use of nevirapine in renal failure but any dose adjustment is unlikely due to nevirapine being predominantly metabolised in the liver, and the inactive metabolites excreted in the urine. Use with caution
- There was a preliminary study in haemodialysis patients in *Nephrol Dial Transplant.* (2001) **16**: 192–3 which showed that a normal dose was not associated with increased side-effects

Nicardipine

Clinical use

Calcium-channel blocker: prophylaxis and treatment of angina; mild to moderate hypertension

Dose in normal renal function

60–120 mg daily given in three divided doses

Pharmacokinetics

Molecular weight (daltons)	516
% Protein binding	98–99
% Excreted unchanged in urine	<1
Volume of distribution (L/kg)	0.7–1.7
Half-life – normal/ESRF (hrs)	5.0–8.6/ unchanged

Dose in renal impairment GFR (mL/min)

20–50	Dose as in normal renal function
10–20	Dose as in normal renal function. Start with small doses
<10	Dose as in normal renal function. Start with small doses

Dose in patients undergoing renal replacement therapies

CAPD	Unlikely to be dialysed. Dose as in GFR = <10 mL/min
HD	Not dialysed. Dose as in GFR = <10 mL/min
CAV/VVHD	Unknown dialysability. Dose as in GFR = 10–20 mL/min

Important drug interactions

POTENTIALLY HAZARDOUS INTERACTIONS WITH OTHER DRUGS

- Ciclosporin: may increase blood ciclosporin concentrations
- Carbamazepine, phenobarbital, phenytoin and primidone may reduce effect of nicardipine
- Alpha-blockers: increased risk of first-dose hypotensive effect
- Antivirals: amprenavir possibly increases plasma concentration
- Rifampicin: reduces plasma concentration
- Digoxin: plasma level may be increased
- Theophylline: levels may increase

Administration

RECONSTITUTION

–

ROUTE

- Oral

RATE OF ADMINISTRATION

–

COMMENTS

- Administration of nicardipine with food appears to reduce the bioavailability and delay the achievement of peak plasma concentrations

Other information

- Nicardipine is extensively metabolised in the liver and is excreted in the urine and faeces, mainly as inactive metabolites
- Nicardipine blood levels may also be elevated in some renally impaired patients. Therefore, start with a low dose and titrate to BP and response. The dose interval may also need to be extended to 12-hourly

Nicorandil

Clinical use

Prevention and treatment of chronic stable angina pectoris

Dose in normal renal function

5–30 mg twice daily

Pharmacokinetics

Molecular weight (daltons)	211.2
% Protein binding	Slightly
% Excreted unchanged in urine	1
Volume of distribution (L/kg)	–
Half-life – normal/ESRF (hrs)	1/unchanged

Dose in renal impairment GFR (mL/min)

20–50	Dose as in normal renal function
10–20	Dose as in normal renal function
<10	Dose as in normal renal function

Dose in patients undergoing renal replacement therapies

CAPD	Unknown dialysability. Dose as in normal renal function
HD	Unknown dialysability. Dose as in normal renal function
CAV/VVHD	Unknown dialysability. Dose as in normal renal function

Important drug interactions

POTENTIALLY HAZARDOUS INTERACTIONS WITH OTHER DRUGS

• Sildenafil: enhanced hypotensive effect, avoid concomitant use

Administration

RECONSTITUTION

–

ROUTE

• Oral

RATE OF ADMINISTRATION

–

COMMENTS

–

Other information

–

Nifedipine

Clinical use

Calcium-channel blocker: prophylaxis and treatment of angina, hypertension, Raynaud's phenomenon

Dose in normal renal function

Oral: 5–20 mg 2–3 times daily
Long acting: 20–90 mg daily

Pharmacokinetics

Molecular weight (daltons)	346.3
% Protein binding	98
% Excreted unchanged in urine	<1
Volume of distribution (L/kg)	0.3–1.2
Half-life – normal/ESRF (hrs)	4–6/5–7

Dose in renal impairment GFR (mL/min)

20–50	Dose as in normal renal function
10–20	Dose as in normal renal function. Start with small doses
<10	Dose as in normal renal function. Start with small doses

Dose in patients undergoing renal replacement therapies

CAPD	Not dialysed. Dose as in GFR = <10 mL/min
HD	Not dialysed. Dose as in GFR = <10 mL/min
CAV/VVHD	Unknown dialysability. Dose as in GFR = 10–20 mL/min

Important drug interactions

POTENTIALLY HAZARDOUS INTERACTIONS WITH OTHER DRUGS

• Ciclosporin: may increase ciclosporin level, but not a problem in practice. Nifedipine concentration may increase

• Phenytoin: plasma concentration increased
• Beta-blockers: occasionally severe hypotension and heart failure
• Digoxin: plasma level may be increased
• Nifedipine may impair glucose tolerance
• Alpha-blockers: increased risk of first-dose hypotensive effect
• Antibacterials: rifampicin reduces plasma concentration. Quinupristin/dalfopristin increases plasma levels
• Theophylline levels may increase
• Magnesium salts: profound hypotension with IV magnesium
• Anti-arrhythmics: plasma concentration of quinidine reduced
• Antivirals: amprenavir possibly increases nifedipine levels
• Tacrolimus: increased tacrolimus levels

Administration

RECONSTITUTION
–

ROUTE
• Oral

RATE OF ADMINISTRATION
–

COMMENTS
–

Other information

• Protein binding decreased in severe renal impairment
• Acute renal dysfunction reported
• Increased incidence of side-effects (headache, flushing, dizziness and peripheral oedema) in patients with ESRD
• For acute use: bite capsule then swallow contents with 10–50 mL water

Nimodipine

Clinical use

Calcium-channel blocker: prevention and treatment of ischaemic neurological deficits following subarachnoid haemorrhage

Dose in normal renal function

Prevention orally: 60 mg every 4 hours (total daily dose – 360 mg)

Treatment via central catheter: 1 mg/hour initially. Increased after 2 hours to 2 mg/hour. If BP unstable, weight <70 kg: start with 0.5 mg/hour or less if necessary

Pharmacokinetics

Molecular weight (daltons)	418
% Protein binding	98
% Excreted unchanged in urine	<10
Volume of distribution (L/kg)	0.9–2.3
Half-life – normal/ESRF (hrs)	1–2.8/22

Dose in renal impairment GFR (mL/min)

20–50	Dose as in normal renal function
10–20	Dose as in normal renal function
<10	Dose as in normal renal function

Dose in patients undergoing renal replacement therapies

CAPD	Not dialysed. Dose as in normal renal function
HD	Not dialysed. Dose as in normal renal function
CAV/VVHD	Unknown dialysability. Dose as in normal renal function

Important drug interactions

POTENTIALLY HAZARDOUS INTERACTIONS WITH OTHER DRUGS

- Anti-epileptics: effect reduced by carbamazepine, phenobarbital, phenytoin and primidone
- Alpha-blockers: increased risk of first-dose hypotensive effect
- Antivirals: amprenavir increases plasma concentration
- Theophylline levels may increase

Administration

RECONSTITUTION

- Nimodipine solution must not be added to an infusion bag or bottle and must not be mixed with other drugs

ROUTE

- Oral, IV

RATE OF ADMINISTRATION

- IV – First 2 hours: 1 mg (5 mL) nimodipine per hour
- After 2 hours: infuse 2 mg (10 mL) nimodipine per hour

COMMENTS

- Nimodipine solution should be administered only via a bypass into a running drip (40 mL/hour) of either sodium chloride 0.9% or glucose 5%
- In the event of nimodipine tablets and solution being administered sequentially, the total duration of treatment should not exceed 21 days

Other information

- Nimodipine solution reacts with PVC. Polyethylene tubes are supplied
- Patients with known renal disease and/or receiving nephrotoxic drugs should have renal function monitored closely during IV treatment

Nisoldipine

Clinical use

Calcium-channel blocker used for hypertension, chronic, stable angina

Dose in normal renal function

10–40 mg daily (varies depending on indication)

Pharmacokinetics

Molecular weight (daltons)	388.4
% Protein binding	>99
% Excreted unchanged in urine	<10
Volume of distribution (L/kg)	2.3–7.1
Half-life – normal/ESRF (hrs)	6–12/unchanged

Dose in renal impairment GFR (mL/min)

20–50	Dose as in normal renal function
10–20	Dose as in normal renal function
<10	Dose as in normal renal function

Dose in patients undergoing renal replacement therapies

CAPD	Not dialysed. Dose as in normal renal function
HD	Not dialysed. Dose as in normal renal function
CAV/VVHD	Not dialysed. Dose as in normal renal function

Important drug interactions

POTENTIALLY HAZARDOUS INTERACTIONS WITH OTHER DRUGS

- Phenytoin: reduces plasma concentration of nisoldipine (avoid concomitant use)
- Quinupristin/dalfopristin: possibly increases metabolism of nisoldipine
- Antihypertensives: enhanced hypotensive effect; increased risk of first-dose hypotensive effect of post-synaptic alpha-blockers like prazosin
- Beta-blockers: occasionally severe hypotension and heart failure
- Anaesthetics: isoflurane enhances the hypotensive effect

Administration

RECONSTITUTION

–

ROUTE

- Oral

RATE OF ADMINISTRATION

–

COMMENTS

–

Other information

–

Nitrazepam

Clinical use

Benzodiazepine: hypnotic

Dose in normal renal function

5–10 mg at bedtime; elderly (or debilitated)
2.5–5 mg

Pharmacokinetics

Molecular weight (daltons)	281
% Protein binding	85
% Excreted unchanged in urine	<5
Volume of distribution (L/kg)	1.9–2.4
Half-life – normal/ESRF (hrs)	18–50/unchanged

Dose in renal impairment GFR (mL/min)

20–50	Dose as in normal renal function
10–20	Dose as in normal renal function
<10	Dose as in normal renal function. Start with small doses

Dose in patients undergoing renal replacement therapies

CAPD	Unlikely to be dialysed. Dose as in GFR < 10 mL/min
HD	Unlikely to be dialysed. Dose as in GFR < 10 mL/min
CAV/VVHD	Unlikely to be dialysed. Dose as in normal renal function

Important drug interactions

POTENTIALLY HAZARDOUS INTERACTIONS WITH OTHER DRUGS

• None known

Administration

RECONSTITUTION

–

ROUTE

• Oral

RATE OF ADMINISTRATION

–

COMMENTS

–

Other information

• Mild to moderate renal insufficiency does not alter the kinetics of nitrazepam
• ESRD patients will be more susceptible to adverse effects (drowsiness, sedation, unsteadiness)

Nitrofurantoin

Clinical use

Antibacterial agent

Dose in normal renal function

Treatment: 50–100 mg every 6 hours

Prophylaxis: 50–100 mg at night

Pharmacokinetics

Molecular weight (daltons)	238
% Protein binding	20–70
% Excreted unchanged in urine	30–40
Volume of distribution (L/kg)	0.3–0.7
Half-life – normal/ESRF (hrs)	0.5/1.0

Dose in renal impairment GFR (mL/min)

20–50	Contra-indicated
10–20	Contra-indicated
<10	Contra-indicated

Dose in patients undergoing renal replacement therapies

CAPD	Dialysed. Avoid – contra-indicated
HD	Dialysed. Avoid – contra-indicated
CAV/VVHD	Dialysed. Avoid – contra-indicated

Important drug interactions

POTENTIALLY HAZARDOUS INTERACTIONS WITH OTHER DRUGS

• None known

Administration

RECONSTITUTION

–

ROUTE

• Oral

RATE OF ADMINISTRATION

–

COMMENTS

• Urine may be coloured a dark yellow or brown
• Macrocrystalline form has slower dissolution and absorption rates, produces lower serum concentration and takes longer to achieve peak concentration in the urine

Other information

• Avoid nitrofurantoin in patients with impaired renal function (GFR < 60 mL/min) as the drug is ineffective due to inadequate urine concentration and toxic plasma concentrations can occur causing adverse effects, e.g. neuropathy, blood dyscrasias
• Nitrofurantoin gives false positive urinary glucose (if testing for reducing substances)

Nizatidine

Clinical use

H_2-receptor antagonist

Dose in normal renal function

Oral: 150–600 mg daily
IV: 300–480 mg daily

Pharmacokinetics

Molecular weight (daltons)	332
% Protein binding	28–35
% Excreted unchanged in urine	54–65
Volume of distribution (L/kg)	0.8–1.3
Half-life – normal/ESRF (hrs)	1.3–1.6/5.3–11.0

Dose in renal impairment GFR (mL/min)

20–50	150 mg daily (50% of normal dose)
<20	150 mg on alternate days (25% of normal dose)

Dose in patients undergoing renal replacement therapies

CAPD	Unknown dialysability. Dose as in GFR < 20 mL/min
HD	Not dialysed. Dose as in GFR < 20 mL/min
CAV/VVHD	Unknown dialysability. Dose as in GFR < 20 mL/min

Important drug interactions

POTENTIALLY HAZARDOUS INTERACTIONS WITH OTHER DRUGS

• None known

Administration

RECONSTITUTION

–

ROUTE

• Oral or IV

RATE OF ADMINISTRATION

• Continuous IV infusion: dilute 300 mg in 150 mL. Rate: 10 mg/hour
• Intermittent IV infusion: dilute 100 mg in 50 mL and infuse over 15 minutes, three times daily

COMMENTS

• Compatible with sodium chloride 0.9% or glucose 5%
• To maintain gastric pH $\geq$ 4, a continuous infusion of 10 mg/hour is recommended
• IV infusion: patients with moderate renal impairment (CL_{CR}: 20–50 mL/min) – the dose should be reduced to 120–150 mg daily. Patients with severe impairment (CL_{CR}: <20 mL/min) – the dose should be reduced to 75 mg daily

Other information

• The effect of haemodialysis is unproven. It is not expected to be efficient since nizatidine has a large Vd

Noradrenaline (norepinephrine)

Clinical use

Hypotension (sympathomimetic)

Dose in normal renal function

1–10 micrograms/minute

Pharmacokinetics

Molecular weight (daltons)	169
% Protein binding	~50
% Excreted unchanged in urine	<10
Volume of distribution (L/kg)	0.09–0.4
Half-life – normal/ESRF (hrs)	0.01–0.05/ unchanged

Dose in renal impairment GFR (mL/min)

20–50	Dose as in normal renal function
10–20	Dose as in normal renal function
<10	Dose as in normal renal function

Dose in patients undergoing renal replacement therapies

CAPD	Not dialysed. Dose as in normal renal function
HD	Not dialysed. Dose as in normal renal function
CAV/VVHD	Not dialysed. Dose as in normal renal function

Important drug interactions

POTENTIALLY HAZARDOUS INTERACTIONS WITH OTHER DRUGS

- Antidepressants: tricyclics may cause hypertension and arrhythmias. MAOIs may cause hypertensive crisis
- Beta-blockers: can cause severe hypertension
- Other sympathomimetics: dopexamine possibly potentiates effect of noradrenaline

Administration

RECONSTITUTION

–

ROUTE

- IV

RATE OF ADMINISTRATION

- According to response

COMMENTS

- Preferably give centrally (low pH)
- Dilute 1–4 mg in 100 mL glucose 5%. Can be given undiluted

Other information

- Do not mix with alkaline drugs/solutions
- The pharmacokinetics of noradrenaline are not significantly affected by renal or hepatic disease

Nortriptyline

Clinical use

Tricyclic antidepressant

Dose in normal renal function

Depression: initially 25–50 mg daily, increased as necessary to 75–100 mg daily in a single dose or divided doses; (maximum 150 mg daily in hospitalised patients)

Pharmacokinetics

Molecular weight (daltons)	263
% Protein binding	95
% Excreted unchanged in urine	<5
Volume of distribution (L/kg)	15–23
Half-life – normal/ESRF (hrs)	25–60/66–200

Dose in renal impairment GFR (mL/min)

20–50	Dose as in normal renal function
10–20	Dose as in normal renal function
<10	Dose as in normal renal function. Start with small dose

Dose in patients undergoing renal replacement therapies

CAPD	Not dialysed. Dose as in normal renal function
HD	Not dialysed. Dose as in normal renal function
CAV/VVHD	Not dialysed. Dose as in normal renal function

Important drug interactions

POTENTIALLY HAZARDOUS INTERACTIONS WITH OTHER DRUGS

- Alcohol: increased sedative effect
- Anti-arrhythmics: increased risk of ventricular arrhythmias with drugs which prolong QT interval – amiodarone, disopyramide, procainamide and quinidine
- Other antidepressants: CNS excitation and hypertension with MAOIs and linezolid. Do not start tricyclic until 2 weeks after stopping MAOI. Do not start MAOI until at least 1 week after stopping tricyclic
- Anti-epileptics: convulsive threshold lowered
- Antihistamines: increased antimuscarinic and sedative effects. Increased risk of ventricular arrhythmias with terfenadine
- Antihypertensives: hypotensive effect increased. Antagonism of effect of adrenergic neurone blockers and of clonidine. Also increased risk of hypertension on clonidine withdrawal
- Anti-malarials: avoid concomitant use with artemether with lumefantrine
- Antipsychotics: increased risk of ventricular arrhythmias with pimozide or thioridazine
- Beta-blockers: sotalol – increased risk of ventricular arrhythmias
- Sibutramine: increased risk of CNS toxicity – avoid concomitant use
- Sympathomimetics: hypertension and arrhythmias with adrenaline. Hypertension with noradrenaline

Administration

RECONSTITUTION

–

ROUTE

- Oral

RATE OF ADMINISTRATION

–

COMMENTS

–

Other information

- Optimal response to nortriptyline associated with plasma concentrations of 50–150 nanograms/mL
- Recommended measure of plasma levels at doses exceeding 100 mg daily
- All metabolites are highly lipophilic

Nystatin mouthwash (suspension) 100,000 units/mL

Clinical use

Antifungal agent

Dose in normal renal function

1–10 mL four times a day

Pharmacokinetics

Molecular weight (daltons)	926
% Protein binding	–
% Excreted unchanged in urine	–
Volume of distribution (L/kg)	–
Half-life – normal/ESRF (hrs)	–

Dose in renal impairment GFR (mL/min)

20–50	Dose as in normal renal function
10–20	Dose as in normal renal function
<10	Dose as in normal renal function

Dose in patients undergoing renal replacement therapies

CAPD	Not dialysed. Dose as in normal renal function
HD	Not dialysed. Dose as in normal renal function
CAV/VVHD	Not dialysed. Dose as in normal renal function

Important drug interactions

POTENTIALLY HAZARDOUS INTERACTIONS WITH OTHER DRUGS

• None known

Administration

RECONSTITUTION

–

ROUTE

• Oral

RATE OF ADMINISTRATION

–

COMMENTS

–

Other information

• Not absorbed from intact skin or mucous membranes

• No significant GI absorption

Octreotide

Clinical use

Relief of symptoms of gastroenteropancreatic
endocrine tumours and acromegaly

Dose in normal renal function

50–600 micrograms daily

Pharmacokinetics

Molecular weight (daltons)	1019.3
% Protein binding	65
% Excreted unchanged in urine	10
Volume of distribution (L/kg)	0.27
Half-life – normal/ESRF (hrs)	1.25–2.0/ prolonged

Dose in renal impairment
GFR (mL/min)

20–50	Dose as in normal renal function
10–20	Dose as in normal renal function
<10	Dose as in normal renal function

Dose in patients undergoing renal replacement therapies

CAPD	Unknown dialysability. Dose as in normal renal function
HD	Dialysed. Dose as in normal renal function
CAV/VVHD	Unknown dialysability. Dose as in normal renal function

Important drug interactions

POTENTIALLY HAZARDOUS INTERACTIONS WITH OTHER DRUGS

• Ciclosporin: absorption of ciclosporin may be reduced

Administration

RECONSTITUTION

• IV: sodium chloride 0.9% to a ratio of not less than 1:1 and not more than 1:9

ROUTE

• SC, IV

RATE OF ADMINISTRATION

• IV bolus with ECG monitoring

COMMENTS

–

Other information

• SC: to reduce local discomfort, warm to room temperature before injection
• For multiple injections, use different sites
• Patients with reduced renal function have been shown to have a reduced clearance of the drug (75 mL/minute vs 175 mL/minute)

Oestrogen, conjugated (unlicensed drug)

Clinical use

Second-line haemostatic agent for uraemic bleeding

Dose in normal renal function

0.6 mg/kg/day IV for 5 days

Pharmacokinetics

Molecular weight (daltons)	–
% Protein binding	–
% Excreted unchanged in urine	–
Volume of distribution (L/kg)	–
Half-life – normal/ESRF (hrs)	–

Dose in renal impairment GFR (mL/min)

20–50	Dose as in normal renal function
10–20	Dose as in normal renal function
<10	Dose as in normal renal function

Dose in patients undergoing renal replacement therapies

CAPD	Unknown dialysability. Dose as in normal renal function
HD	Unknown dialysability. Dose as in normal renal function
CAV/VVHD	Unknown dialysability. Dose as in normal renal function

Important drug interactions

POTENTIALLY HAZARDOUS INTERACTIONS WITH OTHER DRUGS

- Ciclosporin: plasma concentration of ciclosporin increased
- Anticoagulants: antagonism of anticoagulant effect of warfarin, acenocoumarol and phenindione
- Anti-epileptics: accelerate metabolism

Administration

RECONSTITUTION

- To 50 mL with sodium chloride 0.9%

ROUTE

- IV

RATE OF ADMINISTRATION

- Over a minimum of 30 minutes

COMMENTS

–

Other information

- Duration of effect about 14 days
- Used in association with desmopressin (DDAVP) in intractable cases
- Orally 10–20 mg daily for 5–7 days
- Conjugated oestrogens are a mixture of sodium oestrone sulphate and sodium equilin sulphate and other oestrogenic substances of the type excreted by pregnant mares

Ofloxacin

Clinical use

Antibacterial agent

Dose in normal renal function

Oral: 200–400 mg daily, increased if necessary to 400 mg every 12 hours

IV: 200 mg once or twice daily, increased if necessary to 400 mg every 12 hours

Pharmacokinetics

Molecular weight (daltons)	361.4
% Protein binding	<20
% Excreted unchanged in urine	68–90
Volume of distribution (L/kg)	1.0–2.5
Half-life – normal/ESRF (hrs)	5–8/28–37

Dose in renal impairment GFR (mL/min)

20–50	Give normal loading dose then reduce to 100–200 mg daily
10–20	Give normal loading dose then reduce to 100 mg daily
<10	Give normal loading dose then reduce to 100 mg daily

Dose in patients undergoing renal replacement therapies

CAPD	Not significantly dialysed. Dose as in GFR = <10 mL/min
HD	Dialysed. Dose as in GFR = <10 mL/min
CAV/VVHD	Dialysed. Dose as in GFR = 10–20 mL/min

Important drug interactions

POTENTIALLY HAZARDOUS INTERACTIONS WITH OTHER DRUGS

- Ciclosporin: increased risk of nephrotoxicity
- Anticoagulants: effect of acenocoumarol and warfarin enhanced
- Antidiabetics: effect of sulphonylureas enhanced
- NSAIDs: possibly increased risk of convulsions
- Theophylline: possibly increased risk of convulsions

Administration

RECONSTITUTION

–

ROUTE

- Oral, IV

RATE OF ADMINISTRATION

- IV: 200 mg over 30 minutes

COMMENTS

–

Other information

–

Olanzapine

Clinical use

Schizophrenia, moderate to severe mania

Dose in normal renal function

5–20 mg daily

Pharmacokinetics

Molecular weight (daltons)	312.4
% Protein binding	93
% Excreted unchanged in urine	57 (mainly as metabolites)
Volume of distribution (L/kg)	10–20
Half-life – normal/ESRF (hrs)	30–38/37

Dose in renal impairment GFR (mL/min)

20–50	Initial dose 5 mg daily and titrate as necessary
10–20	Initial dose 5 mg daily and titrate as necessary
<10	Initial dose 5 mg daily and titrate as necessary

Dose in patients undergoing renal replacement therapies

CAPD	Not dialysed. Dose as in GFR = <10 mL/min
HD	Not dialysed. Dose as in GFR = <10 mL/min
CAV/VVHD	Unknown dialysability. Dose as in GFR = 10–20 mL/min

Important drug interactions

POTENTIALLY HAZARDOUS INTERACTIONS WITH OTHER DRUGS

- Anaesthetics: enhanced hypotensive effect
- Analgesics: enhanced sedative and hypotensive effects with opioid analgesics
- Antidepressants: fluvoxamine increases plasma concentration of olanzapine
- Anti-epileptics: antagonism (convulsive threshold lowered). Carbamazepine increases metabolism of olanzapine
- Sibutramine: increased risk of CNS toxicity (avoid concomitant use)
- Anti-malarials: manufacturer advises avoid concomitant use with artemether with lumefantrine

Administration

RECONSTITUTION
–

ROUTE
- Oral

RATE OF ADMINISTRATION
–

COMMENTS
–

Other information

–

Olsalazine

Clinical use

Induction and maintenance of remission in ulcerative colitis

Dose in normal renal function

1–3 g daily

Pharmacokinetics

Molecular weight (daltons)	346.2
% Protein binding	99.8
% Excreted unchanged in urine	<10
Volume of distribution (L/kg)	0.1
Half-life – normal/ESRF (hrs)	1/unchanged

Dose in renal impairment GFR (mL/min)

20–50	Caution – use only if necessary. Start with low dose and increase according to response
10–20	Caution – use only if necessary. Start with low dose and increase according to response
<10	Caution – use only if necessary. Start with low dose and increase according to response

Dose in patients undergoing renal replacement therapies

CAPD	Unlikely dialysability. Dose GFR < 10 mL/min
HD	Unlikely dialysability. Dose GFR < 10 mL/min
CAV/VVHD	Unknown dialysability. Dose GFR = 10–20 mL/min

Important drug interactions

POTENTIALLY HAZARDOUS INTERACTIONS WITH OTHER DRUGS

• None known

Administration

RECONSTITUTION

–

ROUTE

• Oral

RATE OF ADMINISTRATION

–

COMMENTS

–

Other information

• Potential to be nephrotoxic due to 5-aminosalicylic acid (5-ASA) component. Both 5-ASA and its acetylated metabolite are rapidly excreted in the urine
• Less than 3% of an oral dose is absorbed before the drug reaches the colon
• It is unlikely that renal dysfunction will have any important effect on the kinetics of the drug
• The manufacturers recommend that the use of olsalazine in patients with significant renal impairment is contra-indicated due to lack of experience of its use in this patient population

Omeprazole

Clinical use

Gastric acid suppression

Dose in normal renal function

Oral: 10–120 mg daily
Intravenous: 40 mg daily for up to 5 days

Pharmacokinetics

Molecular weight (daltons)	345
% Protein binding	95
% Excreted unchanged in urine	minimal
Volume of distribution (L/kg)	0.3–0.4
Half-life – normal/ESRF (hrs)	1/unchanged

Dose in renal impairment GFR (mL/min)

20–50	Dose as in normal renal function
10–20	Dose as in normal renal function
<10	Dose as in normal renal function

Dose in patients undergoing renal replacement therapies

CAPD	Unlikely dialysability. Dose as in normal renal function
HD	Not dialysed. Dose as in normal renal function
CAV/VVHD	Unknown dialysability. Dose as in normal renal function

Important drug interactions

POTENTIALLY HAZARDOUS INTERACTIONS WITH OTHER DRUGS

- Ciclosporin: variable response. Mostly increase in ciclosporin level
- Warfarin: effects of warfarin enhanced
- Phenytoin: effects of phenytoin enhanced

Administration

RECONSTITUTION

- Reconstitute 40-mg vial with 5 mL water for injection. Add to 100 mL sodium chloride 0.9% or glucose 5%

ROUTE

- Oral, IV

RATE OF ADMINISTRATION

- IV: 40 mg over 20–30 minutes

COMMENTS

- IV dosage: 40 mg (single or divided dose) once or twice daily
- Stable for 12 hours in sodium chloride 0.9% as infusion fluid and 3 hours if in glucose 5%
- Use oral dose as soon as possible

Other information

- Omeprazole clearance is not limited by renal disease

Ondansetron

Clinical use

Anti-emetic

Dose in normal renal function

Oral: 4–24 mg daily
IV: 4–32 mg daily

Pharmacokinetics

Molecular weight (daltons)	365.9
% Protein binding	70–75
% Excreted unchanged in urine	<10
Volume of distribution (L/kg)	2.0–2.6
Half-life – normal/ESRF (hrs)	3.5/5–9

Dose in renal impairment GFR (mL/min)

20–50	Dose as in normal renal function
10–20	Dose as in normal renal function
<10	Dose as in normal renal function

Dose in patients undergoing renal replacement therapies

CAPD	Unlikely dialysability. Dose as in normal renal function
HD	Not dialysed. Dose as in normal renal function
CAV/VVHD	Unknown dialysability. Dose as in normal renal function

Important drug interactions

POTENTIALLY HAZARDOUS INTERACTIONS WITH OTHER DRUGS

• None known

Administration

RECONSTITUTION

–

ROUTE

• Oral, IV, IM, rectal

RATE OF ADMINISTRATION

• IV: bolus over 3–5 minutes. IV infusion: not less than 15 minutes or 1 mg/hour

COMMENTS

• Compatible with sodium chloride 0.9% and glucose 5%

Other information

• Renal clearance of ondansetron is low
• Can be used to treat uraemic pruritis

Orphenadrine

Clinical use

Antimuscarinic used for parkinsonism or drug-induced extrapyramidal symptoms

Dose in normal renal function

150–400 mg daily

Pharmacokinetics

Molecular weight (daltons)	269.4
% Protein binding	95
% Excreted unchanged in urine	8
Volume of distribution (L/kg)	–
Half-life – normal/ESRF (hrs)	14/–

Dose in renal impairment GFR (mL/min)

20–50	Dose as in normal renal function
10–20	Dose as in normal renal function
<10	Dose as in normal renal function

Dose in patients undergoing renal replacement therapies

CAPD	Unknown dialysability. Dose as in normal renal function
HD	Unknown dialysability. Dose as in normal renal function
CAV/VVHD	Unknown dialysability. Dose as in normal renal function

Important drug interactions

POTENTIALLY HAZARDOUS INTERACTIONS WITH OTHER DRUGS

• None known

Administration

RECONSTITUTION

–

ROUTE

• Oral

RATE OF ADMINISTRATION

–

COMMENTS

–

Other information

–

Oseltamivir

Clinical use

Treatment and post-exposure prevention of influenza A and B

Dose in normal renal function

Treatment: 75 mg twice daily for 5 days

Post-exposure prevention: 75 mg daily for at least 7 days, longer if epidemic in community

Pharmacokinetics

Molecular weight (daltons)	410.4
% Protein binding	42 (3 as carboxylate)
% Excreted unchanged in urine	Negligible (excreted as carboxylate metabolite in urine)
Volume of distribution (L/kg)	23 litres
Half-life – normal/ESRF (hrs)	1–3, (6–10 as metabolite)/ increased

Dose in renal impairment GFR (mL/min)

30–50	Dose as in normal renal function
10–30	Treatment: 75 mg once daily; prophylaxis: 75 mg every 48 hours
<10	Use with caution. See 'Other information'

Dose in patients undergoing renal replacement therapies

CAPD	Unknown dialysability. Dose as in GFR = <10 mL/min
HD	Unknown dialysability. Dose as in GFR = <10 mL/min
CAV/VVHD	Unknown dialysability. Dose as in GFR = 10–30 mL/min

Important drug interactions

POTENTIALLY HAZARDOUS INTERACTIONS WITH OTHER DRUGS

• None known

Administration

RECONSTITUTION

–

ROUTE

• Oral

RATE OF ADMINISTRATION

–

COMMENTS

–

Other information

• Oseltamivir is a pro-drug extensively metabolised in the liver to the active carboxylate metabolite

• At least 75% of the oral dose reaches the systemic circulation as the carboxylate

• All the active metabolite is excreted in the urine

• There have been no studies done in renal patients but a lower dose may be required due to the active metabolite accumulating in severe renal disease

Oxaliplatin

Clinical use

Treatment of metastatic colorectal cancer in combination with fluorouracil and folinic acid

Dose in normal renal function

85 mg/m², can be repeated at intervals of 2 weeks if toxicity permits

Pharmacokinetics

Molecular weight (daltons)	397.3
% Protein binding	33
% Excreted unchanged in urine	54
Volume of distribution (L/kg)	330 ± 40.9 litres
Half-life – normal/ESRF (hrs)	273/increased

Dose in renal impairment GFR (mL/min)

20–50	Dose as in normal renal function
10–20	Dose as in normal renal function
<10	No information on use, therefore use with great caution and monitor closely

Dose in patients undergoing renal replacement therapies

CAPD	Unlikely to be dialysed. Dose as in GFR < 10 mL/min
HD	Unlikely to be dialysed. Dose as in GFR < 10 mL/min
CAV/VVHD	Unlikely to be dialysed. Dose as in GFR = 10–20 mL/min

Important drug interactions

POTENTIALLY HAZARDOUS INTERACTIONS WITH OTHER DRUGS

• Antibacterials: aminoglycosides, vancomycin and capreomycin increase risk of nephrotoxicity and possibly ototoxicity

Administration

RECONSTITUTION

• Glucose 5% or water for injection to give a concentration of 5 mg/ml

ROUTE

• IV infusion

RATE OF ADMINISTRATION

• 2–6 hours

COMMENTS

• Dilute with 250–500 mL glucose 5% to a concentration not less than 0.2 mg/ml

Other information

• Binds irreversibly to red blood cells, which can prolong the half-life of the drug
• Administer before 5-fluorouracil
• Reduced renal clearance and Vd in renal impairment
• There is a 38–44% reduction of platinum clearance in moderate to severe renal impairment but no increased incidence of side-effects has been reported
• Massari C et al. (2000) Pharmacokinetics of oxaliplatin in patients with normal versus impaired renal function. Cancer Chemother Pharmacol. 45: 157–64
• Graham M et al. (2001) A phase I study of oxaliplatin in cancer patients with impaired renal function. Proceedings of the American Society of Clinical Oncology. 29: 267. 37th annual meeting of American Society of Clinical Oncology, San Francisco, California, 12–15 May 2001

Oxazepam

Clinical use

Anxiolytic

Dose in normal renal function

15–30 mg three or four times a day

Pharmacokinetics

Molecular weight (daltons)	286.7
% Protein binding	97
% Excreted unchanged in urine	<1
Volume of distribution (L/kg)	0.6–1.6
Half-life – normal/ESRF (hrs)	6–25/25–90

Dose in renal impairment GFR (mL/min)

20–50	Dose as in normal renal function
10–20	Dose as in normal renal function
<10	10–20 mg three or four times a day

Dose in patients undergoing renal replacement therapies

CAPD	Not dialysed. Dose as in GFR = <10 mL/min
HD	Not dialysed. Dose as in GFR = <10 mL/min
CAV/VVHD	Unknown dialysability. Dose as in GFR = 10–20 mL/min

Important drug interactions

POTENTIALLY HAZARDOUS INTERACTIONS WITH OTHER DRUGS

• None known

Administration

RECONSTITUTION

–

ROUTE

• Oral

RATE OF ADMINISTRATION

–

COMMENTS

–

Other information

• Protein binding decreased and Vd increased in ESRD
• Inactive glucuronide metabolite accumulates in ESRD. Significance of this unknown

Oxycodone

Clinical use

Opioid analgesic for moderate to severe pain

Dose in normal renal function

5 mg 4–6-hourly, maximum dose 400 mg daily
M/R: 10 mg 12-hourly, maximum dose 200 mg
12-hourly

Pharmacokinetics

Molecular weight (daltons)	351.8
% Protein binding	38
% Excreted unchanged in urine	<10
Volume of distribution (L/kg)	1.2–6.31
Half-life – normal/ESRF (hrs)	2–3 (4.5, M/R)/ 3–4 (5.5, M/R)

Dose in renal impairment GFR (mL/min)

20–50	Dose as in normal renal function
10–20	Dose as in normal renal function
<10	Avoid, see 'Other information'

Dose in patients undergoing renal replacement therapies

CAPD	Unknown dialysability. Dose as in GFR = <10 mL/min
HD	Unknown dialysability. Dose as in GFR = <10 mL/min
CAV/VVHD	Unknown dialysability. Dose as in GFR = 10–20 mL/min

Important drug interactions

POTENTIALLY HAZARDOUS INTERACTIONS WITH OTHER DRUGS

- Anti-arrhythmics: delayed absorption of mexiletine
- MAOIs: CNS excitation or depression. Avoid concomitant use
- Antipsychotics: enhanced sedative and hypotensive effects
- Ritonavir: possibly increased oxycodone concentration

Administration

RECONSTITUTION

–

ROUTE

- Oral

RATE OF ADMINISTRATION

–

COMMENTS

–

Other information

- Has been used in ESRF patients, start with lowest dose and gradually increase dose according to response
- Recommend only using the normal release capsules and extending the dosing interval as long as may be tolerated
- Limited accumulation in renal failure compared with morphine
- Increased Vd in renal failure
- Kirvela et al. (1996) Journal of Clinical Anaesthesia. 8: 13–18

Oxytetracycline

Clinical use

Anti-bacterial agent

Dose in normal renal function

250–500 mg four times a day

Acne: 500 mg twice daily

Pharmacokinetics

Molecular weight (daltons)	460.4
% Protein binding	10–40
% Excreted unchanged in urine	40–70
Volume of distribution (L/kg)	1.5
Half-life – normal/ESRF (hrs)	6–10/66

Dose in renal impairment GFR (mL/min)

20–50	Dose as in normal renal function
10–20	0.5–1 g daily
<10	0.5–1 g every 48 hours

Dose in patients undergoing renal replacement therapies

CAPD	Not dialysed. Dose as in GFR = <10 mL/min
HD	Not dialysed. Dose as in GFR = <10 mL/min
CAV/VVHD	Unknown dialysability. Dose as in GFR = 10–20 mL/min

Important drug interactions

POTENTIALLY HAZARDOUS INTERACTIONS WITH OTHER DRUGS

- Retinoids: possible increased risk of benign intracranial hypertension with tetracyclines and acitretin, isotretinoin and tretinoin; avoid concomitant use
- Other nephrotoxic drugs: avoid concomitant use
- Methoxyflurane: increased risk of nephrotoxicity

Administration

RECONSTITUTION

–

ROUTE

- Oral

RATE OF ADMINISTRATION

–

COMMENTS

–

Other information

- Avoid, if possible, in renal impairment due to its potential nephrotoxicity and increased risk of azotaemia, hyperphosphataemia and acidosis
- May cause an increase in blood urea which is dose related
- Avoid in SLE

Paclitaxel

Clinical use

Treatment of ovarian and breast cancer and non-small-cell lung carcinoma

Dose in normal renal function

135–175 mg/m² every 3 weeks depending on local regimen and duration of infusion

Pharmacokinetics

Molecular weight (daltons)	853.9
% Protein binding	89–98
% Excreted unchanged in urine	1.3–12.6
Volume of distribution (L/kg)	198–688 L/m²
Half-life – normal/ESRF (hrs)	3–52.7

Dose in renal impairment GFR (mL/min)

20–50	Dose as in normal renal function
10–20	Dose as in normal renal function
<10	Dose as in normal renal function

Dose in patients undergoing renal replacement therapies

CAPD	Unlikely dialysability. Dose as in normal renal function
HD	Not dialysed. Dose as in normal renal function
CAV/VVHD	Unknown dialysability. Dose as in normal renal function

Important drug interactions

POTENTIALLY HAZARDOUS INTERACTIONS WITH OTHER DRUGS

• Antidiabetics: metabolism of rosiglitazone possibly inhibited

Administration

RECONSTITUTION

–

ROUTE

• IV

RATE OF ADMINISTRATION

• 3 or 24 hours depending on regimen

COMMENTS

• Dilute to a concentration of 0.3–1.2 mg/mL with sodium chloride 0.9%, glucose 5%, glucose 5% and sodium chloride 0.9% or glucose 5% in Ringer's injection
• Stable for 27 hours at room temperature

Other information

• Administer through a 0.22-micron in-line filter
• Use non-PVC infusion bags

Pamidronate disodium

Clinical use

Bisphosphonate: hypercalcaemia, bone pain,
Paget's disease

Dose in normal renal function

Bone pain: 90 mg every 4 weeks

Paget's disease: 30 mg weekly for 6 weeks or
30 mg first dose then 60 mg every other week

Hypercalcaemia: depends on serum calcium. These
guidelines are based on data on uncorrected
calcium levels, although corrected calcium values
can also be used

Serum calcium (uncorrected) (mmol/L)	Total dose (mg):
up to 3.0	15–30
3.0–3.5	30–60
3.5–4.0	60–90
>4.0	90

Pharmacokinetics

Molecular weight (daltons)	279
% Protein binding	50
% Excreted unchanged in urine	50
Volume of distribution (L/kg)	0.5–0.6
Half-life – normal/ESRF (hrs)	0.5–27/unchanged

Dose in renal impairment GFR (mL/min)

20–50	Dose as in normal renal function
10–20	Dose as in normal renal function
<10	Serum calcium >4.0 give 60 mg. Serum calcium <4.0 give 30 mg

Dose in patients undergoing renal replacement therapies

CAPD	Unknown dialysability. Dose as in GFR = <10 mL/min
HD	Dialysed. Dose as in GFR = <10 mL/min
CAV/VVHD	Unknown dialysability. Dose as in normal renal function

Important drug interactions

POTENTIALLY HAZARDOUS INTERACTIONS WITH
OTHER DRUGS

• None known

Administration

RECONSTITUTION

• 15 mg in 5 mL water for injection
• 30 or 90 mg in 10 mL water for injection
• Final concentration should not exceed 30 mg per
125 mL sodium chloride 0.9%

ROUTE

• IV

RATE OF ADMINISTRATION

• Maximum 20 mg/hour in patients with impaired
renal function

COMMENTS

–

Other information

• If pamidronate is not excreted adequately kidney
stones may be formed
• In dialysis patients there is increased risk of
asymptomatic hypocalcaemia with 90-mg doses
(anecdotal)

Pancreatin

Clinical use

Pancreatic enzyme replacement

Dose in normal renal function

1–2 capsules with meals, adjust according to response
(1 capsule if using the strong preparation)

Pharmacokinetics

Molecular weight (daltons)	No data
% Protein binding	No data
% Excreted unchanged in urine	No data
Volume of distribution (L/kg)	No data
Half-life – normal/ESRF (hrs)	No data

Dose in renal impairment GFR (mL/min)

20–50	Dose as in normal renal function
10–20	Dose as in normal renal function
<10	Dose as in normal renal function

Dose in patients undergoing renal replacement therapies

CAPD	Unlikely dialysability. Dose as in normal renal function
HD	Unlikely dialysability. Dose as in normal renal function
CAV/VVHD	Unlikely dialysability. Dose as in normal renal function

Important drug interactions

POTENTIALLY HAZARDOUS INTERACTIONS WITH OTHER DRUGS

• None known

Administration

RECONSTITUTION

–

ROUTE

• Oral

RATE OF ADMINISTRATION

–

COMMENTS

–

Other information

• Not absorbed from GI tract

Pancuronium

Clinical use

Non-depolarising muscle relaxant of medium
duration

Dose in normal renal function

Initial dose: 50–100 micrograms/kg

Incremental dose: 10–20 micrograms/kg

Pharmacokinetics

Molecular weight (daltons)	732.7
% Protein binding	80–90
% Excreted unchanged in urine	40
Volume of distribution (L/kg)	0.23
Half-life – normal/ESRF (hrs)	1.5–2.2/4.3–8.2

Dose in renal impairment
GFR (mL/min)

20–50	Dose as in normal renal function
10–20	Initial dose: 10–50 micrograms/kg Incremental dose: 5–10 micrograms/kg
<10	Initial dose: 5–25 micrograms/kg Incremental dose: 2.5–5 micrograms/kg

Dose in patients undergoing renal replacement therapies

CAPD	Unknown dialysability. Dose as in GFR = <10 mL/min
HD	Unknown dialysability. Dose as in GFR = <10 mL/min
CAV/VVHD	Unknown dialysability. Dose as in GFR = 10–20 mL/min

Important drug interactions

POTENTIALLY HAZARDOUS INTERACTIONS WITH
OTHER DRUGS

• Effects enhanced by aminoglycosides, azlocillin,
clindamycin, colistin and piperacillin

• Botulinum toxin: neuromuscular block enhanced
(risk of toxicity)

Administration

RECONSTITUTION

–

ROUTE

• IV

RATE OF ADMINISTRATION

• Bolus

COMMENTS

–

Other information

• Active metabolites accumulate in ESRD; duration
of action prolonged

Pantoprazole

Clinical use

Gastric acid suppression

Dose in normal renal function

Oral: 20–40 mg in the morning for 8 weeks
IV: 40 mg daily

Pharmacokinetics

Molecular weight (daltons)	383.4
% Protein binding	98
% Excreted unchanged in urine	80 (as metabolites)
Volume of distribution (L/kg)	0.15
Half-life – normal/ESRF (hrs)	1/2–3

Dose in renal impairment GFR (mL/min)

20–50	Dose as in normal renal function
10–20	Dose as in normal renal function
<10	Dose as in normal renal function

Dose in patients undergoing renal replacement therapies

CAPD	Not dialysed. Dose as in normal renal function
HD	Not dialysed. Dose as in normal renal function
CAV/VVHD	Unknown dialysability. Dose as in normal renal function

Important drug interactions

POTENTIALLY HAZARDOUS INTERACTIONS WITH OTHER DRUGS

• None known

Administration

RECONSTITUTION

• 10 mL sodium chloride 0.9%

ROUTE

• Oral, IV

RATE OF ADMINISTRATION

• 2–15 minutes

COMMENTS

• Use within 3 hours of reconstitution
• Dilute to 100 mL with sodium chloride 0.9% or glucose 5%

Other information

–

Papaveretum

Higher strength (15.4 mg/mL): 1 mL contains 10 mg anhydrous morphine, 1.2 mg papaverine HCl and 1.04 mg codeine HCl

Clinical use

Opiate analgesia

Dose in normal renal function

0.5–1 mL every 4 hours

Pharmacokinetics

	Papaverine	Morphine	Codeine
Molecular weight (daltons)	339	375.8	372
% Protein binding	87	25–35	7
% Excreted unchanged in urine	<1	10	<5
Volume of distribution (L/kg)	0.99–1.52	3.5	3–4
Half-life – normal/ESRF (hrs)	1.5–2.2/–	1–7/ unchanged	2.5–3.5/–

Dose in renal impairment GFR (mL/min)

20–50	Dose as in normal renal function
10–20	0.4–0.75 mL every 6–8 hours
<10	0.25–0.5 mL every 6–8 hours. Avoid if possible

Dose in patients undergoing renal replacement therapies

CAPD	Unknown dialysability. Dose as in GFR = <10 mL/min
HD	Unknown dialysability. Dose as in GFR = <10 mL/min
CAV/VVHD	Unknown dialysability. Dose as in GFR = 10–20 mL/min

Important drug interactions

POTENTIALLY HAZARDOUS INTERACTIONS WITH OTHER DRUGS

- Avoid use with MAOIs
- Hyperpyrexia and CNS toxicity reported with selegiline
- Anti-arrhythmics: delayed absorption of mexiletine
- Antipsychotics: enhanced sedative and hypotensive effect

Administration

RECONSTITUTION

–

ROUTE

- SC or IM or IV

RATE OF ADMINISTRATION

- IV bolus or continuous infusion (1 mg/mL)

COMMENTS

- In general IV dose should be a quarter to half corresponding SC or IM dose

Other information

- As with all opiates, use with extreme caution in patients with impaired renal function
- May cause excessive sedation and respiratory depression
- Contra-indicated in women of child-bearing potential if preparation used contains noscapine (Omnopon)
- Papaveretum 15.4 mg = 1 mL = 10 mg morphine
- Papaveretum paediatric 7.7 mg = 1 mL = 5 mg morphine

Paracetamol

Clinical use

Analgesia and antipyretic

Dose in normal renal function

500 mg – 1 g every 4–6 hours

Pharmacokinetics

Molecular weight (daltons)	151
% Protein binding	20–30
% Excreted unchanged in urine	1–4
Volume of distribution (L/kg)	0.9–1.0
Half-life – normal/ESRF (hrs)	2/unchanged

Dose in renal impairment GFR (mL/min)

20–50	Dose as in normal renal function
10–20	Dose as in normal renal function
<10	500 mg – 1 g every 6–8 hours

Dose in patients undergoing renal replacement therapies

CAPD	Not dialysed. Dose as in GFR = <10 mL/min
HD	Dialysed. Dose as in GFR = <10 mL/min
CAV/VVHD	Unknown dialysability. Dose as in normal renal function

Important drug interactions

POTENTIALLY HAZARDOUS INTERACTIONS WITH OTHER DRUGS

• None known

Administration

RECONSTITUTION

–

ROUTE

• Oral, rectal

RATE OF ADMINISTRATION

–

COMMENTS

–

Other information

• Beware sodium content of soluble tablets (1 tablet ≡ 18.6 mmol sodium)
• Nephrotoxic in overdoses due to a reactive alkylating metabolite
• Metabolites may accumulate in ESRD. Normal doses are very often used in ESRD

Paroxetine

Clinical use

Antidepressant, panic disorders

Dose in normal renal function

Initially 20 mg daily. May be increased by 10-mg increments to a maximum of 50 mg daily

Pharmacokinetics

Molecular weight (daltons)	365.8
% Protein binding	95
% Excreted unchanged in urine	<2
Volume of distribution (L/kg)	17.2
Half-life – normal/ESRF (hrs)	24/30

Dose in renal impairment GFR (mL/min)

10–30	20 mg daily
<10	20 mg daily

Dose in patients undergoing renal replacement therapies

CAPD	Unlikely dialysability. Dose as in GFR = <10 mL/min
HD	Not dialysed. Dose as in GFR = <10 mL/min
CAV/VVHD	Unknown dialysability. Dose as for GFR = 10–30 mL/min

Important drug interactions

POTENTIALLY HAZARDOUS INTERACTIONS WITH OTHER DRUGS

- Anticoagulants: effect of acenocoumarol and warfarin possibly enhanced
- MAOIs: paroxetine should not be started until 2 weeks after stopping MAOI. Conversely, MAOI must not be started until 2 weeks after stopping paroxetine
- Phenytoin and possibly other anti-epileptics reduce plasma levels of paroxetine
- 5HT$_1$ agonists: risk of CNS toxicity increased by sumatriptan (avoid concomitant use)
- Lithium: increased risk of CNS effects (monitor levels)
- Tramadol: increased risk of CNS toxicity
- Antipsychotics: plasma concentration of clozapine increased
- Ritonavir: increased plasma concentration of paroxetine
- Selegilene: hypertension and CNS excitation

Administration

RECONSTITUTION

–

ROUTE

- Oral

RATE OF ADMINISTRATION

–

COMMENTS

–

Other information

- Incremental dosage, if required, should be restricted to lower end of range in patients with CL$_{CR}$ <30 mL/minute

Peginterferon alfa

Clinical use

Treatment of chronic hepatitis C infection with or without ribavirin

Dose in normal renal function

ViraferonPeg: 1.5 micrograms/kg once weekly in combination with ribavirin. Monotherapy: 0.5–1 microgram/kg once weekly
Pegasys: 180 micrograms weekly

Pharmacokinetics

Molecular weight (daltons)	40,000
% Protein binding	–
% Excreted unchanged in urine	30
Volume of distribution (L/kg)	0.99
Half-life – normal/ESRF (hrs)	40–130/increased by about 25–45%

Dose in renal impairment GFR (mL/min)

20–50	Dose as in normal renal function. See 'Other information'
10–20	135 micrograms (Pegasys) once weekly. See 'Other information'
<10	135 micrograms (Pegasys) once weekly. See 'Other information'

Dose in patients undergoing renal replacement therapies

CAPD	Unknown dialysability. Dose as in GFR = <10 mL/min
HD	Dialysed. Dose as in GFR = <10 mL/min
CAV/VVHD	Unknown dialysability. Dose as in GFR = 10–20 mL/min

Important drug interactions

POTENTIALLY HAZARDOUS INTERACTIONS WITH OTHER DRUGS

• Theophylline: inhibits metabolism of theophylline (enhanced effect)

Administration

RECONSTITUTION

• 0.7 mL water for injection or pre-filled syringes

ROUTE

• SC

RATE OF ADMINISTRATION

–

COMMENTS

• Stable for 24 hours at 2–8°C after reconstitution

Other information

• Administer 12 hours after haemodialysis
• ViraferonPeg is contra-indicated once GFR < 50 mL/min
• Monitor closely and reduce dose if required
• In haemodialysis patients, 135 micrograms Pegasys is equivalent to a 180 micrograms dose in the general population
• The kidneys account for approximately 30% of the total clearance of pegylated interferon
• In patients with ESRD undergoing haemodialysis there is a 25–45% reduction in clearance compared with patients with normal renal function

Penicillamine

Clinical use

Rheumatoid arthritis

Dose in normal renal function

125–250 mg daily for first month. Increase by the same amount every 4–12 weeks until remission occurs

Pharmacokinetics

Molecular weight (daltons)	149.2
% Protein binding	80
% Excreted unchanged in urine	10–40
Volume of distribution (L/kg)	0.8
Half-life – normal/ESRF (hrs)	1.5–3/increased

Dose in renal impairment
GFR (mL/min)

20–50	Avoid if possible or reduce dose. 50–125 mg for first 4–8 weeks. Increase by same amount every 4 weeks to a maximum of 1 g daily
10–20	Avoid – nephrotoxic
<10	Avoid – nephrotoxic

Dose in patients undergoing renal replacement therapies

CAPD	Unknown dialysability. Avoid – nephrotoxic
HD	Dialysed. 125–250 mg three times a week after HD
CAV/VVHD	Unknown dialysability. Avoid – nephrotoxic

Important drug interactions

POTENTIALLY HAZARDOUS INTERACTIONS WITH OTHER DRUGS

• None known

Administration

RECONSTITUTION
–

ROUTE

• Oral

RATE OF ADMINISTRATION
–

COMMENTS
–

Other information

• Proteinuria occurs frequently and is partially dose-related. In some patients it may progress to glomerulonephritis or nephrotic syndrome
• Urinalysis should be carried out weekly for the first 2 months of treatment, after any change in dosage and monthly thereafter. Increasing proteinuria may necessitate withdrawal of treatment

Pentamidine

Clinical use

Antibacterial agent. PCP, treatment and prophylaxis

Dose in normal renal function

Nebuliser: 600 mg daily for 3 weeks, then 300 mg every 4 weeks

IV: 4 mg/kg/day for at least 14 days

Pharmacokinetics

Molecular weight (daltons)	340
% Protein binding	69
% Excreted unchanged in urine	<20
Volume of distribution (L/kg)	7–25
Half-life – normal/ESRF (hrs)	6–29/52–118

Dose in renal impairment GFR (mL/min)

20–50	Dose as in normal renal function
10–20	Dose as in normal renal function
<10	Depending on severity of infection: 4 mg/kg/day IV for 7–10 days, then on alternate days to complete minimum 14 doses, or 4 mg/kg on alternate days to complete minimum 14 doses

Dose in patients undergoing renal replacement therapies

CAPD	Not dialysed. Dose as in GFR = <10 mL/min
HD	Not dialysed. Dose as in GFR = <10 mL/min
CAV/VVHD	Unknown dialysability. Dose as in GFR = 10–20 mL/min

Important drug interactions

POTENTIALLY HAZARDOUS INTERACTIONS WITH OTHER DRUGS

- Anti-arrhythmics: increased risk of ventricular arrhythmias with amiodarone
- Antihistamines: increased risk of ventricular arrhythmias with terfenadine
- Antipsychotics: increased risk of ventricular arrhythmias with thioridazine – avoid concomitant use

Administration

RECONSTITUTION

- IV: reconstitute 600 mg with 6 mL water for injection then dilute calculated dose in 50–250 mL sodium chloride 0.9% or glucose 5%
- IM: dilute 300 mg with 3 mL water for injection

ROUTE

- IV, IM, nebulised

RATE OF ADMINISTRATION

- IV: 1 hour

COMMENTS

- Monitor patients closely

Other information

- Patient must be lying down when drug is administered
- If given by IV infusion, patient should be monitored **closely**: heart rate, BP, blood glucose
- IV prophylaxis (unlicensed): 4–5 mg/kg over a minimum of 1 hour every 4 weeks
- Nebulise over 20 minutes using Respigard II or other suitable nebuliser, oxygen flow rate 6–10 L/minute
- 5 mg nebulised salbutamol may be given prior to pentamidine nebulisation to reduce risk of bronchospasm. Do not mix together in nebuliser
- May produce reversible impairment of renal function
- Renal clearance accounts for <5% of the plasma clearance of pentamidine

Perindopril

Clinical use

ACE inhibitor: hypertension, heart failure

Dose in normal renal function

2–8 mg daily

Pharmacokinetics

Molecular weight (daltons)	368.5
% Protein binding	10–20
% Excreted unchanged in urine	80–90
Volume of distribution (L/kg)	0.21
Half-life – normal/ESRF (hrs)	11/26–36

Dose in renal impairment GFR (mL/min)

30–60	2 mg daily
15–30	2 mg alternate days
<15	2 mg alternate days, adjust according to BP response

Dose in patients undergoing renal replacement therapies

CAPD	Unknown dialysability. Dose as in GFR = <15 mL/min
HD	Dialysed. Dose as in GFR = <15 mL/min
CAV/VVHD	Dialysed. Dose as in GFR = 15–30 mL/min

Important drug interactions

POTENTIALLY HAZARDOUS INTERACTIONS WITH OTHER DRUGS

- Ciclosporin: increased risk of hyperkalaemia
- NSAIDs: antagonism of hypotensive effect, increased risk of renal impairment and hyperkalaemia
- Epoetin: antagonism of hypotensive effect, increased risk of hyperkalaemia
- Lithium: increased lithium levels
- Potassium salts: increased risk of hyperkalaemia
- Anaesthetics: enhanced hypotensive effect
- Diuretics: enhanced hypotensive effect; increased risk of hyperkalaemia with potassium-sparing diuretics

Administration

RECONSTITUTION

–

ROUTE

- Oral

RATE OF ADMINISTRATION

–

COMMENTS

–

Other information

- Titrate dose according to response. Normal doses have been used in ESRF
- Small Vd due to low lipophilicity
- Close monitoring of renal function during therapy is necessary in those with renal insufficiency
- Renal failure has been reported in association with ACE inhibitors in patients with renal artery stenosis, post renal transplant and those with severe congestive heart failure
- A high incidence of anaphylactoid reactions has been reported in patients dialysed with high-flux polyacrylonitrile membranes and treated concomitantly with an ACE inhibitor – this combination should therefore be avoided
- Hyperkalaemia and other side-effects are more common in patients with renal impairment

Pethidine

Clinical use

Opiate analgesia

Dose in normal renal function

IV: 25–50 mg every 4 hours
Oral: 50–150 mg every 4 hours
SC, IM: 25–100 mg every 4 hours

Pharmacokinetics

Molecular weight (daltons)	284
% Protein binding	60–80
% Excreted unchanged in urine	0.6–27 depending on urinary pH
Volume of distribution (L/kg)	4–5
Half-life – normal/ESRF (hrs)	2–7/7–32

Dose in renal impairment GFR (mL/min)

20–50	Dose as in normal renal function
10–20	Use small doses. Increase dosing interval to 6 hours and decrease dose by 25%
<10	Avoid if possible. If not, use small doses. Increase dosing interval to 8 hours and decrease dose by 50%

Dose in patients undergoing renal replacement therapies

CAPD	Unknown dialysability. Dose as in GFR = <10 mL/min
HD	Not dialysed. Dose as in GFR = <10 mL/min
CAV/VVHD	Unlikely dialysability. Dose as in GFR = 10–20 mL/min

Important drug interactions

POTENTIALLY HAZARDOUS INTERACTIONS WITH OTHER DRUGS

• Avoid use with MAOIs
• Cimetidine: increases plasma concentration
• Hyperpyrexia and CNS toxicity reported with selegiline
• Anti-arrhythmics: delayed absorption of mexiletine
• Antipsychotics: enhanced sedative and hypotensive effects
• Ritonavir: increased pethidine concentration

Administration

RECONSTITUTION
–

ROUTE
• IV, oral, SC or IM

RATE OF ADMINISTRATION
• IV: bolus 3–4 minutes

COMMENTS
–

Other information

• Risk of CNS and respiratory depression or convulsions, particularly in ESRD patients receiving regular doses, due to accumulation of active metabolite, norpethidine. Norpethidine levels can be measured

Phenelzine

Clinical use

Antidepressant (MAOI)

Dose in normal renal function

15 mg three times daily. Maximum: 30 mg three times daily

Pharmacokinetics

Molecular weight (daltons)	136
% Protein binding	–
% Excreted unchanged in urine	0.25–1.1
Volume of distribution (L/kg)	–
Half-life – normal/ESRF (hrs)	1.5–4/–

Dose in renal impairment GFR (mL/min)

20–50	Dose as in normal renal function
10–20	Dose as in normal renal function
<10	Dose as in normal renal function

Dose in patients undergoing renal replacement therapies

CAPD	Unknown dialysability. Dose as in normal renal function
HD	Unknown dialysability. Dose as in normal renal function
CAV/VVHD	Unknown dialysability. Dose as in normal renal function

Important drug interactions

POTENTIALLY HAZARDOUS INTERACTIONS WITH OTHER DRUGS

• Alcohol: some alcoholic and de-alcoholised drinks contain tyramine which can cause hypertensive crisis
• Analgesics: CNS excitation or depression (hyper- or hypotension) with pethidine, other opioids and nefopam
• Other antidepressants: enhancement of CNS effects and toxicity. Care with all antidepressants including drug-free periods when changing therapies
• Anti-epileptics: antagonism of anticonvulsant effect (convulsive threshold lowered). Avoid carbamazepine with or within 2 weeks of MAOIs
• Antihypertensives: hypotensive effects enhanced. Avoid indoramin
• Antipsychotics: CNS excitation and hypertension with clozapine
• Dopaminergics: hypertensive crisis with levodopa (avoid for at least 2 weeks after stopping MAOI), hypotension with selegiline
• 5HT$_1$ agonists: risk of CNS toxicity (avoid sumatriptan and rizatriptan for 2 weeks after MAOI)
• Sympathomimetics: hypertensive crisis with, for example: dexamphetamine, dexfenfluramine, and other amphetamines; dopamine, dopexamine, ephedrine, phentermine, phenylephrine, propanolamine and pseudoephedrine
• Bupropion: avoid with or for 2 weeks after MAOIs
• Sibutramine: increased risk of CNS toxicity – avoid concomitant use
• Tetrabenazine: CNS excitation and hypertension

Administration

RECONSTITUTION
–
ROUTE
• Oral
RATE OF ADMINISTRATION
–
COMMENTS
–

Other information

–

Phenindione

Clinical use

Anticoagulant

Dose in normal renal function

Day 1: 200 mg

Day 2: 100 mg

Day 3 onwards: according to INR

Pharmacokinetics

Molecular weight (daltons)	222.2
% Protein binding	>97
% Excreted unchanged in urine	–
Volume of distribution (L/kg)	–
Half-life – normal/ESRF (hrs)	5–6/–

Dose in renal impairment GFR (mL/min)

20–50	Dose as in normal renal function
10–20	Dose as in normal renal function
<10	Dose as in normal renal function

Dose in patients undergoing renal replacement therapies

CAPD	Unknown dialysability. Dose as in normal renal function
HD	Unknown dialysability. Dose as in normal renal function
CAV/VVHD	Unknown dialysability. Dose as in normal renal function

Important drug interactions

POTENTIALLY HAZARDOUS INTERACTIONS WITH OTHER DRUGS

• Analgesics: anticoagulant effect enhanced by aspirin; increased risk of haemorrhage with parenteral diclofenac and ketorolac (avoid concomitant use)

• Antiplatelets: anticoagulant effect enhanced by aspirin and dipyridamole

• Clofibrates: enhance anticoagulant effect

• Sex hormones: anticoagulant effect antagonised by oral contraceptives

• Thyroxine: enhanced anticoagulant effect

• Vitamin K: anticoagulant effect reduced

• Anti-arrhythmics: metabolism inhibited by amiodarone

• Antivirals: ritonavir possibly increases plasma concentration

Administration

RECONSTITUTION

–

ROUTE

• Oral

RATE OF ADMINISTRATION

–

COMMENTS

–

Other information

• Titrate dose to end point INR

• Enhanced anticoagulant effect in renal impairment, due to reduced protein binding

• Metabolites of phenindione often colour the urine pink or orange

Phenobarbital (phenobarbitone)

Clinical use

Anti-epileptic agent

Dose in normal renal function

Oral: 60–180 mg at night or 50–100 mg 8–12 hourly

IM: 200 mg repeated after 6 hours if required

Status epilepticus: 10 mg/kg, max 1 g

Pharmacokinetics

Molecular weight (daltons)	232.2 (254.2 as sodium salt)
% Protein binding	15–60
% Excreted unchanged in urine	20–25
Volume of distribution (L/kg)	0.7–1.0
Half-life – normal/ESRF (hrs)	60–150/117–160

Dose in renal impairment GFR (mL/min)

20–50	Dose as in normal renal function
10–20	Dose as in normal renal function, but avoid very large doses
<10	Reduce dose by 25–50% and avoid very large single doses

Dose in patients undergoing renal replacement therapies

CAPD	Dialysed. Dose as in GFR < 10 mL/min
HD	Dialysed. Dose as in GFR < 10 mL/min
CAV/VVHD	Not dialysed. Dose as in GFR = 10–20 mL/min

Important drug interactions

POTENTIALLY HAZARDOUS INTERACTIONS WITH OTHER DRUGS

• Ciclosporin: reduces ciclosporin blood levels
• Anticoagulants: increased metabolism (reduced effect)
• Antidepressants: antagonise anticonvulsant effect. Metabolism of mianserin and some tricyclics accelerated, reduced effect. St John's Wort reduces phenobarbital level

• Antifungals: phenobarbital possibly reduces plasma concentration of voriconazole, avoid concomitant use. Reduces absorption of griseofulvin, reduced effect
• Antipsychotics: antagonise anticonvulsant effect. Phenobarbital accelerates metabolism of haloperidol
• Antivirals: plasma concentration of indinavir, lopinavir, nelfinavir and saquinavir possibly reduced
• Calcium-channel blockers: effect of felodipine, isradipine and probably nicardipine, nifedipine and other dihydropyridines, diltiazem and verapamil reduced
• Corticosteroids: metabolism of corticosteroids accelerated, reduced effect
• Oestrogens and progestogens: metabolism of gestrinone, tibolone and oral contraceptives accelerated, reduced contraceptive effect

Administration

RECONSTITUTION

–

ROUTE

• IV, IM or oral

RATE OF ADMINISTRATION

• IV: not more than 100 mg/min

COMMENTS

• For IV administration dilute injection 1 in 10 with water for injections

Other information

• Aim for plasma concentration of 15–40 mg/L (60–80 µmol/L) for optimum response
• May cause excessive sedation and increased osteomalacia in ESRD
• Charcoal haemoperfusion and haemodialysis more effective than peritoneal dialysis for poisoning
• Up to 50% unchanged drug excreted in urine with alkaline diuresis

Phenoxymethylpenicillin (penicillin V)

Clinical use

Antibacterial agent

Dose in normal renal function

500–1000 mg every 6 hours

Pharmacokinetics

Molecular weight (daltons)	350
% Protein binding	80
% Excreted unchanged in urine	60–90
Volume of distribution (L/kg)	0.2
Half-life – normal/ESRF (hrs)	0.5–1/4

Dose in renal impairment GFR (mL/min)

20–50	Dose as in normal renal function
10–20	Dose as in normal renal function
<10	Dose as in normal renal function

Dose in patients undergoing renal replacement therapies

CAPD	Dialysed. Dose as in normal renal function
HD	Dialysed. Dose as in normal renal function
CAV/VVHD	Dialysed. Dose as in normal renal function

Important drug interactions

POTENTIALLY HAZARDOUS INTERACTIONS WITH OTHER DRUGS

• Reduces excretion of methotrexate

Administration

RECONSTITUTION

–

ROUTE

• Oral

RATE OF ADMINISTRATION

–

COMMENTS

–

Other information

• Potassium salt may produce hyperkalaemia. 250 mg tablet contains 28 mg potassium

• Renal failure prolongs half-life of phenoxymethylpenicillin, but as it has a wide therapeutic index no dose adjustment is necessary

Phentolamine

Clinical use

Alpha-adrenoceptor blocker: hypertensive crisis

Dose in normal renal function

2–60 mg daily

Pharmacokinetics

Molecular weight (daltons)	281
% Protein binding	54
% Excreted unchanged in urine	13
Volume of distribution (L/kg)	–
Half-life – normal/ESRF (hrs)	1.5/–

Dose in renal impairment GFR (mL/min)

20–50	Dose as in normal renal function
10–20	Dose as in normal renal function
<10	Dose as in normal renal function. Titrate dose to end point, i.e. lower BP

Dose in patients undergoing renal replacement therapies

CAPD	Unknown dialysability. Dose as in normal renal function
HD	Unknown dialysability. Dose as in normal renal function
CAV/VVHD	Unknown dialysability. Dose as in normal renal function

Important drug interactions

POTENTIALLY HAZARDOUS INTERACTIONS WITH OTHER DRUGS

- Anaesthetics: enhanced hypotensive effect
- Antidepressants: additive hypotensive effect
- Linezolid: additive hypotensive effect
- Antihypertensives: enhanced hypotensive effect
- Diuretics: enhanced hypotensive effect
- Moxisylyte: possibly severe postural hypotension

Administration

RECONSTITUTION

- Glucose 5% or sodium chloride 0.9%

ROUTE

- IV, IM

RATE OF ADMINISTRATION

- IV bolus: 2–5 mg, repeat if necessary
- IV infusion: 5–60 mg over 10–30 minutes (rate 0.2–2 mg/minute)
- IM bolus: 5–10 mg

COMMENTS

–

Other information

- Titrate according to response
- May increase initial infusion dose to 5 mg/minute for more rapid response

Phenytoin

Clinical use

Anti-epileptic agent

Dose in normal renal function

Oral: 150–600 mg/day or 3–4 mg/kg/day

Pharmacokinetics

Molecular weight (daltons)	252
% Protein binding	90
% Excreted unchanged in urine	up to 5
Volume of distribution (L/kg)	0.7–1.0
Half-life – normal/ESRF (hrs)	10–40/unchanged

Dose in renal impairment GFR (mL/min)

20–50	Dose as in normal renal function
10–20	Dose as in normal renal function
<10	Dose as in normal renal function

Dose in patients undergoing renal replacement therapies

CAPD	Not dialysed. Dose as in normal renal function
HD	Not dialysed. Dose as in normal renal function
CAV/VVHD	Unknown dialysability. Dose as in normal renal function

Important drug interactions

POTENTIALLY HAZARDOUS INTERACTIONS WITH OTHER DRUGS

- Ciclosporin: reduces ciclosporin blood levels
- Analgesics: some NSAIDs increase phenytoin levels
- Anti-arrhythmics: amiodarone increases phenytoin levels. Phenytoin reduces levels of disopyramide, mexiletine and quinidine
- Antibacterials: level increased by chloramphenicol, isoniazid, metronidazole, co-trimoxazole and trimethoprim (increased antifolate effect); levels reduced by rifampicin
- Anticoagulants: increased metabolism (reduced effect)
- Antidepressants: antagonise anticonvulsant effect, fluoxetine and fluvoxamine increase phenytoin level. St John's Wort reduces phenytoin level
- Anti-epileptics: toxicity may be increased without enhanced effect
- Antifungals: levels increased by fluconazole and miconazole. Levels decreased by itraconazole and ketoconazole
- Anti-malarials: antagonise anticonvulsant effect; increased antifolate effect with pyrimethamine
- Antipsychotics: antagonise anticonvulsant effect
- Calcium-channel blockers: levels increased by diltiazem and nifedipine
- Corticosteroids: metabolism accelerated (effect reduced)
- Disulfiram: levels of phenytoin increased
- Sex hormones: metabolism increased – reduced contraceptive effect
- Ulcer-healing drugs: cimetidine inhibits phenytoin metabolism; sucralfate reduces absorption; omeprazole enhances effect of phenytoin
- Uricosurics: sulfinpyrazone increases serum phenytoin levels
- Antivirals: levels possibly reduced by indinavir, lopinavir, nelfinavir and saquinavir. Levels reduced by zidovudine

Administration

RECONSTITUTION

- Dilute in 50–100 mL sodium chloride 0.9%. Final concentration not exceeding 10 mg/mL

ROUTE

- IV, oral

RATE OF ADMINISTRATION

- IV bolus: not greater than 50 mg/minute
- IV infusion: 50–100 mL over 1 hour

COMMENTS

- Give by slow IV injection into large vein followed by sodium chloride 0.9% flush, to avoid irritation. Cardiac monitoring recommended
- With infusion a 0.22–0.5 micron in-line filter should be used

Other information

- Total phenytoin levels must be adjusted for hypoalbuminaemia and uraemia
- Decreased protein binding and Vd in renal failure

- Some useful equations:
  - to correct a phenytoin concentration for low albumin:

$$\text{corrected concentration} = \frac{\text{observed concentration}}{(0.02 \times \text{albumin}) + 0.1}$$

  - to correct for renal failure:

$$\text{corrected concentration} = \frac{\text{observed concentration}}{(0.01 \text{ albumin}) + 0.1}$$

  - from Winters ME (1994) *Basic Clinical Pharmacokinetics* (3e):

$$C_{normal} = \frac{C_{observed}}{[(0.48)(1-0.1) \dfrac{patient's\ albumin]}{4.4\ g/dL} + 0.1}$$

- Free fraction of phenytoin is increased in uraemia to approximately 0.2
- Request **free** phenytoin serum levels, if possible
- Loading dose 15 mg/kg IV or oral, then 5 mg/kg/day. Steady state reached in 3–5 days if loading dose given
- Increase dose gradually (25–50 mg/day at weekly intervals). Demonstrates saturation kinetics
- Phenytoin absorption is markedly reduced by concurrent naso-gastric enteral nutrition administration. Avoid concomitant administration with divalent cations
- May cause folate deficiency

Phosphate supplements

Clinical use

Hypophosphataemia

Dose in normal renal function

Oral: according to response. Maximum oral
dose = 100 mmol in 24 hours

IV: 10–50 mmol/day

Pharmacokinetics

Molecular weight (daltons) (phosphate)	94–97
% Protein binding	–
% Excreted unchanged in urine	High
Volume of distribution (L/kg)	–
Half-life – normal/ESRF (hrs)	–

Dose in renal impairment GFR (mL/min)

20–50	Dose as in normal renal function
10–20	Dose as in normal renal function
<10	Start at one-third of normal dose

Dose in patients undergoing renal replacement therapies

CAPD	Unknown dialysability. Dose as in GFR = <10 mL/min
HD	Not dialysed. Dose as in GFR = <10 mL/min
CAV/VVHD	Dialysed. Dose as in GFR = 10–20 mL/min

Important drug interactions

POTENTIALLY HAZARDOUS INTERACTIONS WITH
OTHER DRUGS

• Avoid insoluble incompatibilities, e.g. calcium salts

Administration

RECONSTITUTION

• Phosphate Polyfusor: give undiluted over
24 hours peripherally

• Addiphos: give each vial (20 mL) diluted to
250–500 mL with glucose 5% over 6–12 hours
peripherally; 20-mL vial made up to 60 mL with
glucose 5% centrally over 6–8 hours via syringe
driver

• Potassium phosphate: each 5-mL ampoule should
be diluted to at least 100 mL with glucose 5%
and given over at least one hour

ROUTE

• IV, oral

RATE OF ADMINISTRATION

• See under 'Reconstitution'

COMMENTS

–

Other information

• Oral dosing: maximum oral dose 100 mmol
phosphate in 24 hours. (i) slow phosphate tablet
(unlicensed product from Ciba) – 3.16 mmol
phosphate/tablet. (ii) Phosphate Sandoz –
16.1 mmol phosphate, 20.4 mmol sodium,
3 mmol potassium/tablet

• IV dosing: (i) Phosphate Polyfusor (500 mL)
containing: 50 mmol phosphate, 81 mmol sodium,
9.5 mmol potassium. (ii) Addiphos (20 mL)
containing: 40 mmol phosphate, 30 mmol sodium,
30 mmol potassium. (iii) Potassium phosphate
8.71% (10 mL) containing: 10 mmol potassium,
5 mmol phosphate. NB: this preparation should
only be used for patients with a high sodium
level. Available from Martindale Pharmaceuticals

• HD patients usually need 15–20 mmol/day in
TPN

• CAV/VVHD patients usually need
30–40 mmol/day

• During IV phosphate replacement, serum
calcium, potassium and phosphate should be
monitored 6–12-hourly to determine the rate of
duration of the infusion. Repeat the dose within
24 hours if an adequate level has not been
achieved. Urinary output should also be
monitored. Excessive doses of phosphates may
cause hypocalcaemia and metastatic calcification

• There is experience giving 15 mmol over 2 hours
up to three times a day

Phytomenadione (vitamin K₁)

Clinical use

Vitamin K deficiency, antidote to oral anticoagulants

Dose in normal renal function

Oral: 10–20 mg daily
IV: 10–40 mg daily

Pharmacokinetics

Molecular weight (daltons)	451
% Protein binding	90
% Excreted unchanged in urine	<10
Volume of distribution (L/kg)	0.05–0.13
Half-life – normal/ESRF (hrs)	1.5–3/unchanged

Dose in renal impairment GFR (mL/min)

20–50	Dose as in normal renal function
10–20	Dose as in normal renal function
<10	Dose as in normal renal function

Dose in patients undergoing renal replacement therapies

CAPD	Unlikely to be dialysed. Dose as in normal renal function
HD	Unlikely to be dialysed. Dose as in normal renal function
CAV/VVHD	Unlikely to be dialysed. Dose as in normal renal function

Important drug interactions

POTENTIALLY HAZARDOUS INTERACTIONS WITH OTHER DRUGS

• Antagonises effect of warfarin, acenocoumarol and phenindione

Administration

RECONSTITUTION

–

ROUTE

• IV, IM, oral

RATE OF ADMINISTRATION

• Konakion – very slow injection (1 mg/min). Konakion MM – dilute each 10 mg with 55 mL of glucose 5% and give by slow infusion over 15–30 minutes

COMMENTS

• Dissolve oral tablets in mouth
• Risk of anaphylaxis if IV injected too rapidly
• Protect infusion from light
• Konakion should not be diluted (non-micellar)
• Only Konakion can be given IM

Other information

• Konakion MM recommended for severe haemorrhage
• Anticoagulation antidote: retest prothrombin time 8–12 hours after Konakion, 3 hours after Konakion MM. Repeat dose if inadequate
• Patients with obstructive jaundice requiring oral phytomenadione should be prescribed the water soluble preparation menadiol sodium diphosphate – dosage range is similar

Pimozide

Clinical use

Antipsychotic

Dose in normal renal function

2–20 mg daily

Pharmacokinetics

Molecular weight (daltons)	461.6
% Protein binding	99
% Excreted unchanged in urine	<1
Volume of distribution (L/kg)	–
Half-life – normal/ESRF (hrs)	55–150/–

Dose in renal impairment GFR (mL/min)

20–50	Dose as in normal renal function
10–20	Dose as in normal renal function
<10	Start with half normal dose

Dose in patients undergoing renal replacement therapies

CAPD	Unknown dialysability. Dose as in GFR = <10 mL/min
HD	Unknown dialysability. Dose as in GFR = <10 mL/min
CAV/VVHD	Unknown dialysability. Dose as in normal renal function

Important drug interactions

POTENTIALLY HAZARDOUS INTERACTIONS WITH OTHER DRUGS

- Do not give with other antipsychotic drugs (including depots) or tricyclic antidepressants which can prolong the QT interval
- Risk of arrhythmias if clarithromycin and possibly erythromycin co-administered
- Do not give with drugs which can cause electrolyte disturbances (especially diuretics)
- Concurrent use of drugs which can prolong the QT interval are not recommended: antifungals, antivirals, quinine, mefloquine, amiodarone, bretylium, disopyramide, procainamide, quinidine, sotalol, terfenadine and sibutramine
- Anaesthetics: enhanced hypotensive effect

Administration

RECONSTITUTION

–

ROUTE

- Oral

RATE OF ADMINISTRATION

–

COMMENTS

–

Other information

- ECG required before treatment. To be repeated annually

Pindolol

Clinical use

Hypertension, angina (beta-blocker)

Dose in normal renal function

7.5–45 mg daily

Pharmacokinetics

Molecular weight (daltons)	248.3
% Protein binding	50
% Excreted unchanged in urine	40
Volume of distribution (L/kg)	1.2
Half-life – normal/ESRF (hrs)	2.5–4/unchanged

Dose in renal impairment GFR (mL/min)

20–50	Dose as in normal renal function
10–20	Dose as in normal renal function
<10	Dose as in normal renal function

Dose in patients undergoing renal replacement therapies

CAPD	Not dialysed. Dose as in normal renal function
HD	Not dialysed. Dose as in normal renal function
CAV/VVHD	Not dialysed. Dose as in normal renal function

Important drug interactions

POTENTIALLY HAZARDOUS INTERACTIONS WITH OTHER DRUGS

- Concurrent use with sympathomimetics may result in severe hypertension
- Care with diltiazem, nifedipine and verapamil because of potential effects on cardiac conduction system and contractility
- Anaesthetics: enhanced hypotensive effect
- Moxisylyte: possibly severe postural hypotension

Administration

RECONSTITUTION

–

ROUTE

- Oral

RATE OF ADMINISTRATION

–

COMMENTS

–

Other information

- The fate of metabolites, even if they are inactive, is unknown
- For dialysis patients and when GFR < 10 mL/min, start with smallest possible dose and titrate to response

Pioglitazone

Clinical use

Combination treatment of type 2 diabetes mellitus

Dose in normal renal function

15–30 mg daily

Pharmacokinetics

Molecular weight (daltons)	392.9
% Protein binding	>99
% Excreted unchanged in urine	Small amount
Volume of distribution (L/kg)	0.25
Half-life – normal/ESRF (hrs)	5–6 (active metabolites: 16–23)

Dose in renal impairment GFR (mL/min)

20–50	Dose as in normal renal function
10–20	Dose as in normal renal function
<10	Dose as in normal renal function

Dose in patients undergoing renal replacement therapies

CAPD	Unlikely dialysability. Dose as in normal renal function and monitor carefully
HD	Unlikely dialysability. Dose as in normal renal function and monitor carefully
CAV/VVHD	Unknown dialysability. Dose as in normal renal function and monitor carefully

Important drug interactions

POTENTIALLY HAZARDOUS INTERACTIONS WITH OTHER DRUGS

• None known

Administration

RECONSTITUTION

–

ROUTE

• Oral

RATE OF ADMINISTRATION

–

COMMENTS

–

Other information

• LFTs should be measured prior to initiation of therapy and then every 2 months for the first 12 months and thereafter at regular intervals

Piperazine

Clinical use

Treatment of threadworm and roundworm infections

Dose in normal renal function

Threadworm: 4 g sachet stirred into a glass of milk or water and drunk immediately, repeat after 14 days

Roundworm: 4 g sachet stirred into a glass of milk or water and drunk immediately, repeat at monthly intervals for up to 3 months if re-infection risk

Pharmacokinetics

Molecular weight (daltons)	202.1
% Protein binding	No data
% Excreted unchanged in urine	15–75
Volume of distribution (L/kg)	No data
Half-life – normal/ESRF (hrs)	No data

Dose in renal impairment GFR (mL/min)

20–50	Dose as in normal renal function
10–20	Dose as in normal renal function
<10	Dose as in normal renal function but avoid repeated administration

Dose in patients undergoing renal replacement therapies

CAPD	Unknown dialysability. Dose as in GFR < 10 mL/min
HD	Unknown dialysability. Dose as in GFR < 10 mL/min
CAV/VVHD	Unknown dialysability. Dose as in GFR = 10–20 mL/min

Important drug interactions

POTENTIALLY HAZARDOUS INTERACTIONS WITH OTHER DRUGS

• Pyrantel: antagonises effect of piperazine

Administration

RECONSTITUTION

–

ROUTE

• Oral

RATE OF ADMINISTRATION

–

COMMENTS

–

Other information

• May accumulate in severe renal impairment causing neurotoxicity

• Acts within the lumen of the GI tract which is independent of any systemic absorption

Piracetam

Clinical use

Myoclonus

Dose in normal renal function

7.2 g daily titrated to a maximum of 20 g

Pharmacokinetics

Molecular weight (daltons)	142.2
% Protein binding	15
% Excreted unchanged in urine	>90
Volume of distribution (L/kg)	0.4
Half-life – normal/ESRF (hrs)	5/–

Dose in renal impairment GFR (mL/min)

40–60	3.6 g daily titrated to a maximum of 10 g
20–40	1.8 g daily titrated to a maximum of 5 g
10–20	Contra-indicated
<10	Contra-indicated

Dose in patients undergoing renal replacement therapies

CAPD	Likely dialysability. Avoid. Contra-indicated
HD	Dialysed. Avoid. Contra-indicated
CAV/VVHD	Unknown dialysability. Avoid. Contra-indicated

Important drug interactions

POTENTIALLY HAZARDOUS INTERACTIONS WITH OTHER DRUGS

• None known

Administration

RECONSTITUTION

–

ROUTE

• Oral

RATE OF ADMINISTRATION

–

COMMENTS

–

Other information

–

Piroxicam

Clinical use

NSAID: anti-inflammatory analgesic

Dose in normal renal function

20 mg daily

Pharmacokinetics

Molecular weight (daltons)	331.4
% Protein binding	99
% Excreted unchanged in urine	10
Volume of distribution (L/kg)	0.12–0.15
Half-life – normal/ESRF (hrs)	41–50/unchanged

Dose in renal impairment GFR (mL/min)

20–50	Dose as in normal renal function, but avoid if possible
10–20	Dose as in normal renal function, but avoid if possible
<10	Only use if ESRD on dialysis, then use normal dose

Dose in patients undergoing renal replacement therapies

CAPD	Not dialysed. Dose as in GFR = <10 mL/min
HD	Not dialysed. Dose as in GFR = <10 mL/min
CAV/VVHD	Not dialysed. Dose as in GFR = 10–20 mL/min

Important drug interactions

POTENTIALLY HAZARDOUS INTERACTIONS WITH OTHER DRUGS

• Ciclosporin: increased risk of nephrotoxicity
• Reduced excretion of lithium
• Cytotoxic agents: reduced excretion of methotrexate
• Anticoagulants: effects of warfarin and acenocoumarol enhanced
• Antidiabetic agents: effects of sulphonylureas enhanced
• Anti-epileptic agents: effects of phenytoin enhanced
• ACE inhibitors and AT-II antagonists: antagonism of hypotensive effects. Increased risk of hyperkalaemia and renal damage
• Probenecid delays excretion of NSAIDs
• Diuretics: increased risk of nephrotoxicity; hyperkalaemia with potassium-sparing diuretics
• Tacrolimus: possibly increased risk of nephrotoxicity
• Analgesics: avoid concomitant use of two or more NSAIDs, increased risk of side-effects
• Quinolones: increased risk of convulsions

Administration

RECONSTITUTION
–

ROUTE
• Oral, IM, PR, topical

RATE OF ADMINISTRATION
–

COMMENTS
–

Other information

• Inhibition of renal prostaglandin synthesis by NSAIDs may interfere with renal function, especially in the presence of existing renal disease. Avoid if possible. If not, check serum creatinine 48–72 hours after starting NSAID. If serum creatinine increased, stop NSAID
• Use normal doses in patients with ESRD on dialysis
• Use with caution in renal transplant recipients – can reduce intra-renal autocoid synthesis
• Water soluble inactive metabolites may be removed by HD and CAPD

Potassium chloride

Clinical use

Hypokalaemia

Dose in normal renal function

2–4 g (25–50 mmol) daily

Pharmacokinetics

Molecular weight (daltons)	75
% Protein binding	N/A
% Excreted unchanged in urine	N/A
Volume of distribution (L/kg)	N/A
Half-life – normal/ESRF (hrs)	N/A

Dose in renal impairment GFR (mL/min)

20–50	According to response
10–20	According to response
<10	According to response

Dose in patients undergoing renal replacement therapies

CAPD	Dialysed. Dose according to response
HD	Dialysed. Dose according to response
CAV/VVHD	Dialysed. Dose according to response

Important drug interactions

POTENTIALLY HAZARDOUS INTERACTIONS WITH OTHER DRUGS

- Ciclosporin: increased risk of hyperkalaemia
- ACE inhibitors and AT-II antagonists: hyperkalaemia
- Potassium-sparing diuretics: hyperkalaemia
- Tacrolimus: increased risk of hyperkalaemia

Administration

RECONSTITUTION

–

ROUTE

- Oral, or IV peripherally

RATE OF ADMINISTRATION

- Infusion up to 20 mmol potassium per hour except in extreme hypokalaemic emergency where some units give up to 40 mmol/hour with cardiac monitoring

COMMENTS

- Give IV solution well diluted not exceeding 40 mmol/500 mL for peripheral administration. **Mix IV solutions thoroughly to avoid layering effect**
- Some units give more concentrated solution centrally, 100–200 mmol/100 mL sodium chloride 0.9% or glucose 5%, but at a rate no more than 20 mmol/hour. Cardiac monitoring mandatory

Other information

- Potassium chloride injection **must not** be injected undiluted
- Monitor potassium levels
- Sando K: 12 mmol potassium per tablet
- Slow K: 8 mmol potassium per tablet
- Potassium chloride strong 15% injection: 20 mmol potassium/10 mL

Pravastatin

Clinical use

HMG CoA reductase inhibitor; used for hypercholesterolaemia

Dose in normal renal function

10–40 mg daily at night

Pharmacokinetics

Molecular weight (daltons)	446.5
% Protein binding	approx 50
% Excreted unchanged in urine	20
Volume of distribution (L/kg)	0.9
Half-life – normal/ESRF (hrs)	1.5–2/unchanged

Dose in renal impairment GFR (mL/min)

20–50	Dose as in normal renal function
10–20	Dose as in normal renal function
<10	Dose as in normal renal function

Dose in patients undergoing renal replacement therapies

CAPD	Unlikely dialysability. Dose as in normal renal function
HD	Not dialysed. Dose as in normal renal function
CAV/VVHD	Unlikely dialysability. Dose as in normal renal function

Important drug interactions

POTENTIALLY HAZARDOUS INTERACTIONS WITH OTHER DRUGS

- Amprenavir: possibly an increased risk of myopathy
- Other lipid-regulating drugs: increased risk of myopathy with fibrates and nicotinic acid
- Ciclosporin: increased risk of myopathy

Administration

RECONSTITUTION

–

ROUTE

- Oral

RATE OF ADMINISTRATION

–

COMMENTS

–

Other information

- Rhabdomyolysis with ARF secondary to statin-induced myoglobinaemia has been reported
- Inactive polar metabolite accumulates but is readily removed by haemodialysis

Praziquantel (unlicensed product)

Clinical use

Treatment of tapeworm, *Schistosoma haematobium* worms and *S. japonicum* infections

Dose in normal renal function

Tapeworm: 10–20 mg/kg after a light breakfast

Hymenolepis nana: 25 mg/kg

Schistosoma haematobium: 40 mg/kg in two divided doses 4–6 hours apart in 1 day

S. japonicum: 60 mg/kg in three divided doses in 1 day

Pharmacokinetics

Molecular weight (daltons)	312.4
% Protein binding	80
% Excreted unchanged in urine	Mainly as metabolites
Volume of distribution (L/kg)	No data
Half-life – normal/ESRF (hrs)	0.8–1.5 (metabolites 4 hours)/slightly increased

Dose in renal impairment GFR (mL/min)

20–50	Dose as in normal renal function
10–20	Dose as in normal renal function
<10	Dose as in normal renal function. Use lower dose with caution

Dose in patients undergoing renal replacement therapies

CAPD	Not dialysed. Dose as in GFR < 10 mL/min
HD	Not dialysed. Dose as in GFR < 10 mL/min
CAV/VVHD	Not dialysed. Dose as in GFR = 10–20 mL/min

Important drug interactions

POTENTIALLY HAZARDOUS INTERACTIONS WITH OTHER DRUGS

• Carbamazepine, phenytoin, chloroquine: reduce bioavailability of praziquantel
• Cimetidine: increases bioavailability

Administration

RECONSTITUTION

–

ROUTE

• Oral

RATE OF ADMINISTRATION

–

COMMENTS

–

Other information

• Available on a 'named patient' basis from Merck (Cysticide)
• One study did not show any adverse effects in a haemodialysis patient

Prazosin

Clinical use

Alpha-adrenoceptor blocker: hypertension,
congestive heart failure, Raynaud's syndrome

Dose in normal renal function

500 micrograms – 20 mg daily

Pharmacokinetics

Molecular weight (daltons)	419.9
% Protein binding	97
% Excreted unchanged in urine	<5
Volume of distribution (L/kg)	0.6–1.1
Half-life – normal/ESRF (hrs)	2.9/unchanged

Dose in renal impairment
GFR (mL/min)

20–50	Dose as in normal renal function
10–20	Dose as in normal renal function
<10	Dose as in normal renal function

Dose in patients undergoing renal replacement therapies

CAPD	Not dialysed. Dose as in normal renal function
HD	Not dialysed. Dose as in normal renal function
CAV/VVHD	Not dialysed. Dose as in normal renal function

Important drug interactions

POTENTIALLY HAZARDOUS INTERACTIONS WITH OTHER DRUGS

- Anaesthetics: enhanced hypotensive effect
- NSAIDs: antagonism of hypotensive effect
- Antidepressants: enhanced hypotensive effect, especially with MAOIs and linezolid
- Beta-blockers: increased risk of first-dose hypotensive effect
- Calcium-channel blockers: increased risk of first-dose hypotensive effect
- Diuretics: enhanced hypotensive effect
- Moxisylyte: possibly severe postural hypotension

Administration

RECONSTITUTION

–

ROUTE

- Oral

RATE OF ADMINISTRATION

–

COMMENTS

–

Other information

–

Prednisolone

Clinical use

Corticosteroid: immunosuppression, inflammation

Dose in normal renal function

Variable

Pharmacokinetics

Molecular weight (daltons)	361
% Protein binding	70–95 saturable
% Excreted unchanged in urine	7–34
Volume of distribution (L/kg)	0.3–0.7
Half-life – normal/ESRF (hrs)	2.2–3.5/ unchanged

Dose in renal impairment GFR (mL/min)

20–50	Dose as in normal renal function
10–20	Dose as in normal renal function
<10	Dose as in normal renal function

Dose in patients undergoing renal replacement therapies

CAPD	Not dialysed. Dose as in normal renal function
HD	Not dialysed. Dose as in normal renal function. Give dose after HD
CAV/VVHD	Unknown dialysability. Dose as in normal renal function

Important drug interactions

POTENTIALLY HAZARDOUS INTERACTIONS WITH OTHER DRUGS

- Ciclosporin increases plasma levels of prednisolone; increased ciclosporin levels reported with prednisolone
- Metabolism accelerated by rifampicin, phenytoin, carbamazepine, phenobarbital and primidone
- Antagonises effects of hypoglycaemic agents
- Increased risk of hypokalaemia with amphotericin
- Anticoagulants: anticoagulant effect enhanced

Administration

RECONSTITUTION

–

ROUTE

- Oral, IV, rectal

RATE OF ADMINISTRATION

–

COMMENTS

–

Other information

- Evidence of unpredictable bioavailability from enteric-coated tablets. Avoid if possible
- Methylprednisolone anecdotally exhibits less mineralocorticoid activity compared with prednisolone in equipotent glucocorticoid activity doses

Primaquine

Clinical use

Treatment and prophylaxis of malaria in combination with chloroquine (*Plasmodium vivax* and *Plasmodium ovale*)

Treatment, in combination with clindamycin, for PCP

Dose in normal renal function

15–30 mg once daily for 14 days

or

4 mg once a week for 8 weeks

Pharmacokinetics

Molecular weight (daltons)	455.3 (as phosphate)
% Protein binding	–
% Excreted unchanged in urine	<1
Volume of distribution (L/kg)	269 ± 120.9 litres
Half-life – normal/ESRF (hrs)	4–7/unknown

Dose in renal impairment GFR (mL/min)

20–50	Dose as in normal renal function
10–20	Dose as in normal renal function
<10	Dose as in normal renal function

Dose in patients undergoing renal replacement therapies

CAPD	Unknown dialysability. Dose as in normal renal function
HD	Unknown dialysability. Dose as in normal renal function
CAV/VVHD	Unknown dialysability. Dose as in normal renal function

Important drug interactions

POTENTIALLY HAZARDOUS INTERACTIONS WITH OTHER DRUGS

• Gold preparations – avoid concomitant use, increased risk of blood dyscrasias

Administration

RECONSTITUTION

–

ROUTE

• Oral

RATE OF ADMINISTRATION

–

COMMENTS

–

Other information

• Primaquine base 7.5 mg is approximately equivalent to 13.2 mg primaquine phosphate

• Major metabolite, 8-(3-carboxyl-1-methylpropylamino)-6-methoxyquinolone possesses less anti-malarial activity than the parent compound

• Contra-indicated in acutely ill patients with rheumatoid arthritis or SLE – increased risk of developing granulocytopenia

• Risk of haemolytic anaemia in patients with G-6-PD deficiency. Haemolysis generally appears 2–3 days after primaquine administration

• Risk of methaemoglobinaemia at high doses

Primaxin (imipenem/cilastatin)

Clinical use

Antibacterial agent

Dose in normal renal function

Mild infection: 250 mg every 6 hours

Moderate infection: 500 mg every 8 hours

Severe, fully susceptible infection:
500 mg every 6 hours

Severe pseudomonal infection or other less
susceptible infection: 1 g every 6–8 hours

IM, mild-moderate infections: 500–750 mg
every 12 hours

Pharmacokinetics

Molecular weight (daltons)	Imipenem: 317; cilastatin: 380
% Protein binding	Imipenem: 13–21; cilastatin: 35
% Excreted unchanged in urine	Imipenem: 20–70; cilastatin: 60–70
Volume of distribution (L/kg)	Imipenem: 0.17–0.30; cilastatin: 0.22
Half-life – normal/ESRF (hrs)	Imipenem: 1/4; cilastatin: 1/15–24

Dose in renal impairment GFR (mL/min)

31–70	500 mg – 1 g every 8 hours
21–30	500 mg – 1 g every 12 hours
<20	250 mg (or 3.5 mg/kg whichever is **lower**) every 12 hours

Dose in patients undergoing renal replacement therapies

CAPD	Dialysed. Dose as in GFR = <20 mL/min
HD	Dialysed. Dose as in GFR = <20 mL/min
CAV/VVHD	Dialysed. Dose as in GFR = 21–30 mL/min

Important drug interactions

POTENTIALLY HAZARDOUS INTERACTIONS WITH
OTHER DRUGS

• Ciclosporin: variable reports of increase/no
change in ciclosporin levels and of neurotoxicity

• Convulsions reported with concomitant
administration of ganciclovir

Administration

RECONSTITUTION

• 250 mg with 50 mL, 500 mg with 100 mL sodium
chloride 0.9% (in some units 500 mg with 50 mL)

• IM: 2 mL lidocaine 1%

ROUTE

• IM, IV peripherally or centrally (500 mg/50 mL –
given centrally)

RATE OF ADMINISTRATION

• 250 or 500 mg dose over 20–30 minutes

• 1 g over 40–60 minutes

COMMENTS

–

Other information

• Risk of adverse neurological effects, e.g.
convulsions. Extreme caution required in patients
with history of CNS disease

• Cilastatin can accumulate in patients with
impaired renal function

• Sodium content 2.8 mmol/g

• Imipenem is administered with cilastatin to
prevent metabolism of imipenem within the
kidney

• Non-renal clearance in ARF is less than in CRF

• Patients with GFR < 5 mL/min should not receive
drug unless HD is started within 48 hours

Prochlorperazine

Clinical use

Nausea and vomiting, labyrinthine disorders,
psychoses

Dose in normal renal function

Oral: 5–10 mg 2–3 times daily

IM/IV: 12.5 mg (unlicensed IV)

PR: 25 mg followed if necessary after 6 hours by
an oral dose; or migraine 5 mg three times daily

Psychoses: orally, 75–100 mg daily; IM, 12.5–25 mg
2–3 times daily

Pharmacokinetics

Molecular weight (daltons)	373.9
% Protein binding	96
% Excreted unchanged in urine	0.005–0.04
Volume of distribution (L/kg)	23
Half-life – normal/ESRF (hrs)	3–13/–

Dose in renal impairment
GFR (mL/min)

20–50	Dose as in normal renal function
10–20	Dose as in normal renal function
<10	Start with small doses, i.e. 6.25 mg IM or 5 mg orally

Dose in patients undergoing renal replacement therapies

CAPD	Unlikely dialysability. Dose as in GFR = <10 mL/min
HD	Unlikely dialysability. Dose as in GFR = <10 mL/min
CAV/VVHD	Unlikely dialysability. Dose as in GFR = 10–20 mL/min

Important drug interactions

POTENTIALLY HAZARDOUS INTERACTIONS WITH
OTHER DRUGS

- Anaesthetics: enhanced hypotensive effect
- Anti-arrhythmics: increased risk of ventricular
  arrhythmias with drugs which prolong QT
  interval, e.g. quinidine, procainamide,
  disopyramide, amiodarone and sotalol
- Antidepressants: increase plasma concentrations
  and additive antimuscarinic effects notably with
  tricyclics
- Anti-epileptics: antagonised (convulsive threshold
  lowered)
- Mizolastine/terfenadine: increased risk of
  arrhythmias
- Avoid desferrioxamine
- Possible severe postural hypotension with ACE
  inhibitors and AT-II antagonists

Administration

RECONSTITUTION

–

ROUTE

- IM, or IV (unlicensed), oral, PR

RATE OF ADMINISTRATION

- IM or IV over 3–4 minutes

COMMENTS

- **Unlicensed** IV administration methods:
  - Either: dilute injection to give in 5 times its own
    volume with water for injection and administer
    slowly over not less than 5 minutes
  - Or: dilute to 1 mg/mL and administer at rate
    not greater than 1 mg/minute

Other information

- Increased CNS sensitivity in severe renal
  impairment

Procyclidine

Clinical use

Control of extrapyramidal symptoms

Dose in normal renal function

2.5–10 mg three times a day

Pharmacokinetics

Molecular weight (daltons)	323.9
% Protein binding	–
% Excreted unchanged in urine	<5
Volume of distribution (L/kg)	1.0
Half-life – normal/ESRF (hrs)	12/–

Dose in renal impairment GFR (mL/min)

20–50	Dose as in normal renal function
10–20	Dose as in normal renal function
<10	Dose as in normal renal function

Dose in patients undergoing renal replacement therapies

CAPD	Unknown dialysability. Dose as in normal renal function
HD	Not dialysed. Dose as in normal renal function
CAV/VVHD	Unknown dialysability. Dose as in normal renal function

Important drug interactions

POTENTIALLY HAZARDOUS INTERACTIONS WITH OTHER DRUGS

• None known

Administration

RECONSTITUTION

• N/A

ROUTE

• IV, IM, oral

RATE OF ADMINISTRATION

• Bolus over 3–5 minutes

COMMENTS

–

Other information

–

Proguanil

Clinical use

Malaria chemoprophylaxis

Dose in normal renal function

200 mg daily

Pharmacokinetics

Molecular weight (daltons)	290.2
% Protein binding	75
% Excreted unchanged in urine	60
Volume of distribution (L/kg)	–
Half-life – normal/ESRF (hrs)	20/–

Dose in renal impairment GFR (mL/min)

20–60	100 mg daily
10–20	50 mg every 48 hours
<10	50 mg weekly

Dose in patients undergoing renal replacement therapies

CAPD	Removal unlikely. Dose as in GFR < 10 mL/min
HD	Removal unlikely. Dose as in GFR < 10 mL/min
CAV/VVHD	Unknown dialysability. Dose as in GFR = 10–20 mL/min

Important drug interactions

POTENTIALLY HAZARDOUS INTERACTIONS WITH OTHER DRUGS

• Anticoagulants: effect of warfarin possibly enhanced

Administration

RECONSTITUTION

–

ROUTE

• Oral

RATE OF ADMINISTRATION

–

COMMENTS

–

Other information

• Rare reports of haematological changes, e.g. megaloblastic anaemia and pancytopenia, in patients with severe renal impairment

Promethazine

Clinical use

Antihistamine

Dose in normal renal function

25 mg at night increasing to 25 mg twice daily or
10–20 mg 2–3 times a day
Slow IV/IM: 25–100 mg

Pharmacokinetics

Molecular weight (daltons)	320.9
% Protein binding	93
% Excreted unchanged in urine	0
Volume of distribution (L/kg)	13.5
Half-life – normal/ESRF (hrs)	12/–

Dose in renal impairment GFR (mL/min)

20–50	Dose as in normal renal function
10–20	Dose as in normal renal function
<10	Dose as in normal renal function

Dose in patients undergoing renal replacement therapies

CAPD	Unknown dialysability. Dose as in normal renal function
HD	Not dialysed. Dose as in normal renal function
CAV/VVHD	Unknown dialysability. Dose as in normal renal function

Important drug interactions

POTENTIALLY HAZARDOUS INTERACTIONS WITH OTHER DRUGS

• None known

Administration

RECONSTITUTION

–

ROUTE

• IV, IM, oral

RATE OF ADMINISTRATION

• Bolus over 3–5 minutes

COMMENTS

• Administer as a solution of 25 mg/mL of water for slow IV injection

Other information

–

Propiverine hydrochloride

Clinical use

Treatment of urinary frequency, urgency and incontinence, neurogenic bladder instability

Dose in normal renal function

15 mg 1–3 times daily (maximum four times a day)

Pharmacokinetics

Molecular weight (daltons)	403.9
% Protein binding	90
% Excreted unchanged in urine	<20
Volume of distribution (L/kg)	125–473 litres (average: 253 litres)
Half-life – normal/ESRF (hrs)	20/–

Dose in renal impairment GFR (mL/min)

20–50	Dose as in normal renal function
10–20	Dose as in normal renal function
<10	Avoid

Dose in patients undergoing renal replacement therapies

CAPD	Unknown dialysability. Avoid
HD	Unknown dialysability. Avoid
CAV/VVHD	Unknown dialysability. Avoid

Important drug interactions

POTENTIALLY HAZARDOUS INTERACTIONS WITH OTHER DRUGS

• None known

Administration

RECONSTITUTION

–

ROUTE

• Oral

RATE OF ADMINISTRATION

–

COMMENTS

–

Other information

–

Propofol

Clinical use

- Induction and maintenance of general anaesthesia
- Sedation of ventilated patients for up to 3 days

Dose in normal renal function

Induction: 1.5–2.5 mg/kg

Maintenance: 4–12 mg/kg/hour

Sedation: 0.3–4 mg/kg/hour

Pharmacokinetics

Molecular weight (daltons)	178.3
% Protein binding	>95
% Excreted unchanged in urine	<0.3
Volume of distribution (L/kg)	3.0–14.4
Half-life – normal/ESRF (hrs)	3–4.5/unchanged

Dose in renal impairment GFR (mL/min)

20–50	Dose as in normal renal function
10–20	Dose as in normal renal function
<10	Dose as in normal renal function

Dose in patients undergoing renal replacement therapies

CAPD	Unlikely dialysability. Dose as in normal renal function
HD	Unlikely dialysability. Dose as in normal renal function
CAV/VVHD	Unknown dialysability. Dose as in normal renal function

Important drug interactions

POTENTIALLY HAZARDOUS INTERACTIONS WITH OTHER DRUGS

- ACE inhibitors and AT-II antagonists: enhanced hypotensive effect
- Calcium-channel blockers: enhanced hypotensive effect
- Beta-blockers: enhanced hypotensive effect
- Antipsychotics: enhanced hypotensive effect

Administration

RECONSTITUTION

–

ROUTE

- IV

RATE OF ADMINISTRATION

- See local protocols

COMMENTS

–

Other information

–

Propranolol

Clinical use

Beta-adrenoceptor blocker: hypertension, angina, arrhythmias, anxiety, migraine prophylaxis

Dose in normal renal function

30–320 mg daily

Pharmacokinetics

Molecular weight (daltons)	259
% Protein binding	80–95
% Excreted unchanged in urine	1–4
Volume of distribution (L/kg)	2.3–5.5
Half-life – normal/ESRF (hrs)	2–6/unchanged

Dose in renal impairment GFR (mL/min)

20–50	Dose as in normal renal function
10–20	Start with small doses
<10	Start with small doses

Dose in patients undergoing renal replacement therapies

CAPD	Not dialysed. Dose as in GFR = <10 mL/min
HD	Not dialysed. Dose as in GFR = <10 mL/min
CAV/VVHD	Unknown dialysability. Dose as in GFR = 10–20 mL/min

Important drug interactions

POTENTIALLY HAZARDOUS INTERACTIONS WITH OTHER DRUGS

- Anaesthetics: enhanced hypotensive effect, risk of bupivacaine toxicity increased
- Anti-arrhythmics: increased risk of myocardial depression and bradycardia, risk of lidocaine toxicity increased. Propafenone increases plasma concentration
- Amiodarone: increased risk of bradycardia and AV block
- Antihypertensives: enhanced effect
- Calcium-channel blockers: increased risk of bradycardia and AV block with diltiazem
- Chlorpromazine: plasma concentration increased
- Sympathomimetics: severe hypertension
- Antidepressants: enhanced hypotensive effect with MAOIs and linezolid. Fluvoxamine increases levels
- Moxisylyte: possibly severe postural hypotension

Administration

RECONSTITUTION

–

ROUTE

- Oral, IV

RATE OF ADMINISTRATION

–

COMMENTS

–

Other information

- Avoid use. Non-selective. Active metabolites accumulate in renal impairment. Consider metoprolol or atenolol
- May reduce renal blood flow in severe renal impairment

Propylthiouracil

Clinical use

Hyperthyroidism

Dose in normal renal function

Maintenance dose: 50–150 mg daily – oral

Pharmacokinetics

Molecular weight (daltons)	170.2
% Protein binding	80
% Excreted unchanged in urine	<10
Volume of distribution (L/kg)	0.3–0.4
Half-life – normal/ESRF (hrs)	1–2/8.5

Dose in renal impairment GFR (mL/min)

20–50	Dose as in normal renal function
10–20	75% of normal dose
<10	50% of normal dose

Dose in patients undergoing renal replacement therapies

CAPD	Unknown dialysability. Dose as in GFR = <10 mL/min
HD	Unknown dialysability. Dose as in GFR = <10 mL/min
CAV/VVHD	Unknown dialysability. Dose as in GFR = 10–20 mL/min

Important drug interactions

POTENTIALLY HAZARDOUS INTERACTIONS WITH OTHER DRUGS

• None known

Administration

RECONSTITUTION

–

ROUTE

• Oral

RATE OF ADMINISTRATION

–

COMMENTS

–

Other information

• Renally impaired patients are at a greater risk of cardiotoxicity and leucopenia

Protamine

Clinical use

Counteract anticoagulant effect of heparin

Dose in normal renal function

Depends on time since stopping IV/subcutaneous heparin and dose of heparin

Pharmacokinetics

Molecular weight (daltons)	Approx 4500
% Protein binding	I
% Excreted unchanged in urine	–
Volume of distribution (L/kg)	–
Half-life – normal/ESRF (hrs)	–

Dose in renal impairment GFR (mL/min)

20–50	Dose as in normal renal function
10–20	Dose as in normal renal function
<10	Dose as in normal renal function

Dose in patients undergoing renal replacement therapies

CAPD	Unknown dialysability. Dose as in normal renal function
HD	Unknown dialysability. Dose as in normal renal function
CAV/VVHD	Unknown dialysability. Dose as in normal renal function

Important drug interactions

POTENTIALLY HAZARDOUS INTERACTIONS WITH OTHER DRUGS

• None known

Administration

RECONSTITUTION

–

ROUTE

–

RATE OF ADMINISTRATION

• Slow IV injection over 10 minutes

COMMENTS

–

Other information

• In general, 1 mg of protamine sulphate will neutralise approximately 90 units of heparin sodium derived from bovine lung tissue, and 100 units of heparin calcium or 115 units of heparin sodium derived from porcine intestinal mucosa

• Most clinicians recommend a dose of 1.0–1.5 mg protamine sulphate for each 100 units heparin given

• May be used topically for bleeding fistulas

Pseudoephedrine

Clinical use

Decongestant (nasal)

Dose in normal renal function

60 mg four times a day

Pharmacokinetics

Molecular weight (daltons)	201.7
% Protein binding	–
% Excreted unchanged in urine	90–98
Volume of distribution (L/kg)	2.7
Half-life – normal/ESRF (hrs)	5.5 (depends on pH of urine)

Dose in renal impairment GFR (mL/min)

20–50	Dose as in normal renal function
10–20	Dose as in normal renal function
<10	Dose as in normal renal function

Dose in patients undergoing renal replacement therapies

CAPD	Unlikely dialysability. Dose as in normal renal function
HD	5–20% removed. Dose as in normal renal function
CAV/VVHD	Unknown dialysability. Dose as in normal renal function

Important drug interactions

POTENTIALLY HAZARDOUS INTERACTIONS WITH OTHER DRUGS

• MAOIs and linezolid: risk of hypertensive crisis
• Beta-blockers: risk of severe hypertension

Administration

RECONSTITUTION

–

ROUTE

• Oral

RATE OF ADMINISTRATION

–

COMMENTS

–

Other information

–

Pyrazinamide

Clinical use

Antimicrobial agent for tuberculosis

Dose in normal renal function

20–35 mg/kg/day (usually 1.5–2.0 g per day)

Pharmacokinetics

Molecular weight (daltons)	123.1
% Protein binding	5
% Excreted unchanged in urine	1–3
Volume of distribution (L/kg)	0.75–1.3
Half-life – normal/ESRF (hrs)	9/26

Dose in renal impairment GFR (mL/min)

20–50	Dose as in normal renal function
10–20	Dose as in normal renal function
<10	Dose as in normal renal function

Dose for patients undergoing renal replacement therapies

CAPD	Unknown dialysability. Dose as in normal renal function
HD	50–100% dialysed. Dose as in normal renal function
CAV/VVHD	Unknown dialysability. Dose as in normal renal function

Important drug interactions

POTENTIALLY HAZARDOUS INTERACTIONS WITH OTHER DRUGS

• Ciclosporin: on limited evidence, pyrazinamide appears to reduce ciclosporin levels

Administration

RECONSTITUTION

–

ROUTE

• Oral

RATE OF ADMINISTRATION

–

COMMENTS

–

Other information

–

Pyridostigmine

Clinical use

Myasthenia gravis

Dose in normal renal function

60 mg – 1.2 g per day in divided doses

Pharmacokinetics

Molecular weight (daltons)	261.1
% Protein binding	–
% Excreted unchanged in urine	80–90
Volume of distribution (L/kg)	0.8–1.4
Half-life – normal/ESRF (hrs)	1.5–2/6

Dose in renal impairment GFR (mL/min)

20–50	35% of daily dose
10–20	35% of daily dose
<10	20% of daily dose

Dose in patients undergoing renal replacement therapies

CAPD	Unknown dialysability. Dose as in GFR = <10 mL/min
HD	Unknown dialysability. Dose as in GFR = <10 mL/min
CAV/VVHD	Unknown dialysability. Dose as in GFR = 10–20 mL/min

Important drug interactions

POTENTIALLY HAZARDOUS INTERACTIONS WITH OTHER DRUGS

• Aminoglycosides, clindamycin and colistin antagonise effects of pyridostigmine

Administration

RECONSTITUTION

–

ROUTE

• Oral

RATE OF ADMINISTRATION

–

COMMENTS

–

Other information

–

Pyridoxine

Clinical use

Vitamin B$_6$

Dose in normal renal function

25–150 mg daily

Pharmacokinetics

Molecular weight (daltons)	205.6
% Protein binding	High (as pyridoxal and pyridoxal phosphate)
% Excreted unchanged in urine	–
Volume of distribution (L/kg)	–
Half-life – normal/ESRF (hrs)	15–20 days

Dose in renal impairment GFR (mL/min)

20–50	Dose as in normal renal function
10–20	Dose as in normal renal function
<10	Dose as in normal renal function

Dose in patients undergoing renal replacement therapies

CAPD	Unknown dialysability. Dose as in normal renal function
HD	Dialysed. Dose as in normal renal function
CAV/VVHD	Unknown dialysability. Dose as in normal renal function

Important drug interactions

POTENTIALLY HAZARDOUS INTERACTIONS WITH OTHER DRUGS

• None known

Administration

RECONSTITUTION

–

ROUTE

• Oral

RATE OF ADMINISTRATION

–

COMMENTS

–

Other information

–

Pyrimethamine

Clinical use

Antiprotozoal agent

Dose in normal renal function

50–75 mg per day

Pharmacokinetics

Molecular weight (daltons)	248.7
% Protein binding	80–90
% Excreted unchanged in urine	16–30
Volume of distribution (L/kg)	2.9
Half-life – normal/ESRF (hrs)	80/unchanged

Dose in renal impairment GFR (mL/min)

20–50	Dose as in normal renal function
10–20	Dose as in normal renal function
<10	Dose as in normal renal function

Dose in patients undergoing renal replacement therapies

CAPD	Not dialysed. Dose as in normal renal function
HD	Not dialysed. Dose as in normal renal function
CAV/VVHD	Not dialysed. Dose as in normal renal function

Important drug interactions

POTENTIALLY HAZARDOUS INTERACTIONS WITH OTHER DRUGS

• Increased antifolate effect with cotrimoxazole, trimethoprim, phenytoin and methotrexate

Administration

RECONSTITUTION

–

ROUTE

• Oral

RATE OF ADMINISTRATION

–

COMMENTS

–

Other information

–

Quetiapine fumarate

Clinical use

Treatment of schizophrenia

Dose in normal renal function

150–750 mg daily in two divided doses

Pharmacokinetics

Molecular weight (daltons)	883.1
% Protein binding	83
% Excreted unchanged in urine	5
Volume of distribution (L/kg)	10 ± 4
Half-life – normal/ESRF (hrs)	6–7/unchanged

Dose in renal impairment GFR (mL/min)

20–50	Initial dose 25 mg/day and increase in increments of 25–50 mg/day according to response
10–20	Initial dose 25 mg/day and increase in increments of 25–50 mg/day according to response
<10	Initial dose 25 mg/day and increase in increments of 25–50 mg/day according to response

Dose in patients undergoing renal replacement therapies

CAPD	Unknown dialysability. Dose as in GFR = <10 mL/min
HD	Unknown dialysability. Dose as in GFR = <10 mL/min
CAV/VVHD	Unknown dialysability. Dose as in GFR = 10–20 mL/min

Important drug interactions

POTENTIALLY HAZARDOUS INTERACTIONS WITH OTHER DRUGS

- Anaesthetics: enhanced hypotensive effect
- Analgesics: enhanced sedative and hypotensive effect with opioid analgesics
- Anti-epileptics: antagonism of convulsive threshold; phenytoin increases clearance of quetiapine
- Anti-malarials: manufacturer advises avoid use with artemether with lumefantrine
- Antivirals: ritonavir possibly increases plasma concentration
- Thioridazine: increased clearance of quetiapine
- Sibutramine: increased risk of CNS toxicity (avoid concomitant use)

Administration

RECONSTITUTION

–

ROUTE

- Oral

RATE OF ADMINISTRATION

–

COMMENTS

–

Other information

- Plasma clearance is reduced by 25% in severe renal impairment
- Absorption is increased by food so it should be taken consistently either with or without food

Quinagolide

Clinical use

Hyperprolactinaemia

Dose in normal renal function

75–150 micrograms daily

Pharmacokinetics

Molecular weight (daltons)	432
% Protein binding	90
% Excreted unchanged in urine	Very little, most is excreted as metabolites in faeces and urine
Volume of distribution (L/kg)	100 litres
Half-life – normal/ESRF (hrs)	17/–

Dose in renal impairment GFR (mL/min)

20–50	Use with caution
10–20	Use with caution
<10	Use with caution

Dose in patients undergoing renal replacement therapies

CAPD	Unknown dialysability. Dose as in GFR = <10 mL/min
HD	Unknown dialysability. Dose as in GFR = <10 mL/min
CAV/VVHD	Unknown dialysability. Dose as in GFR = 10–20 mL/min

Important drug interactions

POTENTIALLY HAZARDOUS INTERACTIONS WITH OTHER DRUGS

• None known

Administration

RECONSTITUTION

–

ROUTE

• Oral

RATE OF ADMINISTRATION

–

COMMENTS

–

Other information

• Manufacturer advises to avoid use in renal impairment due to lack of data
• Renally excreted metabolites (glucuronide and sulphate) are inactive. Monitor patients carefully

Quinapril

Clinical use

ACE inhibitor: hypertension, heart failure

Dose in normal renal function

10–80 mg daily

Pharmacokinetics

Molecular weight (daltons)	475
% Protein binding	97
% Excreted unchanged in urine	30
Volume of distribution (L/kg)	1.5
Half-life – normal/ESRF (hrs)	1–2/6–15

Dose in renal impairment GFR (mL/min)

20–50	75–100% of normal dose
10–20	75–100% of normal dose
<10	50% of normal dose

Dose in patients undergoing renal replacement therapies

CAPD	Not dialysed. Dose as in GFR = <10 mL/min
HD	25% dialysed. Dose as in GFR = 10–20 mL/min
CAV/VVHD	Unknown dialysability. Dose as in GFR = 10–20 mL/min

Important drug interactions

POTENTIALLY HAZARDOUS INTERACTIONS WITH OTHER DRUGS

- Ciclosporin: increased risk of hyperkalaemia and nephrotoxicity
- Anaesthetics: enhanced hypotensive effect
- NSAIDs: antagonism of hypotensive effects, hyperkalaemia, risk of renal impairment
- Diuretics: enhanced hypotensive effects, increased risk of hyperkalaemia with potassium-sparing diuretics
- Epoetin: increased risk of hyperkalaemia
- Lithium: reduced excretion of lithium – increased plasma levels
- Potassium salts: increased risk of hyperkalaemia
- Tacrolimus: increased risk of hyperkalaemia and nephrotoxicity

Administration

RECONSTITUTION

–

ROUTE

- Oral

RATE OF ADMINISTRATION

–

COMMENTS

–

Other information

- Renal failure has been reported with ACE inhibitors mainly in patients with renal artery stenosis, post renal transplant or those with severe congestive heart failure
- A high incidence of anaphylactoid reactions has been reported in patients dialysed with high-flux polyacrylonitrile membranes and treated concomitantly with an ACE inhibitor – this combination should be avoided
- Hyperkalaemia and other side-effects more common in patients with renal impairment
- Close monitoring of renal function during therapy is necessary in those patients with known renal insufficiency

Quinidine bisulphate

Clinical use

Supraventricular tachycardias and ventricular arrhythmias

Dose in normal renal function

200–400 mg 3–4 times daily
Modified release: 500 mg 12-hourly

Pharmacokinetics

Molecular weight (daltons)	422.5
% Protein binding	70–95
% Excreted unchanged in urine	20
Volume of distribution (L/kg)	2–3.5
Half-life – normal/ESRF (hrs)	6/4–14

Dose in renal impairment GFR (mL/min)

20–50	Dose as in normal renal function
10–20	Dose as in normal renal function
<10	Dose as in normal renal function

Dose in patients undergoing renal replacement therapies

CAPD	Not dialysed. Dose as in normal renal function
HD	Dialysed. Dose as in normal renal function
CAV/VVHD	Dialysed. Dose as in normal renal function

Important drug interactions

POTENTIALLY HAZARDOUS INTERACTIONS WITH OTHER DRUGS

• Increased risk of myocardial depression with anti-arrhythmics. Amiodarone increases plasma levels of quinidine – increased risk of ventricular arrhythmias
• Antibacterials: increased risk of arrhythmias with quinupristin/dalfopristin – avoid concomitant use. Rifamycins reduce plasma levels

• Antifungals: plasma levels increased by itraconazole and miconazole, increased risk of ventricular arrhythmias – avoid concomitant use
• Antivirals: increased risk of ventricular arrhythmias with nelfinavir and ritonavir
• Increased risk of ventricular arrhythmias with tricyclic antidepressants
• Terfenadine and mizolastine: increased risk of ventricular arrhythmias
• Mefloquine: increased risk of ventricular arrhythmias
• Phenothiazines: increased risk of ventricular arrhythmias
• Sotalol: increased risk of ventricular arrhythmias – avoid concomitant use
• Calcium-channel blockers: nifedipine decreases plasma levels of quinidine; verapamil increases plasma levels of quinidine
• Plasma levels of digoxin increased – halve dose of digoxin
• Diuretics: quinidine toxicity enhanced by hypokalaemia, e.g. with acetazolamide, loop and thiazide diuretics
• Muscle relaxants: effects enhanced by quinidine
• Cimetidine: inhibits metabolism of quinidine, hence increases plasma levels

Administration

RECONSTITUTION

–

ROUTE

• Oral

RATE OF ADMINISTRATION

–

COMMENTS

–

Other information

–

Quinine dihydrochloride injection

Clinical use

Treatment of severe and complicated falciparum malaria

Dose in normal renal function

Quinine salt (not bisulphate): loading dose 20 mg/kg to maximum 1.4 g, then after 8–12 hours, maintenance 10 mg/kg (up to maximum 700 mg) 8–12 hourly, reduced to 5–7 mg/kg if parenteral treatment required for more than 48 hours

Pharmacokinetics

Molecular weight (daltons)	397
% Protein binding	70–90
% Excreted unchanged in urine	<20
Volume of distribution (L/kg)	1.5 (healthy subjects), 1.2 (severe malaria)
Half-life – normal/ESRF (hrs)	9 (healthy), 18 (malaria)/ unchanged

Dose in renal impairment GFR (mL/min)

20–50	5–10 mg/kg every 8 hours
10–20	5–10 mg/kg every 8–12 hours
<10	5–10 mg/kg every 24 hours

Dose in patients undergoing renal replacement therapies

CAPD	Not dialysed. Dose as in GFR = <10 mL/min
HD	Dialysed. Dose as in GFR = <10 mL/min
CAV/VVHD	Probably dialysed. Dose as in GFR = 10–20 mL/min

Important drug interactions

POTENTIALLY HAZARDOUS INTERACTIONS WITH OTHER DRUGS

- Ciclosporin: decreased ciclosporin levels reported
- Anti-arrhythmics: flecainide levels increased; increased risk of ventricular arrhythmias with amiodarone – avoid concomitant use
- Antipsychotics: increased risk of ventricular arrhythmias with pimozide or thioridazine – avoid concomitant use
- Digoxin: plasma levels of digoxin increased (halve maintenance dose)
- Cimetidine: may increase plasma levels of quinine
- Mefloquine: do not give mefloquine with quinine or other drugs which may induce arrhythmias (CSM advice)
- Mizolastine and terfenadine: increased risk of ventricular arrhythmias
- Rifampicin: may decrease quinine levels
- Warfarin: effect may be increased

Administration

RECONSTITUTION

- Add to sodium chloride 0.9% or glucose 5% for infusion

ROUTE

- IV infusion

RATE OF ADMINISTRATION

- 4 hours

COMMENTS

- Loading dose of 20 mg/kg may be required in some cases (refer to specialist treatment). Not to be given if patient has had quinine, quinidine or mefloquine in previous 12–24 hours

Other information

- Quinine dihydrochloride injection is available as a special order
- Monitor for signs of cardiotoxicity
- Give doses after haemodialysis on dialysis days

Quinine sulphate, bisulphate or hydrochloride

Clinical use

Nocturnal cramp

Dose in normal renal function

200–300 mg at night

Pharmacokinetics

Molecular weight (daltons)	397
% Protein binding	70–90
% Excreted unchanged in urine	5–20
Volume of distribution (L/kg)	1.5
Half-life – normal/ESRF (hrs)	7–11/unchanged

Dose in renal impairment GFR (mL/min)

20–50	Dose as in normal renal function
10–20	Dose as in normal renal function
<10	Dose as in normal renal function

Dose in patients undergoing renal replacement therapies

CAPD	Unknown dialysability. Dose as in normal renal function
HD	Dialysed. Dose as in normal renal function
CAV/VVHD	Dialysed. Dose as in normal renal function

Important drug interactions

POTENTIALLY HAZARDOUS INTERACTIONS WITH OTHER DRUGS

• Ciclosporin: decreased ciclosporin levels reported

• Anti-arrhythmics: flecainide levels increased; increased risk of ventricular arrhythmias with amiodarone – avoid concomitant use
• Antipsychotics: increased risk of ventricular arrhythmias with pimozide or thioridazine – avoid concomitant use
• Digoxin: plasma levels of digoxin increased (halve maintenance dose)
• Cimetidine: may increase plasma levels of quinine
• Mefloquine: do not give mefloquine with quinine or other drugs which may induce arrhythmias (CSM advice)
• Mizolastine and terfenadine: increased risk of ventricular arrhythmias
• Rifampicin: may decrease quinine levels
• Warfarin: effect may be increased

Administration

RECONSTITUTION

–

ROUTE

• Oral

RATE OF ADMINISTRATION

–

COMMENTS

–

Other information

• Monitor quinine levels if patient exhibits any symptoms of toxicity
• Give dose after haemodialysis on dialysis days

Rabeprazole

Clinical use

Gastric acid suppression

Dose in normal renal function

10–20 mg in the morning before eating

Pharmacokinetics

Molecular weight (daltons)	381.43
% Protein binding	97
% Excreted unchanged in urine	0 (90 as metabolites)
Volume of distribution (L/kg)	0.34
Half-life – normal/ESRF (hrs)	0.7–1.5/ unchanged

Dose in renal impairment GFR (mL/min)

20–50	Dose as in normal renal function
10–20	Dose as in normal renal function
<10	Dose as in normal renal function

Dose in patients undergoing renal replacement therapies

CAPD	Unlikely dialysability. Dose as in normal renal function
HD	Not dialysed. Dose as in normal renal function
CAV/VVHD	Unlikely dialysability. Dose as in normal renal function

Important drug interactions

POTENTIALLY HAZARDOUS INTERACTIONS WITH OTHER DRUGS

• Ketoconazole: 33% reduction in ketoconazole levels
• Digoxin: 22% increase in digoxin trough level

Administration

RECONSTITUTION
–

ROUTE

• Oral

RATE OF ADMINISTRATION
–

COMMENTS
–

Other information

–

Raloxifene

Clinical use

Treatment and prevention of osteoporosis in post-menopausal women

Dose in normal renal function

60 mg daily

Pharmacokinetics

Molecular weight (daltons)	510
% Protein binding	98–99
% Excreted unchanged in urine	<0.2
Volume of distribution (L/kg)	2348
Half-life – normal/ESRF (hrs)	15.8–86.6 (average 32.5)/ unchanged

Dose in renal impairment GFR (mL/min)

20–50	Dose as in normal renal function
10–20	Dose as in normal renal function
<10	Use with caution

Dose in patients undergoing renal replacement therapies

CAPD	Unlikely dialysability. Use with caution
HD	Unlikely dialysability. Use with caution
CAV/VVHD	Unlikely dialysability. Use with caution

Important drug interactions

POTENTIALLY HAZARDOUS INTERACTIONS WITH OTHER DRUGS

• Colestyramine: reduced absorption of raloxifene – avoid concomitant use
• Anticoagulants: antagonism of anticoagulant effect of warfarin and acenocoumarol

Administration

RECONSTITUTION
–

ROUTE
• Oral

RATE OF ADMINISTRATION
–

COMMENTS
–

Other information

• Manufacturer advises use is contra-indicated in severe renal impairment due to lack of data rather than known toxicity
• <6% of dose is excreted in the urine

Raltitrexed

Clinical use

Treatment of colorectal cancer when fluorouracil and folinic acid cannot be used

Dose in normal renal function

3 mg/m² every 3 weeks

Pharmacokinetics

Molecular weight (daltons)	458.5
% Protein binding	93
% Excreted unchanged in urine	40–50
Volume of distribution (L/kg)	548 litres
Half-life – normal/ESRF (hrs)	198/increased

Dose in renal impairment
GFR (mL/min)

55–65	Use 75 % of the dose every 4 weeks
25–54	Use 50 % of the dose every 4 weeks
<25	Avoid – see 'Other information'

Dose in patients undergoing renal replacement therapies

CAPD	Unlikely dialysability. Dose as in GFR < 25 mL/min
HD	Unlikely dialysability. Dose as in GFR < 25 mL/min
CAV/VVHD	Unlikely dialysability. Dose as in GFR < 25 mL/min

Important drug interactions

POTENTIALLY HAZARDOUS INTERACTIONS WITH OTHER DRUGS

• Folic and folinic acid: impairs cytotoxic action

Administration

RECONSTITUTION

• With 4 mL water for injection

ROUTE

• IV infusion

RATE OF ADMINISTRATION

• Over 15 minutes

COMMENTS

• Dilute in 50–250 mL sodium chloride 0.9% or glucose 5%
• Stable for 24 hours at 2–8°C

Other information

• Doses above 3 mg/m² have an increased incidence of life-threatening/fatal toxicity
• Increased risk of treatment-related toxicity if CL_{CR} <65 mL/min
• Anecdotal reports of using 30–40% of the dose every 4 weeks and closely monitoring haematological parameters in patients with severe renal impairment. Risk of severe and prolonged side-effects. Use if risk of not treating the patient outweighs the risk of adverse effects

Ramipril

Clinical use

ACE inhibitor. Hypertension, secondary prevention of MI, congestive heart failure

Dose in normal renal function

1.25–10 mg once a day

Pharmacokinetics

Molecular weight (daltons)	388*
% Protein binding	50–60*
% Excreted unchanged in urine	10–21
Volume of distribution (L/kg)	430* litres
Half-life – normal/ESRF (hrs)	3/15*

Dose in renal impairment GFR (mL/min)

20–50	Dose as in normal renal function
10–20	1.25–5 mg daily
<10	1.25–2.5 mg daily

Dose in patients undergoing renal replacement therapies

CAPD	Unknown dialysability. Dose as in GFR = <10 mL/min
HD	Dialysed. Dose as in GFR = <10 mL/min
CAV/VVHD	Dialysed. Dose as in GFR = 10–20 mL/min

Important drug interactions

POTENTIALLY HAZARDOUS INTERACTIONS WITH OTHER DRUGS

- Ciclosporin: increased risk of hyperkalaemia and nephrotoxicity
- Potassium supplements: increased risk of hyperkalaemia
- Lithium levels may be increased

- NSAIDs: risk of renal impairment, antagonism of hypotensive effects, increased risk of hyperkalaemia
- Anaesthetics: enhanced hypotensive effect
- Diuretics: enhanced hypotensive effect, increased risk of hyperkalaemia with potassium-sparing diuretics
- Epoetin: increased risk of hyperkalaemia
- Tacrolimus: increased risk of hyperkalaemia and nephrotoxicity

Administration

RECONSTITUTION

–

ROUTE

- Oral

RATE OF ADMINISTRATION

–

COMMENTS

–

Other information

- * Refers to active metabolite ramiprilat
- Renal failure has been reported in association with ACE inhibitors in patients with renal artery stenosis, post renal transplant, or those with congestive heart failure
- A high incidence of anaphylactoid reactions has been reported in patients dialysed with high-flux polyacrylonitrile membranes and treated concomitantly with an ACE inhibitor – this combination should therefore be avoided
- Hyperkalaemia and other side-effects more common in patients with impaired renal function
- Close monitoring of renal function during therapy is necessary in those patients with known renal insufficiency
- Normal doses have been used in ESRD

Ranitidine

Clinical use

H_2-antagonist. Conditions associated with hyperacidity

Dose in normal renal function

Oral: 150–300 mg once or twice daily

Zollinger-Ellison: 150 mg three times daily up to 6 g/day

IM/Slow IV injection: 50 mg every 6–8 hours

IV infusion: 25 mg/hour for 2 hours, 6–8 hourly; or for stress ulceration prophylaxis 125–250 micrograms/kg/hour

Pharmacokinetics

Molecular weight (daltons)	314
% Protein binding	15
% Excreted unchanged in urine	Oral: 30–70 IV: 70–80
Volume of distribution (L/kg)	1–2
Half-life – normal/ESRF (hrs)	2–3/6–9

Dose in renal impairment GFR (mL/min)

20–50	Dose as in normal renal function
10–20	Dose as in normal renal function
<10	50–100% of normal dose

Dose in patients undergoing renal replacement therapies

CAPD	Unknown dialysability. Dose as in GFR = <10 mL/min
HD	Dialysed. Dose as in GFR = <10 mL/min
CAV/VVHD	Probably dialysed. Dose as in GFR = 10–20 mL/min

Important drug interactions

POTENTIALLY HAZARDOUS INTERACTIONS WITH OTHER DRUGS

• Ciclosporin: may increase or not change ciclosporin levels. Nephrotoxicity, additive hepatotoxicity and thrombocytopenia reported

Administration

RECONSTITUTION

• Compatible with sodium chloride 0.9%, glucose 5% and other fluids

ROUTE

• Oral or IV peripherally. IM (undiluted)

RATE OF ADMINISTRATION

• Bolus: 50 mg made up to 20 mL over at least 2 minutes
• Intermittent infusion: 50 mg to 100 mL of appropriate intravenous solution run over 2 hours
• Continuous infusion: required dose in 250 mL of intravenous fluid over 24 hours

COMMENTS

• Admixtures stable for 24 hours

Other information

• Use in preference to cimetidine in the elderly, those who have side-effects to cimetidine and those in whom drug interactions may be a problem

Reboxetine

Clinical use

Antidepressant

Dose in normal renal function

4–5 mg twice daily; maximum 12 mg daily

Pharmacokinetics

Molecular weight (daltons)	409.5
% Protein binding	97 (92% in elderly)
% Excreted unchanged in urine	10
Volume of distribution (L/kg)	0.38–0.92
Half-life – normal/ESRF (hrs)	13/26

Dose in renal impairment GFR (mL/min)

20–50	Dose as in normal renal function
10–20	2 mg twice daily, adjust according to response
<10	2 mg twice daily, adjust according to response

Dose in patients undergoing renal replacement therapies

CAPD	Unknown dialysability. Dose as in GFR = <10 mL/min
HD	Unknown dialysability. Dose as in GFR = <10 mL/min
CAV/VVHD	Unknown dialysability. Dose as in GFR = 10–20 mL/min

Important drug interactions

POTENTIALLY HAZARDOUS INTERACTIONS WITH OTHER DRUGS

- Ciclosporin: use with caution as high concentrations of reboxetine inhibit CYP 3A4 and CYP 2D6
- Antibacterials: avoid concomitant use with macrolides and linezolid
- Antidepressants: MAOIs – risk of increased toxicity with concomitant use; avoid concomitant use with fluvoxamine; use with caution with tricyclics
- Antifungals: avoid concomitant use with imidazoles and triazoles
- Anti-malarials: avoid concomitant use with artemether with lumefantrine
- Sibutramine: increased risk of CNS toxicity (avoid concomitant use)

Administration

RECONSTITUTION

–

ROUTE

- Oral

RATE OF ADMINISTRATION

–

COMMENTS

–

Other information

–

Remifentanil

Clinical use

Analgesic, induction of anaesthesia

Dose in normal renal function

Induction: 0.5–1 microgram/kg/min

Maintenance:

- Ventilated patients:
  0.05–2 micrograms/kg/min
- Spontaneous respiration:
  0.025–0.1 micrograms/kg/min

Pharmacokinetics

Molecular weight (daltons)	412.9
% Protein binding	70
% Excreted unchanged in urine	95 (as metabolites)
Volume of distribution (L/kg)	0.35
Half-life – normal/ESRF (hrs)	3–10 minutes (biological activity). Terminal elimination 10–20 minutes/ unchanged

Dose in renal impairment GFR (mL/min)

20–50	Dose as in normal renal function
10–20	Dose as in normal renal function
<10	Dose as in normal renal function

Dose in patients undergoing renal replacement therapies

CAPD	Unknown dialysability. Dose as in normal renal function
HD	Dialysed. Dose as in normal renal function
CAV/VVHD	Unknown dialysability. Dose as in normal renal function

Important drug interactions

POTENTIALLY HAZARDOUS INTERACTIONS WITH OTHER DRUGS

- Anti-arrhythmics: delayed absorption of mexiletine
- Inhaled and IV anaesthetics, benzodiazepine: doses should be reduced
- Antidepressants: possible CNS excitation or depression (hypertension or hypotension) with MAOIs – avoid concomitant use
- Antipsychotics: enhanced sedative and hypotensive effect
- Antivirals: plasma concentration of remifentanil may be increased by ritonavir (risk of toxicity) – avoid

Administration

RECONSTITUTION

- To 1 mg/ml with infusion fluid

ROUTE

- IV

RATE OF ADMINISTRATION

- Dependent on indication

COMMENTS

- Dilute to 20–250 micrograms/mL with glucose 5%, sodium chloride 0.9% or water for injection. Usually 50 micrograms/mL for general anaesthesia

Other information

- Half-life of metabolites are increased to 30 hours in renal failure compared with 90 minutes in patients with normal renal function
- Metabolite is essentially inactive
- Remifentanil would be expected to be metabolised before patient needs to be dialysed
- The metabolites have a dialysis extraction of 30%

Repaglinide

Clinical use

Type 2 diabetes mellitus

Dose in normal renal function

500 micrograms – 16 mg daily, doses given
15–30 minutes before a meal

Pharmacokinetics

Molecular weight (daltons)	452.6
% Protein binding	>98
% Excreted unchanged in urine	<8 (mainly as metabolites)
Volume of distribution (L/kg)	30 litres
Half-life – normal/ESRF (hrs)	0.5–1/slightly increased

Dose in renal impairment GFR (mL/min)

30–80	Dose as in normal renal function
5–29	Start at a low dose and gradually increase according to response
<5	Start at a low dose and gradually increase according to response

Dose in patients undergoing renal replacement therapies

CAPD	Unlikely to be dialysed. Dose as in GFR = <5 mL/min
HD	Not dialysed. Dose as in GFR = <5 mL/min
CAV/VVHD	Unlikely to be dialysed. Dose as in GFR = 5–29 mL/min

Important drug interactions

POTENTIALLY HAZARDOUS INTERACTIONS WITH OTHER DRUGS

• Rifampicin: reduction in repaglinide levels

Administration

RECONSTITUTION

–

ROUTE

• Oral

RATE OF ADMINISTRATION

–

COMMENTS

–

Other information

• Major route of elimination is hepatic metabolism to inactive metabolites

Reteplase

Clinical use

Thrombolytic, used for acute myocardial infarction

Dose in normal renal function

10 units over 2 minutes, second dose of 10 units given 30 minutes later

Pharmacokinetics

Molecular weight (daltons)	39,571.1
% Protein binding	No data
% Excreted unchanged in urine	Negligible
Volume of distribution (L/kg)	6–6.5 litres
Half-life – normal/ESRF (hrs)	Fibrinolytic half-life is 1.6 hrs/increased
	Dominant (α) half-life is 14.6 ± 6.7 mins
	Terminal (β) half-life is 1.6 hrs ± 39 mins

Dose in renal impairment GFR (mL/min)

20–50	Dose as in normal renal function
10–20	Dose as in normal renal function
<10	Use with caution

Dose in patients undergoing renal replacement therapies

CAPD	Unknown dialysability. Use as in GFR < 10 mL/min
HD	Unknown dialysability. Use as in GFR < 10 mL/min
CAV/VVHD	Unknown dialysability. Use as in GFR = 10–20 mL/min

Important drug interactions

POTENTIALLY HAZARDOUS INTERACTIONS WITH OTHER DRUGS

• Antiplatelets, heparin, vitamin K antagonists: increased risk of bleeding

Administration

RECONSTITUTION

• With diluent provided

ROUTE

• Slow IV

RATE OF ADMINISTRATION

• Over not more than 2 minutes

COMMENTS

• Use immediately once reconstituted
• Do not mix with heparin in the same line

Other information

• Heparin and aspirin should be given before and after reteplase therapy to reduce the risk of re-thrombosis but may increase the risk of bleeding
• The half-life is increased in severe renal failure in animal models
• Possible increased risk of bleeding complications in severe renal impairment

Ribavirin (tribavirin)

Clinical use

(1) Antiviral agent for treatment of severe respiratory syncytial virus bronchiolitis

(2) Treatment of chronic hepatitis C in combination with interferon alfa-2b therapy or interferon alfa or peginterferon alfa-2b

Dose in normal renal function

(1) 6 g nebulised daily for 3–7 days

(2) <65 kg: 400 mg twice daily;

65–85 kg: 400 mg in the morning and 600 mg at 6 pm;

>85 kg: 600 mg twice daily

Pharmacokinetics

Molecular weight (daltons)	244
% Protein binding	0
% Excreted unchanged in urine	10–40
Volume of distribution (L/kg)	Nebulised: 647 litres; Oral: 5000 litres
Half-life – normal/ESRF (hrs)	Nebulised: 9/– Oral: 79/increased

Dose in renal impairment GFR (mL/min)

20–50	Dose as in normal renal function. Avoid oral, see 'Other information'
10–20	Dose as in normal renal function. Avoid oral, see 'Other information'
<10	Dose as in normal renal function. Avoid oral, see 'Other information'

Dose in patients undergoing renal replacement therapies

CAPD	Unknown dialysability. Dose as in GFR < 10 mL/min
HD	Not dialysed. Dose as in GFR < 10 mL/min
CAV/VVHD	Unknown dialysability. Dose as in GFR = 10–20 mL/min

Important drug interactions

POTENTIALLY HAZARDOUS INTERACTIONS WITH OTHER DRUGS

• Ribavirin may antagonise the effects of zidovudine and stavudine

Administration

RECONSTITUTION

• Dissolve contents of one vial in water for injection and further dilute to a volume of 300 mL

ROUTE

• Nebulised, oral

RATE OF ADMINISTRATION

• Administer over 12–18 hours per day

COMMENTS

• Treatment should be carried out for at least 3 days and no more than 7 days

Other information

• Ribavirin is also available as an intravenous infusion (on a 'named patient' basis). Available from ICN Pharmaceuticals (24 hour on-call line 01256 707744 or main switchboard). Refer to product literature for dosage reduction in renal failure

Oral:

• Administer ribavirin with interferon alfa-2b 3 MIU three times a week or peginterferon alfa-2b 1.5 micrograms/kg/week

• Take with food

• Contra-indicated by the company due to reduced clearance leading to increased side-effects

• Ribavirin is metabolised by reversible phosphorylation and a degradative pathway involving deribosylation and amide hydrolysis to produce renally excreted active metabolites

• There are a couple of studies using ribavirin in combination with interferon in haemodialysis and peritoneal dialysis patients. In these studies a dose of 200–400 mg a day of ribavirin was used. Anaemia was one of the main problems, resulting in either increased doses of erythropoietin or discontinuation of ribavirin therapy. Most patients were stabilised on a dose of 200 mg daily or 200 mg three times a week. A dose of 200 mg daily gave comparable troughs when compared with patients with normal renal function at a dose of 1200 mg daily. (*J Viral Hepat.* (2001) **8**: 287–92 and *Nephrol Dial Transplant.* (2001) **16**: 193–5)

• After stopping therapy the half-life was approximately 298 hours, due to slow elimination from non-plasma compartments

Rifampicin

Clinical use

Antibacterial agent for tuberculosis and staphylococcal infection

Dose in normal renal function

Oral or IV: 450–1200 mg daily

Pharmacokinetics

Molecular weight (daltons)	823
% Protein binding	60–90
% Excreted unchanged in urine	15–30
Volume of distribution (L/kg)	0.9
Half-life – normal/ESRF (hrs)	1.5–5/1.8–11

Dose in renal impairment GFR (mL/min)

20–50	Dose as in normal renal function
10–20	Dose as in normal renal function
<10	50–100% of normal dose

Dose in patients undergoing renal replacement therapies

CAPD	Not dialysed. Dose as in GFR = <10 mL/min
HD	Not dialysed. Dose as in GFR = <10 mL/min
CAV/VVHD	Unknown dialysability. Dose as in normal renal function

Important drug interactions

POTENTIALLY HAZARDOUS INTERACTIONS WITH OTHER DRUGS

- Ciclosporin: markedly reduced plasma levels (danger of transplant rejection); ciclosporin dose may need increasing 5-fold or more
- Tacrolimus: reduced tacrolimus concentration
- Sirolimus: reduced sirolimus concentration
- Indinavir: increases rifampicin levels
- Drugs metabolised by the CYP 450 3A system
- Reduced plasma concentration of chloramphenicol and dapsone
- Reduced anticoagulant effect of warfarin
- Reduced antidiabetic effect of chlorpropamide and tolbutamide
- Reduced plasma concentration of phenytoin
- Reduced plasma concentration of fluconazole, itraconazole, ketaconazole and terbinafine
- Reduced plasma level of corticosteroids. Double steroid dose. Give as twice-daily dosage
- Increased metabolism of azathioprine – reduced plasma levels
- Reduced plasma levels of combined and progestogen-only oral contraceptive
- Rifampicin also accelerates the metabolism of the following drugs (possible reduced effect): antivirals, atovaquone, methadone, disopyramide, mexiletine, propafenone, quinidine, tricyclic antidepressants, haloperidol, benzodiazepines, bisoprolol, propranolol, diltiazem, verapamil, isradipine, nifedipine, digitoxin, fluvastatin

Administration

RECONSTITUTION

- Use solvent provided. Dilute in 500 mL glucose 5% or sodium chloride 0.9%

ROUTE

- IV peripherally or orally

RATE OF ADMINISTRATION

- 2–3 hours

COMMENTS

- For central administration, 600 mg in 100 mL glucose 5% over 0.5–2 hours has been used (unlicensed). Stable for up to 24 hours at room temperature

Other information

- Some units give dose in concentrations up to 60 mg/mL over 10 minutes in its own solvent on prescriber's responsibility
- May cause acute interstitial nephritis, potassium wasting or renal tubular defects
- Reduce dose if LFT is abnormal or patient <45 kg
- Absorption from GI tract can be reduced by up to 80% by the presence of food in the GI tract
- CAPD exit site infections, 300 mg twice daily for 4 weeks has been used
- Rifampicin is excreted into CAPD fluid causing an orange/yellow colour
- Monitor rifampicin levels if necessary

Risedronate

Clinical use

Treatment and prevention of post-menopausal osteoporosis (including corticosteroid induced) and Paget's disease

Dose in normal renal function

Post-menopausal osteoporosis: 5 mg daily or 35 mg weekly

Paget's disease: 30 mg daily for 2 months

Pharmacokinetics

Molecular weight (daltons)	305.1
% Protein binding	24
% Excreted unchanged in urine	50
Volume of distribution (L/kg)	6.3
Half-life – normal/ESRF (hrs)	480/increased

Dose in renal impairment GFR (mL/min)

20–50	Dose as in normal renal function
10–20	Use 50% of the dose
<10	Avoid. See 'Other information'

Dose in patients undergoing renal replacement therapies

CAPD	Unknown dialysability. Dose as in GFR < 10 mL/min
HD	Unknown dialysability. Dose as in GFR < 10 mL/min
CAV/VVHD	Unknown dialysability. Dose as in GFR = 10–20 mL/min

Important drug interactions

POTENTIALLY HAZARDOUS INTERACTIONS WITH OTHER DRUGS

• Calcium-containing substances: avoid for 2 hours before and after administration

Administration

RECONSTITUTION

–

ROUTE

• Oral

RATE OF ADMINISTRATION

–

COMMENTS

–

Other information

• Swallow whole with a glass of water 30 minutes before food. Sit or stand upright for 30 minutes after administration

• Renal clearance is decreased by 70% in patients with CL_{CR} < 30 mL/min

• No data, but one paper suggests using a decreased dose when GFR < 20 mL/min. Mitchell D et al. (2000) British Journal of Clinical Pharmacology. **49**: 215–22

• Examples of use in other units:
  • Normal doses
  • 5 mg once weekly in dialysis patients

Risperidone

Clinical use

Treatment of schizophrenia and psychoses

Dose in normal renal function

• Oral: 2–10 mg daily in divided doses
• IM: 25–50 mg every 2 weeks

Pharmacokinetics

Molecular weight (daltons)	410.5
% Protein binding	88
% Excreted unchanged in urine	70
Volume of distribution (L/kg)	1–1.5
Half-life – normal/ESRF (hrs)	24/increased

Dose in renal impairment GFR (mL/min)

20–50	Initially 0.5 mg twice daily increasing by 0.5 mg BD to 1–2 mg twice daily. Use with caution. See 'Other information' for IM dosing
10–20	Initially 0.5 mg twice daily increasing by 0.5 mg BD to 1–2 mg twice daily. Use with caution. See 'Other information' for IM dosing
<10	Initially 0.5 mg twice daily increasing by 0.5 mg BD to 1–2 mg twice daily. Use with caution. See 'Other information' for IM dosing

Dose in patients undergoing renal replacement therapies

CAPD	Unlikely dialysability. Dose as in GFR < 10 mL/min
HD	Dialysed. Dose as in GFR < 10 mL/min
CAV/VVHD	Unlikely dialysability. Dose as in GFR = 10–20 mL/min

Important drug interactions

POTENTIALLY HAZARDOUS INTERACTIONS WITH OTHER DRUGS

• Fluoxetine, haloperidol: increased risperidone levels
• Anaesthetics: enhanced hypotensive effect
• Analgesics: enhanced sedative and hypotensive effects with opioids
• Antidepressants: increased risk of arrhythmias with tricyclics
• Anti-epileptics: antagonism, convulsive threshold may be lowered, carbamazepine lowers plasma concentration of risperidone
• Anti-malarials: avoid concomitant use with artemether with lumefantrine
• Antivirals: ritonavir may increase plasma concentration of risperidone
• Sibutramine: increased risk of CNS toxicity (avoid concomitant use)

Administration

RECONSTITUTION

• With solvent provided

ROUTE

• Oral, deep IM

RATE OF ADMINISTRATION

–

COMMENTS

–

Other information

• At a dose of 3 mg twice daily, 1.5 mg of risperidone is removed after a 5-hour dialysis session with a dialysate flow of 500 mL/min
• In overdose, rare cases of QT prolongation have been reported
• Clearance of risperidone and active metabolites decreased by 60% in severe renal impairment
• If a dose of 2 mg daily orally is tolerated then a dose of 25 mg IM every 2 weeks can be used initially in renal impairment

Ritonavir

Clinical use

Protease inhibitor for the treatment of HIV-1 infected adults with advanced or progressive immunodeficiency, in combination with nucleoside reverse transcriptase inhibitor

Dose in normal renal function

600 mg twice daily

Pharmacokinetics

Molecular weight (daltons)	720.9
% Protein binding	98–99
% Excreted unchanged in urine	3.5
Volume of distribution (L/kg)	20–40 litres
Half-life – normal/ESRF (hrs)	3–5/unchanged

Dose in renal impairment GFR (mL/min)

20–50	Dose as in normal renal function
10–20	Dose as in normal renal function
<10	Dose as in normal renal function

Dose in patients undergoing renal replacement therapies

CAPD	Not dialysed. Dose as in normal renal function
HD	Not dialysed. Dose as in normal renal function
CAV/VVHD	Unlikely to be dialysed. Dose as in normal renal function

Important drug interactions

POTENTIALLY HAZARDOUS INTERACTIONS WITH OTHER DRUGS

- Ciclosporin: levels possibly increased by ritonavir
- Amfebutamone (bupropion): amfebutamone levels increased – risk of toxicity, avoid
- Analgesics: opioid and NSAID plasma levels may be increased, risk of toxicity (avoid dextropropoxyphene, pethidine, piroxicam); methadone levels reduced
- Anti-arrhythmics: increased plasma concentrations of amiodarone, flecainide, propafenone and quinidine, increased risk of ventricular arrhythmias (avoid concomitant use); possible increased risk of arrhythmias with disopyramide and mexiletine
- Antibacterials: rifabutin plasma concentration increased, risk of uveitis, avoid; plasma concentration of clarithromycin and other macrolides increased, reduce dose of clarithromycin in renal impairment
- Anticoagulants: plasma concentration of warfarin and other anticoagulants possibly increased
- Antidepressants: SSRIs and tricyclic concentrations possibly increased; St John's Wort may reduce ritonavir plasma concentrations
- Anti-epileptics: carbamazepine plasma concentrations may be increased
- Antifungals: imidazole and triazole plasma concentrations possibly increased
- Antihistamines: increased risk of arrhythmias with terfenadine – avoid. Plasma concentrations of other non-sedating antihistamines possibly increased
- Antipsychotics: plasma concentrations of pimozide, clozapine and possibly other antipsychotics may be increased, risk of toxicity, avoid concomitant use
- Antivirals: levels of both nelfinavir and ritonavir may be increased if used in combination; combination with amprenavir may increase plasma concentration of both drugs; indinavir and saquinavir levels increased. Increased risk of toxicity with efavirenz (monitor LFTs)
- Anxiolytics and hypnotics: plasma levels of many of them increased – risk of extreme sedation and respiratory depression (avoid alprazolam, clorazepate, diazepam, flurazepam, midazolam, zolpidem)
- Calcium-channel blockers: plasma levels of calcium-channel blockers possibly increased
- Ergotamine and ergometrine: risk of ergotism, avoid
- Lipid-lowering drugs – increased risk of myopathy with simvastatin, avoid
- Oestrogens and progestogens: metabolism accelerated, combined OCP contraceptive effect reduced
- $5HT_1$ agonists: plasma concentration of eletriptan increased – avoid
- Sildenafil: plasma concentrations of sildenafil significantly increased, avoid
- Theophylline: metabolism accelerated, plasma theophylline levels reduced
- Tacrolimus: levels possibly increased by ritonavir

Administration

RECONSTITUTION

–

ROUTE

• Oral

RATE OF ADMINISTRATION

–

COMMENTS

–

Other information

• Administer with food
• Renal clearance is by glomerular filtration

Rituximab

Clinical use

Monoclonal antibody used to treat stage III–IV follicular lymphoma, and for diffuse large B-cell non-Hodgkin's lymphoma in combination with other chemotherapy

Dose in normal renal function

375 mg/m^2 weekly for 4 weeks

Pharmacokinetics

Molecular weight (daltons)	144,000
% Protein binding	No data
% Excreted unchanged in urine	No data
Volume of distribution (L/kg)	No data
Half-life – normal/ESRF (hrs)	68.1 (after 1st infusion)
	189.9 (after 4th infusion)

Dose in renal impairment GFR (mL/min)

20–50	Use with caution
10–20	Use with caution
<10	Use with caution

Dose in patients undergoing renal replacement therapies

CAPD	Removal unlikely. Use with caution
HD	Removal unlikely. Use with caution
CAV/VVHD	Unknown dialysability. Use with caution

Important drug interactions

POTENTIALLY HAZARDOUS INTERACTIONS WITH OTHER DRUGS

• None known

Administration

RECONSTITUTION

–

ROUTE

• IV infusion

RATE OF ADMINISTRATION

• 1st dose: 50 mg/hour then increase the rate every 30 minutes by 50 mg/hour to achieve a maximum rate of 400 mg/hour

• Further doses: 100 mg an hour increasing the rate by 100 mg/hour every 30 minutes to achieve a maximum rate of 400 mg/hour

COMMENTS

• Add to sodium chloride 0.9% or glucose 5% and gently invert to prevent foaming to achieve a concentration of 1 to 4 mg/mL

• Use immediately after dilution. Infusion solution is stable for 12 hours at room temperature

• Prepared solution has 24 hours chemical stability at 2–8°C

Other information

• Always give a pre-medication of paracetamol and an antihistamine before infusion

• Patients with high tumour burden or malignant cells >50,000 mm^3 may be at risk of severe cytokine release syndrome which may be associated with acute renal failure. Treat with caution

Rivastigmine

Clinical use

Treatment of mild–moderate dementia in Alzheimer's disease

Dose in normal renal function

3–6 mg twice daily (initially 1.5 mg twice daily)

Pharmacokinetics

Molecular weight (daltons)	250.3 (400.4 as hydrogen tartrate)
% Protein binding	40
% Excreted unchanged in urine	0 (>90 as pharmacologically inactive metabolites)
Volume of distribution (L/kg)	1.8–2.7
Half-life – normal/ESRF (hrs)	1/–

Dose in renal impairment GFR (mL/min)

20–50	Start at a low dose and gradually increase
10–20	Use with caution
<10	Use with caution

Dose in patients undergoing renal replacement therapies

CAPD	Likely to be dialysed. Start at low dose and titrate according to tolerability
HD	Likely to be dialysed. Start at low dose and titrate according to tolerability
CAV/VVHD	Likely to be dialysed. Start at low dose and titrate according to tolerability

Important drug interactions

POTENTIALLY HAZARDOUS INTERACTIONS WITH OTHER DRUGS

• Muscle relaxants: enhances effect of suxamethonium, antagonises effect of non-depolarising muscle relaxants

Administration

RECONSTITUTION

–

ROUTE

• Oral

RATE OF ADMINISTRATION

–

COMMENTS

–

Other information

• Administer with food. Swallow whole

Rizatriptan

Clinical use

Acute treatment of migraine

Dose in normal renal function

10 mg, maximum of two doses in 24 hours at least 2 hours apart

Pharmacokinetics

Molecular weight (daltons)	391.5
% Protein binding	14
% Excreted unchanged in urine	14
Volume of distribution (L/kg)	110 litres (females), 140 litres (males)
Half-life – normal/ESRF (hrs)	2–3/unchanged

Dose in renal impairment GFR (mL/min)

20–50	5 mg, then 5 mg. Maximum 10 mg in 24 hours
10–20	5 mg, then 5 mg. Maximum 10 mg in 24 hours
<10	Use with caution. Maximum 5 mg daily

Dose in patients undergoing renal replacement therapies

CAPD	Unknown dialysability. Maximum 5 mg, monitor closely
HD	Unknown dialysability. Maximum 5 mg, monitor closely
CAV/VVHD	Unknown dialysability. Dose as in GFR = 10–20 mL/min

Important drug interactions

POTENTIALLY HAZARDOUS INTERACTIONS WITH OTHER DRUGS

• Antidepressants: risk of CNS toxicity with MAOIs and linezolid (avoid for 2 weeks after discontinuation of MAOI); avoid St John's Wort – increased serotonergic effects

• Ergotamine: increased risk of vasospasm (avoid for 6 hours after rizatriptan, and avoid rizatriptan for 24 hours after ergotamine)

• Propranolol: plasma rizatriptan levels increased, reduce dose of rizatriptan to 5 mg (max 10 mg in 24 hours)

Administration

RECONSTITUTION

–

ROUTE

• Oral

RATE OF ADMINISTRATION

–

COMMENTS

–

Other information

• Administration with food delays absorption by approximately 1 hour

• Metabolised to mainly inactive metabolites

• <1% excreted in the urine as active N-monodesmethyl metabolite

• AUC increases by 44% in haemodialysis patients

Rocuronium bromide

Clinical use

Muscle relaxant in general anaesthesia

Dose in normal renal function

IV injection: intubation dose = 0.6 mg/kg; maintenance = 0.15 mg/kg

IV infusion: 0.6 mg/kg loading dose, followed by 0.3–0.6 mg/kg/hour

Pharmacokinetics

Molecular weight (daltons)	610
% Protein binding	25–30
% Excreted unchanged in urine	13–30
Volume of distribution (L/kg)	0.21
Half-life – normal/ESRF (hrs)	1.5/2

Dose in renal impairment GFR (mL/min)

20–50	Dose as in normal renal function
10–20	Dose as in normal renal function
<10	Dose as in normal renal function

Dose in patients undergoing renal replacement therapies

CAPD	Unknown dialysability. Dose as in normal renal function
HD	Unknown dialysability. Dose as in normal renal function
CAV/VVHD	Unknown dialysability. Dose as in normal renal function

Important drug interactions

POTENTIALLY HAZARDOUS INTERACTIONS WITH OTHER DRUGS

- Effects of rocuronium enhanced by quinidine and aminoglycoside and polypeptide antibiotics
- Botulinum toxin: neuromuscular block enhanced (risk of toxicity)

Administration

RECONSTITUTION

–

ROUTE

- IV

RATE OF ADMINISTRATION

- Slow bolus or continuous infusion

COMMENTS

- Compatible with sodium chloride 0.9% and glucose 5%

Other information

- Use with caution in renal failure. Prolongation of action may be seen
- There are no clinically active metabolites of rocuronium

Rofecoxib

Clinical use

COX-2 inhibitor, used for symptomatic treatment
of osteoarthritis and rheumatoid arthritis, acute
pain including dysmenorrhoea, dental and
orthopaedic surgery

Dose in normal renal function

OA: 12.5–25 mg once daily

RA: 25 mg once daily

Acute pain: 25–50 mg daily

Pharmacokinetics

Molecular weight (daltons)	314.4
% Protein binding	85
% Excreted unchanged in urine	1
Volume of distribution (L/kg)	Approx 1.55
Half-life – normal/ESRF (hrs)	17/unchanged

Dose in renal impairment GFR (mL/min)

20–50	Dose as in normal renal function. Use with caution
10–20	Dose as in normal renal function, but avoid if possible
<10	Dose as in normal renal function, but only use if ESRD on dialysis

Dose in patients undergoing renal replacement therapies

CAPD	Unlikely dialysability. Start with low doses
HD	Not dialysed. Start with low doses
CAV/VVHD	Unknown dialysability. Start with low doses

Important drug interactions

POTENTIALLY HAZARDOUS INTERACTIONS WITH
OTHER DRUGS

- Ciclosporin: potential for increased risk of
nephrotoxicity
- Cytotoxic agents: reduced excretion of
methotrexate, possible increased risk of toxicity
- ACE inhibitors and AT-II antagonists: antagonism
of hypotensive effect; increased risk of renal
damage and hyperkalaemia
- Analgesics: avoid use of two or more NSAIDs,
including aspirin (increased side-effects)
- Antibacterials: possible increased risk of
convulsions with quinolones
- Anticoagulants: anticoagulant effect of warfarin
and acenocoumarol enhanced
- Antidiabetics: effect of sulphonylureas possibly
enhanced
- Anti-epileptics: phenytoin effects enhanced
- Antivirals: increased risk of haematological
toxicity with zidovudine; NSAID plasma
concentrations possibly increased by ritonavir
- Diuretics: risk of NSAID nephrotoxicity
increased, possible antagonism of diuretic effect,
increased risk of hyperkalaemia with potassium-
sparing diuretics
- Lithium: reduced lithium excretion, risk of
toxicity
- Tacrolimus: increased risk of nephrotoxicity

Administration

RECONSTITUTION

–

ROUTE

- Oral

RATE OF ADMINISTRATION

–

COMMENTS

–

Other information

- Clinical trials have shown renal effects similar to
those observed with comparator NSAIDs.
Monitor patient for deterioration in renal
function and fluid retention
- Inhibition of renal prostaglandin synthesis by
NSAIDs may interfere with renal function,
especially in the presence of existing renal
disease. Avoid if possible; if not, check serum
creatinine 48–72 hours after starting NSAID. If
raised, discontinue NSAID therapy
- Use normal doses in patients with ESRD on
dialysis
- Use with caution in renal transplant recipients –
can reduce intra-renal autocoid synthesis
- Rofecoxib should be used with caution in
uraemic patients predisposed to GI bleeding or
uraemic coagulopathies

Ropinirole

Clinical use

Parkinson's disease

Dose in normal renal function

0.25–3 mg three times a day

Maximum 24 mg in 24 hours

Pharmacokinetics

Molecular weight (daltons)	260.4
% Protein binding	10–40
% Excreted unchanged in urine	<10
Volume of distribution (L/kg)	8
Half-life – normal/ESRF (hrs)	6/–

Dose in renal impairment GFR (mL/min)

30–50	Dose as in normal renal function
10–30	Dose as in normal renal function – use with caution
<10	Dose as in normal renal function – use with caution

Dose in patients undergoing renal replacement therapies

CAPD	Unlikely dialysability. Dose as in GFR < 10 mL/min
HD	Unlikely dialysability. Dose as in GFR < 10 mL/min
CAV/VVHD	Unlikely dialysability. Dose as in GFR = 10–30 mL/min

Important drug interactions

POTENTIALLY HAZARDOUS INTERACTIONS WITH OTHER DRUGS

- Antipsychotics: antagonism of antiparkinsonian effect of ropinirole (avoid concomitant use)
- Metoclopramide: antagonism of antiparkinsonian effect of ropinirole (avoid concomitant use)
- Oestrogens and progestogens: plasma concentration increased by oestrogens

Administration

RECONSTITUTION

–

ROUTE

- Oral

RATE OF ADMINISTRATION

–

COMMENTS

–

Other information

- If administered with levodopa, decrease the dose of levodopa by 20%
- Take with meals to improve GI tolerance, but T_{max} increases by 2.5 hours
- No data in renal impairment
- Ropinirole is hepatically metabolised to inactive metabolites

Rosiglitazone

Clinical use

Type 2 diabetes in combination with other oral antidiabetic medication

Dose in normal renal function

4 mg per day in one or two divided doses

In combination with metformin, dose can be increased to 8 mg per day

Pharmacokinetics

Molecular weight (daltons)	357.4 (473.5 as maleate)
% Protein binding	99.8
% Excreted unchanged in urine	None (66% as metabolites)
Volume of distribution (L/kg)	14 litres
Half-life – normal/ESRF (hrs)	3–4/unchanged

Dose in renal impairment GFR (mL/min)

20–50	Dose as in normal renal function
10–20	Dose as in normal renal function
<10	Dose as in normal renal function

Dose in patients undergoing renal replacement therapies

CAPD	Unlikely to be dialysed. Dose as in normal renal function
HD	Not dialysed. Dose as in normal renal function
CAV/VVHD	Unlikely to be dialysed. Dose as in normal renal function

Important drug interactions

POTENTIALLY HAZARDOUS INTERACTIONS WITH OTHER DRUGS

• None known

Administration

RECONSTITUTION

–

ROUTE

• Oral

RATE OF ADMINISTRATION

–

COMMENTS

–

Other information

• Measure liver function prior to initiating therapy, and then every 2 months thereafter for 12 months, and then at regular intervals

• Rosiglitazone is extensively metabolised in the liver. Some of the metabolites are active, and are largely excreted in the urine

• Rosiglitazone is contra-indicated for co-administration with insulin

Salbutamol

Clinical use

Beta$_2$-adrenoceptor agonist: reversible airways disease

Dose in normal renal function

Oral: 4 mg 3–4 times daily

SC/IM: 500 micrograms repeated 4-hourly if necessary

IV: 250 micrograms/5 mL slow bolus

Infusion: start with 5 micrograms/minute, adjust according to response, usually 3–20 micrograms/minute

Aerosol: 100–200 micrograms (1–2 puffs) four times daily

Powder: 200–400 micrograms four times daily

Nebulisation: 2.5–5 mg four times daily or more frequently

Pharmacokinetics

Molecular weight (daltons)	239.3
% Protein binding	10
% Excreted unchanged in urine	51–64
Volume of distribution (L/kg)	2.8–4.0
Half-life – normal/ESRF (hrs)	2.7–5/unchanged

Dose in renal impairment GFR (mL/min)

20–50	Dose as in normal renal function
10–20	Dose as in normal renal function
<10	Dose as in normal renal function

Dose in patients undergoing renal replacement therapies

CAPD	Unknown dialysability. Dose as in normal renal function
HD	Unknown dialysability. Dose as in normal renal function
CAV/VVHD	Unknown dialysability. Dose as in normal renal function

Important drug interactions

POTENTIALLY HAZARDOUS INTERACTIONS WITH OTHER DRUGS

- Increased risk of hypokalaemia when diuretics, theophylline or large doses of corticosteroids are given with high doses of salbutamol
- Antihypertensives: acute hypotension with methyldopa

Administration

RECONSTITUTION

- Infusion: dilute 10 mL to 500 mL with sodium chloride 0.9% or glucose 5% (20 micrograms/mL)
- Via syringe pump: dilute 10 mL to 50 mL with sodium chloride 0.9% or glucose 5% (200 micrograms/mL)

ROUTE

- IV, SC, IM, oral, inhaled, nebulised

RATE OF ADMINISTRATION

- IV slow bolus; IV infusion 3–20 micrograms/minute

COMMENTS

–

Other information

- Monitor ECG/BP/pulse
- Nebulised salbutamol may be prescribed for hypokalaemic effect in acute hyperkalaemia (unlicensed)

Saquinavir

Clinical use

HIV protease inhibitor for the treatment of HIV-infected patients with advanced or progressive immunodeficiency, in combination with other antiviral drugs

Dose in normal renal function

Invirase: 600 mg three times a day

Fortovase: 1200 mg three times a day

Pharmacokinetics

Molecular weight (daltons)	670.8 (saquinavir), 766.9 (Fortovase)
% Protein binding	98
% Excreted unchanged in urine	<4
Volume of distribution (L/kg)	700 litres
Half-life – normal/ESRF (hrs)	13.2/–

Dose in renal impairment GFR (mL/min)

20–50	Dose as in normal renal function
10–20	Dose as in normal renal function
<10	Dose as in normal renal function

Dose in patients undergoing renal replacement therapies

CAPD	Unlikely dialysability. Dose as in normal renal function
HD	Unlikely dialysability. Dose as in normal renal function
CAV/VVHD	Unknown dialysability. Dose as in normal renal function

Important drug interactions

POTENTIALLY HAZARDOUS INTERACTIONS WITH OTHER DRUGS

- Rifampicin, rifabutin: can reduce saquinavir levels by 80%, 40% respectively (metabolism accelerated)
- Anti-epileptics: carbamazepine, phenobarbital and phenytoin can reduce saquinavir levels
- Terfenadine: can increase the risk of arrhythmias
- Antivirals: nevirapine and efavirenz can reduce saquinavir levels. Nelfinavir can cause an increase in levels of both nelfinavir and saquinavir. Indinavir and ritonavir can increase saquinavir levels
- Antidepressants: plasma concentration reduced by St John's Wort – avoid
- Antipsychotics: risk of arrythmias with pimozide – avoid; saquinavir possibly increases plasma concentration of thioridazine
- Anxiolytics and hypnotics: midazolam plasma concentration possibly increased (prolonged sedation – avoid)
- Ergotamine and ergometrine: risk of ergotism – avoid
- Lipid-lowering drugs: increased risk of myopathy with simvastatin – avoid

Administration

RECONSTITUTION

–

ROUTE

- Oral

RATE OF ADMINISTRATION

–

COMMENTS

- Administer within 2 hours after meal

Other information

- TDM is available from HIV Focus Roche Products UK and the University of Liverpool, but this service is not available to all patients

Senna (sennoside B)

Clinical use

Constipation

Dose in normal renal function

15–30 mg (2–4 tablets) at night

Pharmacokinetics

Molecular weight (daltons)	862.7
% Protein binding	Systemic bioavailability less than 5%
% Excreted unchanged in urine	–
Volume of distribution (L/kg)	–
Half-life – normal/ESRF (hrs)	–

Dose in renal impairment GFR (mL/min)

20–50	Dose as in normal renal function
10–20	Dose as in normal renal function
<10	Dose as in normal renal function

Dose in patients undergoing renal replacement therapies

CAPD	Unknown dialysability. Dose as in normal renal function
HD	Unknown dialysability. Dose as in normal renal function
CAV/VVHD	Unknown dialysability. Dose as in normal renal function

Important drug interactions

POTENTIALLY HAZARDOUS INTERACTIONS WITH OTHER DRUGS

• None known

Administration

RECONSTITUTION

–

ROUTE

• Oral

RATE OF ADMINISTRATION

–

COMMENTS

–

Other information

• Acts in 8–12 hours
• Syrup available, 1 tablet = 5 mL
• Granules available, 1 x 5 mL spoonful = 2 tablets
• Diabetic patients should use the tablets as these have a negligible sugar content

Sertraline

Clinical use

SSRI antidepressant, used for post-traumatic stress disorder

Dose in normal renal function

50 mg daily (maximum 200 mg for 8 weeks only)

Pharmacokinetics

Molecular weight (daltons)	342.7
% Protein binding	>98
% Excreted unchanged in urine	0
Volume of distribution (L/kg)	>20
Half-life – normal/ESRF (hrs)	26/probably unchanged

Dose in renal impairment GFR (mL/min)

20–50	Dose as in normal renal function
10–20	Dose as in normal renal function
<10	Dose as in normal renal function

Dose in patients undergoing renal replacement therapies

CAPD	Unknown dialysability. Dose as in normal renal function
HD	Not dialysed. Dose as in normal renal function
CAV/VVHD	Unknown dialysability. Dose as in normal renal function

Important drug interactions

POTENTIALLY HAZARDOUS INTERACTIONS WITH OTHER DRUGS

• Effect of warfarin and acenocoumarol possibly enhanced
• Increased risk of toxic CNS effects of MAOIs; sertraline and MAOIs should not be prescribed within a 2-week period of each other
• Lithium: increased risk of CNS effects – lithium toxicity reported
• Analgesics: increased risk of CNS toxicity with tramadol
• Antipsychotics: increased plasma concentrations with clozapine
• Ritonavir: possibly increases sertraline concentration
• Dopaminergics: hypertension and CNS excitation
• Sibutramine: increased risk of CNS toxicity – avoid concomitant use
• Linezolid: use with caution
• Anti-malarials: manufacturer advises avoid concomitant use with artemether with lumefantrine

Administration

RECONSTITUTION

–

ROUTE

• Oral

RATE OF ADMINISTRATION

–

COMMENTS

–

Other information

• Sertraline is extensively metabolised by the liver. It can be used in renal failure at normal doses with caution

Sevelamer (Renagel)

Clinical use

Phosphate-binding agent

Dose in normal renal function

1–10 capsules (if using 403 mg capsules), 1–5 (if using 800 mg tablets) three times a day with meals, dose is adjusted according to serum phosphate level

(Average 6–12 of 403 mg, 3–6 of 800 mg)

Pharmacokinetics

Molecular weight (daltons)	Large
% Protein binding	–
% Excreted unchanged in urine	–
Volume of distribution (L/kg)	–
Half-life – normal/ESRF (hrs)	–

Dose in renal impairment GFR (mL/min)

20–50	Dose as in normal renal function
10–20	Dose as in normal renal function
<10	Dose as in normal renal function

Dose in patients undergoing renal replacement therapies

CAPD	Unlikely dialysability. Dose as in normal renal function
HD	Unlikely dialysability. Dose as in normal renal function
CAV/VVHD	Unlikely dialysability. Dose as in normal renal function

Important drug interactions

POTENTIALLY HAZARDOUS INTERACTIONS WITH OTHER DRUGS

• None known

Administration

RECONSTITUTION

–

ROUTE

• Oral

RATE OF ADMINISTRATION

–

COMMENTS

–

Other information

• Do not use if the patient has swallowing disorders, or untreated or severe gastroparesis

• Renagel is not systemically absorbed

• One capsule = 403 mg of poly(allylamine hydrochloride) polymer

• One tablet = 800 mg of poly(allylamine hydrochloride) polymer

• At present only licensed for haemodialysis patients

Sibutramine

Clinical use

Treatment of obesity for patients who have not responded to appropriate weight-reducing methods

Dose in normal renal function

10–15 mg daily

Pharmacokinetics

Molecular weight (daltons)	334.3
% Protein binding	97
% Excreted unchanged in urine	Only inactive metabolites
Volume of distribution (L/kg)	No data
Half-life – normal/ESRF (hrs)	14–16/–

Dose in renal impairment GFR (mL/min)

20–50	Dose as in normal renal function. Use with caution
10–20	Dose as in normal renal function. Use with caution
<10	Dose as in normal renal function. Use with caution

Dose in patients undergoing renal replacement therapies

CAPD	Unlikely dialysability. Dose as in GFR = <10 mL/min
HD	Unlikely dialysability. Dose as in GFR = <10 mL/min
CAV/VVHD	Unknown dialysability. Dose as in GFR = 10–20 mL/min

Important drug interactions

POTENTIALLY HAZARDOUS INTERACTIONS WITH OTHER DRUGS

• Antidepressants: increased risk of CNS toxicity; avoid concomitant administration with MAOIs and avoid MAOIs for at least 2 weeks after stopping sibutramine
• Antipsychotics: increased risk of CNS toxicity (avoid concomitant use)
• Avoid use with drugs which increase heart rate or BP
• Drugs which are metabolised by CYP 3A4 may affect plasma sibutramine concentration

Administration

RECONSTITUTION

–

ROUTE

• Oral

RATE OF ADMINISTRATION

–

COMMENTS

–

Other information

• Do not use in patients with uncontrolled hypertension, i.e. BP > 145/90 mmHg
• Initiation of therapy is associated with a mean increase in resting systolic and diastolic BP of 2–3 mmHg

Sildenafil

Clinical use

Treatment of erectile dysfunction

Dose in normal renal function

25–100 mg half to 4 hours (ideally approximately 1 hour) before sexual intercourse. No more than 1 dose per day

Pharmacokinetics

Molecular weight (daltons)	666.7
% Protein binding	96
% Excreted unchanged in urine	<2
Volume of distribution (L/kg)	1–2
Half-life – normal/ESRF (hrs)	3–5/increased

Dose in renal impairment GFR (mL/min)

30–50	Dose as in normal renal function
10–30	Initial dose 25 mg and increase if required
<10	Initial dose 25 mg and increase if required

Dose in patients undergoing renal replacement therapies

CAPD	Unlikely to be dialysed. Dose as in GFR = <10 mL/min
HD	Unlikely to be dialysed. Dose as in GFR = <10 mL/min
CAV/VVHD	Unlikely to be dialysed. Dose as in GFR = 10–20 mL/min

Important drug interactions

POTENTIALLY HAZARDOUS INTERACTIONS WITH OTHER DRUGS

• Antivirals: ritonavir significantly increases plasma-sildenafil concentrations (avoid concomitant use); saquinavir and possibly amprenavir, indinavir and nelfinavir increase plasma-sildenafil concentration (reduce dose of sildenafil)

• Nicorandil: enhanced hypotensive effect (avoid concomitant use)

• Nitrates: enhanced hypotensive effect (absolutely contra-indicated)

• CYP 3A4 inhibitors: increases levels of sildenafil so use 25 mg

Administration

RECONSTITUTION

–

ROUTE

• Oral

RATE OF ADMINISTRATION

–

COMMENTS

–

Other information

• Dialysis is not expected to increase clearance as sildenafil is highly protein bound

• Patients should seek prompt medical advice if their erections last for more than 4 hours

• Recommend use on non-dialysis days. Need to evaluate timing of sildenafil in haemodialysis patients. In peritoneal dialysis, treatment with sildenafil is well tolerated

• Anecdotally it has been used at Guy's Hospital, London, for diabetic gastroparesis at a dose of 25 mg three times a day

• The use of sildenafil is potentially hazardous in patients with active coronary ischaemia, those with congestive heart failure and those with complicated multi-drug antihypertensive therapy regimens

• In nine patients on maintenance haemodialysis, sildenafil 50 mg appeared to produce firmer erections and greater sexual satisfaction, but the effects were prolonged for up to 48 hours after administration

Simple linctus

Clinical use

Relief of dry, irritating coughs

Dose in normal renal function

5–10 mL 3–4 times daily

Pharmacokinetics

Molecular weight (daltons)	210.1 (citric acid monohydrate)
% Protein binding	–
% Excreted unchanged in urine	–
Volume of distribution (L/kg)	–
Half-life – normal/ESRF (hrs)	–

Dose in renal impairment GFR (mL/min)

20–50	Dose as in normal renal function
10–20	Dose as in normal renal function
<10	Dose as in normal renal function

Dose in patients undergoing renal replacement therapies

CAPD	Unknown dialysability. Dose as in normal renal function
HD	Unknown dialysability. Dose as in normal renal function
CAV/VVHD	Unknown dialysability. Dose as in normal renal function

Important drug interactions

POTENTIALLY HAZARDOUS INTERACTIONS WITH OTHER DRUGS

• None known

Administration

RECONSTITUTION
–

ROUTE

• Oral

RATE OF ADMINISTRATION
–

COMMENTS
–

Other information

• Sugar content has not been found to alter diabetics' insulin requirements. Use diabetic cough preparations wherever possible

Simvastatin

Clinical use

HMG CoA reductase inhibitor: primary
hypercholesterolaemia

Dose in normal renal function

10–80 mg at night

Pharmacokinetics

Molecular weight (daltons)	418
% Protein binding	>94
% Excreted unchanged in urine	13
Volume of distribution (L/kg)	54
Half-life – normal/ESRF (hrs)	1.9/–

Dose in renal impairment GFR (mL/min)

20–50	Dose as in normal renal function
10–20	Dose as in normal renal function
<10	10 mg daily*

Dose in patients undergoing renal replacement therapies

CAPD	Unlikely dialysability. Dose as in GFR = <10 mL/min
HD	Unlikely dialysability. Dose as in GFR = <10 mL/min
CAV/VVHD	Unknown dialysability. Dose as in normal renal function

Important drug interactions

POTENTIALLY HAZARDOUS INTERACTIONS WITH OTHER DRUGS

- Ciclosporin: increased risk of myopathy.
  Maximum recommended dosage of simvastatin is
  10 mg/day
- Warfarin effect potentiated
- Increased risk of myopathy if prescribed
  concomitantly with fibrates
- Antibiotics: increased risk of myopathy with
  clarithromycin and erythromycin – avoid
  concomitant use
- Antifungals: increased risk of myopathy – avoid
  concomitant use
- Antivirals: increased risk of myopathy – avoid
  concomitant use

Administration

RECONSTITUTION

–

ROUTE

- Oral

RATE OF ADMINISTRATION

–

COMMENTS

–

Other information

- * In severe renal impairment doses above 10 mg
  should be used with caution

Sirolimus

Clinical use

Immunosuppressant: used for prophylaxis of transplant allograft rejection

Dose in normal renal function

6 mg loading dose followed by 2 mg daily, the dose is adjusted according to levels – see 'Other information'

Pharmacokinetics

Molecular weight (daltons)	914.2
% Protein binding	92
% Excreted unchanged in urine	2.2
Volume of distribution (L/kg)	12 ± 4.6
Half-life – normal/ESRF (hrs)	57–63/unchanged

Dose in renal impairment GFR (mL/min)

20–50	Dose as in normal renal function
10–20	Dose as in normal renal function
<10	Dose as in normal renal function

Dose in patients undergoing renal replacement therapies

CAPD	Unlikely dialysability. Dose as in normal renal function
HD	Not dialysed. Dose as in normal renal function
CAV/VVHD	Unlikely dialysability. Dose as in normal renal function

Important drug interactions

POTENTIALLY HAZARDOUS INTERACTIONS WITH OTHER DRUGS

- Ciclosporin: increased absorption of sirolimus, give sirolimus 4 hours after ciclosporin; sirolimus concentration increased

- Sirolimus levels increased by: fluconazole, itraconazole, ketoconazole, clarithromycin, erythromycin, metoclopramide, cimetidine, nicardipine, verapamil, diltiazem, danazol, protease inhibitors, grapefruit juice, bromocriptine
- Sirolimus levels decreased by: rifampicin, carbamazepine, phenobarbital, phenytoin

Administration

RECONSTITUTION

–

ROUTE

- Oral

RATE OF ADMINISTRATION

–

COMMENTS

–

Other information

- Aim for trough levels of 4–12 nanograms/mL where sirolimus is used in combination with low dose ciclosporin
- In cases of delayed graft function or where a calcineurin inhibitor is not tolerated or contra-indicated, sirolimus may be used with steroids alone. Here, recommend a loading dose of 10–15 mg, followed by a maintenance dose of 3–6 mg daily and adjust according to levels. Aim for trough levels of 8–20 nanograms/mL
- May be used in combination with MMF, but can lead to delayed wound healing post surgery. Sirolimus can increase levels of mycophenolic acid, leading to anaemia
- Some centres successfully using level-controlled sirolimus in conjunction with low dose tacrolimus
- Anecdotally has been used for sclerosing peritonitis in a CAPD patient at Guy's Hospital, London. Acts by interfering with various growth factors and its effect on impairing wound healing

Sodium bicarbonate

Clinical use

Metabolic acidosis, alkalinisation of urine

Dose in normal renal function

Oral: 600 mg – 1.8 g three times daily (or more may be required)

IV: 8.4%: 60–120 mL per hour; 4.2%: up to 120 mL per hour

Pharmacokinetics

Molecular weight (daltons)	84
% Protein binding	0
% Excreted unchanged in urine	–
Volume of distribution (L/kg)	Dependent on the physical state of the patient at the time
Half-life – normal/ESRF (hrs)	–

Dose in renal impairment GFR (mL/min)

20–50	Dose as in normal renal function
10–20	Dose as in normal renal function
<10	Use with caution

Dose in patients undergoing renal replacement therapies

CAPD	Dialysed. Dose as in GFR = <10 mL/min
HD	Dialysed. Dose as in GFR = <10 mL/min
CAV/VVHD	Dialysed. Dose as in normal renal function

Important drug interactions

POTENTIALLY HAZARDOUS INTERACTIONS WITH OTHER DRUGS

• Increases lithium excretion

Administration

RECONSTITUTION

–

ROUTE

• Oral, IV, central administration for undiluted infusion

RATE OF ADMINISTRATION

–

COMMENTS

–

Other information

• Caution – may result in sodium retention and oedema

• 8.4% ≡ 1 mmol bicarbonate per mL + 1 mmol sodium per mL

• 600 mg sodium bicarbonate contains ≡ 7 mmol sodium + 7 mmol bicarbonate

• Sodium bicarbonate reduces serum potassium concentrations by inducing a shift of potassium ions into the cell

Sodium chloride

Clinical use

Treatment and prophylaxis of sodium chloride deficiency

Dose in normal renal function

Oral: Prophylaxis: 40–80 mmol sodium daily, up to a maximum of 200 mmol sodium daily

• 100–160 mmol sodium orally after haemodialysis

Pharmacokinetics

Molecular weight (daltons)	58.5
% Protein binding	0
% Excreted unchanged in urine	–
Volume of distribution (L/kg)	Dependent on the physiological state of the patient at the time
Half-life – normal/ESRF (hrs)	–

Dose in renal impairment GFR (mL/min)

20–50	Dose as in normal renal function
10–20	Dose as in normal renal function
<10	Dose as in normal renal function

Dose in patients undergoing renal replacement therapies

CAPD	Dialysed. Dose as in normal renal function
HD	Dialysed. Dose as in normal renal function
CAV/VVHD	Dialysed. Dose as in normal renal function

Important drug interactions

POTENTIALLY HAZARDOUS INTERACTIONS WITH OTHER DRUGS

• May impair the efficacy of antihypertensive drugs in CRF

Administration

RECONSTITUTION

–

ROUTE

• Oral, IV

RATE OF ADMINISTRATION

–

COMMENTS

–

Other information

• Other regimens: for acute muscular cramps post haemodialysis 10 mL sodium chloride 30% injection diluted in 100 mL sodium chloride 0.9% and infused over 30 minutes or in dialysis washback

• Sodium salts should be administered with caution to patients with congestive heart failure, peripheral or pulmonary oedema, or impaired renal function

• Slow Sodium 600 mg tablet contains approximately 10 mmol Na^+ and 10 mmol Cl^-

Sodium nitroprusside

Clinical use

Hypertensive crisis, cardiac failure

Dose in normal renal function

IV: 0.3–8.0 micrograms/kg/minute
Range: 10–400 micrograms/minute

Pharmacokinetics

Molecular weight (daltons)	298
% Protein binding	0
% Excreted unchanged in urine	<10
Volume of distribution (L/kg)	0.2
Half-life – normal/ESRF (hrs)	2–10 minutes/ unchanged

Dose in renal impairment GFR (mL/min)

20–50	Dose as in normal renal function
10–20	Dose as in normal renal function. Avoid prolonged use
<10	Dose as in normal renal function. Avoid prolonged use

Dose in patients undergoing renal replacement therapies

CAPD	Dialysed. Dose as in GFR = <10 mL/min
HD	Dialysed. Dose as in GFR = <10 mL/min
CAV/VVHD	Unknown dialysability. Dose as in GFR = 10–20 mL/min

Important drug interactions

POTENTIALLY HAZARDOUS INTERACTIONS WITH OTHER DRUGS

• Anaesthetics: enhanced hypotensive effect

Administration

RECONSTITUTION

• 2 mL glucose 5%, then dilute to 50–200 micrograms/mL with glucose 5%

ROUTE

• IV

RATE OF ADMINISTRATION

• 10–400 micrograms/minute adjusted according to response

COMMENTS

• Wrap syringes and lines in foil to protect from light
• For peripheral use dilute 50 mg to 250 mL (200 micrograms/mL)

Other information

• Sodium nitroprusside is rapidly metabolised to cyanogen which is converted to thiocyanate
• Avoid prolonged use in renal impairment. Accumulation of thiocyanate (toxic), which is dialysable
• Monitor thiocyanate and cyanide levels
• Do not stop infusion abruptly – tail off over 10–30 minutes

Sodium valproate

Clinical use

All forms of epilepsy

Dose in normal renal function

Oral: 600 mg – 2.5 g daily in divided doses

IV: For continuation of therapy give existing oral dose. **Initiation:** 400–800 mg (up to 10 mg/kg), then further doses up to 2.5 g daily

Pharmacokinetics

Molecular weight (daltons)	166
% Protein binding	90
% Excreted unchanged in urine	3–7
Volume of distribution (L/kg)	0.1–0.4
Half-life – normal/ESRF (hrs)	6–15/unchanged

Dose in renal impairment
GFR (mL/min)

20–50	Dose as in normal renal function
10–20	Dose as in normal renal function
<10	Dose as in normal renal function

Dose in patients undergoing renal replacement therapies

CAPD	Unknown dialysability. Dose as in normal renal function
HD	Not dialysed. Dose as in normal renal function
CAV/VVHD	Unknown dialysability. Dose as in normal renal function

Important drug interactions

POTENTIALLY HAZARDOUS INTERACTIONS WITH OTHER DRUGS

• Ciclosporin: variable ciclosporin blood level response

• Antidepressants, antipsychotics and anti-malarials: antagonise anticonvulsant effect

• Other anti-epileptics: enhance toxicity and possibly reduce plasma concentrations

Administration

RECONSTITUTION

• IV: use solvent provided

ROUTE

• IV, oral

RATE OF ADMINISTRATION

• 3–5 minute bolus, or continuous infusion

COMMENTS

–

Other information

• Available as enteric-coated, controlled-release and crushable tablets; liquid and syrup

• Increases ketones in urine. May give false positive urine tests for ketones

• Sodium valproate serum levels do not correlate with anti-epileptic activity

• Monitor serum levels to ensure not greater than 100 micrograms/mL, or if non-compliance is suspected

• In severe renal insufficiency it may be necessary to alter doses according to **free** serum levels

• Suppositories are available on a 'named patient' basis

Sotalol

Clinical use

Beta-adrenoceptor blocker: treatment of life-threatening ventricular arrhythmias; prophylaxis of SVT

Dose in normal renal function

Oral: 80–640 mg per day in single or divided doses
IV: 0.5–1.5 mg/kg every 6 hours

Pharmacokinetics

Molecular weight (daltons)	309
% Protein binding	0
% Excreted unchanged in urine	>90%
Volume of distribution (L/kg)	1–2
Half-life – normal/ESRF (hrs)	7–15/56

Dose in renal impairment
GFR (mL/min)

20–50	50% of normal dose
10–20	25% of normal dose
<10	Avoid or use with caution

Dose in patients undergoing renal replacement therapies

CAPD	Unlikely dialysability. Dose as in GFR = <10 mL/min
HD	Dialysed. Dose as in GFR = <10 mL/min
CAV/VVHD	Unknown dialysability. Dose as in GFR = 10–20 mL/min

Important drug interactions

POTENTIALLY HAZARDOUS INTERACTIONS WITH OTHER DRUGS

- Anti-arrhythmics: increased risk of bradycardia and AV block with amiodarone
- Calcium-channel blockers: increased risk of bradycardia and AV block with diltiazem and verapamil
- Mefloquine may increase risk of bradycardia
- Risk of ventricular arrhythmias associated with sotalol increased by tricyclic antidepressants, mizolastine, terfenadine, erythromycin, phenothiazines, pimozide
- Anaesthetics: enhanced hypotensive effect
- NSAIDs: antagonise hypotensive effect
- MAOIs: enhanced hypotensive effect
- Moxisylyte: possibly severe postural hypotension
- Sympathomimetics: severe hypertension

Administration

RECONSTITUTION
–

ROUTE
- IV, oral

RATE OF ADMINISTRATION
- Slow IV bolus with ECG monitoring, over 10 minutes
- Infusion: 0.2–0.5 mg/kg/hour

COMMENTS
–

Other information

- Sotalol prolongs the QT interval, which predisposes to the development of torsades de pointes
- If used in haemodialysis, give lowest possible dose, after dialysis

Stavudine

Clinical use

Nucleoside reverse transcriptase inhibitor for the treatment of HIV-infected adults and children with progressive or advanced immunodeficiency in combination with other drugs

Dose in normal renal function

<60 kg: 30 mg twice daily
>60 kg: 40 mg twice daily

Pharmacokinetics

Molecular weight (daltons)	224.2
% Protein binding	<1
% Excreted unchanged in urine	35–40
Volume of distribution (L/kg)	0.53
Half-life – normal/ESRF (hrs)	1–1.5/8

Dose in renal impairment GFR (mL/min)

26–50   <60 kg: 15 mg twice daily
>60 kg: 20 mg twice daily
<25   <60 kg: 15 mg daily
>60 kg: 20 mg daily

Dose in patients undergoing renal replacement therapies

CAPD	Unknown dialysability. Dose as in GFR = <25 mL/min
HD	Dialysed. Dose as in GFR = <25 mL/min
CAV/VVHD	Unknown dialysability. Dose as in GFR = 26–50 mL/min

Important drug interactions

POTENTIALLY HAZARDOUS INTERACTIONS WITH OTHER DRUGS

• Other antivirals: zidovudine may inhibit intracellular activation of stavudine (avoid concomitant use)

Administration

RECONSTITUTION

–

ROUTE

• Oral

RATE OF ADMINISTRATION

–

COMMENTS

• Administer at least an hour before food

Other information

• Clearance by haemodialysis is 120 mL/min
• Patients on haemodialysis should take stavudine after the completion of haemodialysis **and** at the same time on non-dialysis days
• Lactic acidosis, sometimes fatal, has been reported with the use of nucleoside analogues

Streptokinase

Clinical use

Fibrinolytic: thrombolysis in DVT, PE, acute arterial thromboembolism, acute MI, thrombosed arterio-venous (HD) shunts

Dose in normal renal function

Loading dose: 250,000 IU followed by 100,000 IU/hour for 72 hours (refer to data sheet)

Myocardial infarction (MI): 1.5 MIU followed by aspirin

Thrombolysed HD shunts: 10–25,000 IU sealed in shunt and repeated after 30–45 minutes

Pharmacokinetics

Molecular weight (daltons)	47,408
% Protein binding	–
% Excreted unchanged in urine	0
Volume of distribution (L/kg)	0.02–0.08
Half-life – normal/ESRF (hrs)	18–20 minutes/–

Dose in renal impairment GFR (mL/min)

20–50	Dose as in normal renal function
10–20	Dose as in normal renal function
<10	Dose as in normal renal function

Dose in patients undergoing renal replacement therapies

CAPD	Not dialysed. Dose as in normal renal function
HD	Not dialysed. Dose as in normal renal function
CAV/VVHD	Not dialysed. Dose as in normal renal function

Important drug interactions

POTENTIALLY HAZARDOUS INTERACTIONS WITH OTHER DRUGS

- Anticoagulants should not be given with streptokinase
- Heparin infusions should be stopped 4 hours before streptokinase infusion. If this is not possible, protamine sulphate should be used to neutralise the heparin
- Heparin infusions can be restarted 4 hours post streptokinase infusion followed by oral anticoagulants

Administration

RECONSTITUTION

- See manufacturers' literature

ROUTE

- IV

RATE OF ADMINISTRATION

- Give loading dose of 250,000 IU in 100 mL fluid over 30 minutes, followed by an appropriate volume for the maintenance dose
- Give 1.5 MIU for acute MI in 50–200 mL fluid over 1 hour

COMMENTS

- For occluded HD shunts, add 100,000 IU to 100 mL sodium chloride 0.9% and put 10–25 mL into the clotted portion of the shunt

Other information

- There are no significant changes in pharmacokinetics in patients with renal insufficiency. Dosage reduction is therefore not necessary

Streptomycin

Clinical use

Aminoglycoside, effective in the treatment of tuberculosis, endocarditis, plague, mycobacterial infections, tularaemia and brucella infections

Dose in normal renal function

0.5–4.0 g/day in 1–4 divided doses, or
7.5 mg/kg twice a day

Pharmacokinetics

Molecular weight (daltons)	1457.38
% Protein binding	34
% Excreted unchanged in urine	89
Volume of distribution (L/kg)	0.26
Half-life – normal/ESRF (hrs)	1.9–4.7/100

Dose in renal impairment GFR (mL/min)

20–50	7.5–15.0 mg/kg every 24 hours
10–20	7.5–15.0 mg/kg every 24–72 hours
<10	7.5–15.0 mg/kg every 72–96 hours – see 'Other information'

Dose in patients undergoing renal replacement therapies

CAPD	Dialysed. Dose as for GFR < 10 mL/min
HD	Dialysed. Dose as for GFR < 10 mL/min
CAV/VVHD	Dialysed. Dose as for GFR = 10–20 mL/min

Important drug interactions

POTENTIALLY HAZARDOUS INTERACTIONS WITH OTHER DRUGS

- Increased risk of neuromuscular blockade and respiratory paralysis, when given after anaesthetic agents or muscle relaxants
- Avoid concomitant use of other potentially ototoxic or nephrotoxic agents, e.g. loop diuretics, aminoglycosides, carboplatin, cidofovir, ciclosporin, tacrolimus

Administration

RECONSTITUTION

–

ROUTE

- IM, IV

RATE OF ADMINISTRATION

- In 100 mL sodium chloride 0.9% or glucose 5% over 30 minutes

COMMENTS

- In patients who experience tingling sensations or dizziness during administration, increase the infusion time to 60 minutes

Other information

- Due to the efficacy of twice-weekly therapy, it is recommended that patients with severe renal impairment be given a dose of 750 mg 2–3 times a week for the first 2 months of treatment for tuberculosis. Trough levels should not exceed 4 mg/L (Ellard GA et al. (1993) Am Rev Respir Dis. 148: 650–5)
- Peak serum concentrations in individuals with renal impairment should not exceed 20–25 micrograms/mL
- The risk of severe neurotoxicity, irreversible vestibular damage and cochlear reactions is sharply increased in patients with impaired renal function. Optic nerve dysfunction, peripheral neuritis, arachnoiditis and encephalopathy may also occur

Sucralfate (aluminium sucrose sulphate)

Clinical use

Treatment of peptic ulcer and chronic gastritis; prophylaxis of stress ulceration in seriously ill patients

Dose in normal renal function

4 g daily in 2–4 divided doses. Maximum 8 g daily

Prophylaxis of stress ulceration: 1 g six times daily

Pharmacokinetics

Molecular weight (daltons)	2087
% Protein binding	–
% Excreted unchanged in urine	3–5
Volume of distribution (L/kg)	–
Half-life – normal/ESRF (hrs)	–

Dose in renal impairment GFR (mL/min)

20–50	4 g daily
10–20	2–4 g daily
<10	2–4 g daily

Dose in patients undergoing renal replacement therapies

CAPD	Not dialysed. Dose as in GFR = <10 mL/min
HD	Not dialysed. Dose as in GFR = <10 mL/min
CAV/VVHD	Not dialysed. Dose as in GFR = 10–20 mL/min

Important drug interactions

POTENTIALLY HAZARDOUS INTERACTIONS WITH OTHER DRUGS

- Absorption of digoxin, tetracyclines, ciprofloxacin, warfarin and phenytoin reduced – give 2 hours after sucralfate

Administration

RECONSTITUTION

- Tablets may be dispersed in 10–15 mL of water

ROUTE

- Oral

RATE OF ADMINISTRATION

–

COMMENTS

- Sucralfate exerts its action at the site of the ulcer and is minimally absorbed (3–5%) from the GI tract as sucrose sulphate
- In normal renal function any aluminium which is absorbed is excreted in the urine

Other information

- Sucralfate should be used with caution in renal impairment as aluminium may be absorbed and accumulate
- In severe renal impairment and patients receiving dialysis, sucralfate should be used with extreme caution and only for short periods
- Absorbed aluminium is bound to plasma proteins and is not dialysable
- Use of other aluminium-containing products with sucralfate can increase the total body burden of aluminium

Sulfadiazine

Clinical use

Antimicrobial agent used for UTIs, toxoplasmosis (unlicensed product) in AIDS patients, malaria, meningococcal meningitis

Dose in normal renal function

Oral:

• Loading dose: 2–4 g

• Maintenance dose: 2–4 g daily in 4–6 divided doses. In toxoplasmosis, doses up to 8 g daily have been used

IV:

• Loading dose 2–3 g

• Maintenance dose: 1 g four times daily

Pharmacokinetics

Molecular weight (daltons)	272.3
% Protein binding	20–55
% Excreted unchanged in urine	57% – see 'Other information'
Volume of distribution (L/kg)	0.29
Half-life – normal/ESRF (hrs)	7–16/prolonged

Dose in renal impairment GFR (mL/min)

20–50	Dose as in normal renal function
10–20	Use 50% dose and monitor levels
<10	Use 25% dose and monitor levels

Dose in patients undergoing renal replacement therapies

CAPD	Unknown dialysability
HD	Dialysed. Dose as in GFR < 10 mL/min
CAV/VVHD	Dialysed. Dose as in GFR = 10–20 mL/min

Important drug interactions

POTENTIALLY HAZARDOUS INTERACTIONS WITH OTHER DRUGS

• Ciclosporin: sulfadiazine causes reduced levels of ciclosporin

• Phenytoin: sulfadiazine increases phenytoin half-life by 80% and reduces clearance by 45%

Administration

RECONSTITUTION

–

ROUTE

• Oral, IV

RATE OF ADMINISTRATION

–

COMMENTS

• Give by IV infusion or slow IV bolus injection, of a solution containing up to 5% sulfadiazine in sodium chloride 0.9%

Other information

• Penetrates into the CSF within 4 hours of oral administration to produce therapeutic concentrations which may be more than half those in the blood

• Metabolised in the liver to the acetylated form, with elimination predominantly via the kidneys

• The urinary excretion of sulfadiazine and its acetyl derivative is dependent on pH. About 30% is excreted unchanged in both fast and slow acetylators when the urine is acidic, whereas about 75% is excreted unchanged by slow acetylators when the urine is alkaline

• Crystalluria may be avoided by adequate hydration and alkalinising the urine to a pH >7.15

• Blood concentrations of 100–150 micrograms/mL are desirable

• For treatment of toxoplasmosis, use sulfadiazine in conjunction with pyrimethamine 25–100 mg daily

• IM injections are painful, cause sloughing and necrosis, and should be avoided

Sulfasalazine (sulphasalazine)

Clinical use

Ulcerative colitis, Crohn's disease, rheumatoid arthritis

Dose in normal renal function

1–2 g four times daily reduced to 0.5 g four times daily

Rheumatoid arthritis: 0.5 g daily increased to 1.5 g twice daily

Pharmacokinetics

Molecular weight (daltons)	398.4
% Protein binding	95–99
% Excreted unchanged in urine	10–15
Volume of distribution (L/kg)	–
Half-life – normal/ESRF (hrs)	6–17/–

Dose in renal impairment GFR (mL/min)

20–50	Dose as in normal renal function. Use with caution
10–20	Dose as in normal renal function. Use with caution
<10	Avoid

Dose in patients undergoing renal replacement therapies

CAPD	Unknown dialysability. Dose as in GFR = <10 mL/min
HD	Unknown dialysability. Dose as in GFR = <10 mL/min
CAV/VVHD	Unknown dialysability. Dose as in GFR = 10–20 mL/min

Important drug interactions

POTENTIALLY HAZARDOUS INTERACTIONS WITH OTHER DRUGS

• None known

Administration

RECONSTITUTION

–

ROUTE

• Oral, rectal

RATE OF ADMINISTRATION

–

COMMENTS

–

Other information

• 20–30% of a dose of sulfasalazine is absorbed in the small intestine and becomes highly bound to plasma proteins. The remainder is split into sulphapyridine and 5-ASA by colonic bacteria. Sulphapyridine is rapidly absorbed from the colon, whereas 5-ASA is poorly absorbed

• Most of a dose of sulfasalazine is excreted in the urine. Unchanged sulfasalazine accounts for 15% of the original dose, sulphapyridine and its metabolites 60% and 5-ASA and its metabolites 20–33%

• Up to 5% of a dose is excreted in the faeces, mainly as sulphapyridine metabolites

Sulindac

Clinical use

NSAID: pain and inflammation in musculoskeletal disorders, acute gout

Dose in normal renal function

200 mg twice daily

Pharmacokinetics

Molecular weight (daltons)	356
% Protein binding	93
% Excreted unchanged in urine	–
Volume of distribution (L/kg)	–
Half-life – normal/ESRF (hrs)	8/17 (metabolite)

Dose in renal impairment GFR (mL/min)

20–50	Dose as in normal renal function. Avoid if possible
10–20	Give 50–100% of normal dose. Avoid if possible
<10	Give 50–100% of normal dose. Avoid if possible

Dose in patients undergoing renal replacement therapies

CAPD	Unknown dialysability. Dose as in GFR = <10 mL/min
HD	Not dialysed. Dose as in GFR = <10 mL/min
CAV/VVHD	Unknown dialysability. Dose as in GFR = 10–20 mL/min

Important drug interactions

POTENTIALLY HAZARDOUS INTERACTIONS WITH OTHER DRUGS

- Ciclosporin: increased risk of nephrotoxicity
- Excretion of lithium reduced
- Cytotoxic agents: reduced excretion of methotrexate
- Anticoagulants: effects of acenocoumarol and warfarin enhanced
- Antidiabetic agents: effects of sulphonylureas enhanced
- Anti-epileptic agents: effects of phenytoin enhanced
- ACE inhibitors and AT-II antagonists: antagonism of hypotensive effect; increased risk of hyperkalaemia and renal damage
- Uricosurics: probenecid delays excretion of NSAIDs
- Diuretics: increased risk of nephrotoxicity. Hyperkalaemia with potassium-sparing diuretics
- Tacrolimus: increased risk of nephrotoxicity
- Other analgesics: increased risk of side-effects with two or more NSAIDs
- Antibacterials: increased risk of convulsions with quinolones

Administration

RECONSTITUTION

–

ROUTE

- Oral

RATE OF ADMINISTRATION

–

COMMENTS

–

Other information

- Sulindac has become the NSAID of choice in some centres for patients with renal impairment. This is due to reports of renal-sparing effects. There is evidence that this sparing effect is dose-related and is lost if doses above 100 mg twice daily are used
- Inhibition of renal prostaglandin synthesis by NSAIDs may interfere with renal function, especially in the presence of existing renal disease. Avoid NSAIDs if possible; if not, check serum creatinine 48–72 hours after starting NSAID. If increased, discontinue therapy
- Use normal doses in patients with ESRD on dialysis
- Use with caution in renal transplant recipients as can reduce intra-renal autocoid synthesis

Sulpiride

Clinical use

Antipsychotic: acute and chronic schizophrenia

Dose in normal renal function

400–800 mg daily increasing to maximum 1.2 g twice daily

Pharmacokinetics

Molecular weight (daltons)	341.4
% Protein binding	14–40
% Excreted unchanged in urine	90–95
Volume of distribution (L/kg)	0.65–1.4
Half-life – normal/ESRF (hrs)	6–8/26

Dose in renal impairment GFR (mL/min)

20–50	Give 70% of normal dose, or increase dosing interval by factor of 1.5
10–20	Give 50% of normal dose, or increase dosing interval by factor of 2
<10	Give 30% of normal dose, or increase dosing interval by factor of 3

Dose in patients undergoing renal replacement therapies

CAPD	Removal likely. Dose as in GFR = <10 mL/min
HD	Removal likely. Dose as in GFR = <10 mL/min
CAV/VVHD	Unknown dialysability. Dose as in GFR = 10–20 mL/min

Important drug interactions

POTENTIALLY HAZARDOUS INTERACTIONS WITH OTHER DRUGS

- Anaesthetics: enhanced hypotensive effect
- Analgesics: enhanced sedative and hypotensive effect with opioid analgesics
- Anti-epileptics: antagonism (convulsive threshold lowered)
- Sibutramine: increased risk of CNS toxicity – avoid concomitant use

Administration

RECONSTITUTION

–

ROUTE

- Oral

RATE OF ADMINISTRATION

–

COMMENTS

–

Other information

- Sulpiride is almost entirely excreted in the urine as unchanged drug. Administer with caution and decrease the dose in renal impairment

Sumatriptan

Clinical use

Acute relief of migraine

Dose in normal renal function

Oral: 50–100 mg, maximum 300 mg in 24 hours

SC: 6 mg, maximum 12 mg in 24 hours

Intranasally: 20 mg, maximum 40 mg in 24 hours

Pharmacokinetics

Molecular weight (daltons)	413.5
% Protein binding	14–21
% Excreted unchanged in urine	<20
Volume of distribution (L/kg)	170 litres
Half-life – normal/ESRF (hrs)	2/probably unchanged

Dose in renal impairment GFR (mL/min)

20–50	Dose as in normal renal function
10–20	Dose as in normal renal function. Use with caution
<10	Dose as in normal renal function. Use with caution

Dose in patients undergoing renal replacement therapies

CAPD	Unknown dialysability. Dose as in normal renal function. Use with caution
HD	Unknown dialysability. Dose as in normal renal function. Use with caution
CAV/VVHD	Unknown dialysability. Dose as in normal renal function. Use with caution

Important drug interactions

POTENTIALLY HAZARDOUS INTERACTIONS WITH OTHER DRUGS

• MAOIs, SSRIs, St John's Wort and lithium: risk of CNS toxicity

• Ergotamine: increased risk of vasospasm

Administration

RECONSTITUTION

• Injection is pre-filled into syringes ready for administration

ROUTE

• Oral, SC, nasal spray

RATE OF ADMINISTRATION

–

COMMENTS

–

Other information

• Non-renal clearance accounts for about 80% of the total clearance. The remaining 20% is excreted in urine, mainly as metabolites and involving active renal tubular secretion

Suxamethonium

Clinical use

Depolarising muscle relaxant used in short procedures and ECT

Dose in normal renal function

IV injection: initially 1 mg/kg; maintenance: 0.5–1 mg/kg at 5–10 minute intervals, maximum 500 mg per hour; or as an IV infusion

Pharmacokinetics

Molecular weight (daltons)	361
% Protein binding	70
% Excreted unchanged in urine	<10
Volume of distribution (L/kg)	–
Half-life – normal/ESRF (hrs)	3 minutes/–

Dose in renal impairment GFR (mL/min)

20–50	Dose as in normal renal function
10–20	Dose as in normal renal function
<10	Dose as in normal renal function. Use with caution. See 'Other information'

Dose in patients undergoing renal replacement therapies

CAPD	Unknown dialysability. Dose as in GFR = <10 mL/min
HD	Unknown dialysability. Dose as in GFR = <10 mL/min
CAV/VVHD	Dose as in normal renal function

Important drug interactions

POTENTIALLY HAZARDOUS INTERACTIONS WITH OTHER DRUGS

- Neuromuscular blockade may be enhanced by certain antibiotics, local anaesthetics, quinidine, calcium-channel blockers, lithium, cimetidine
- Procainamide, quinidine, lithium, cyclophosphamide and thiotepa enhance muscle relaxant effect
- Increased risk of cardiac arrhythmias if suxamethonium given with digoxin

Administration

RECONSTITUTION

- For continuous infusion add 10 mL to 500 mL glucose 5% or sodium chloride 0.9% = 0.1% solution

ROUTE

- IV

RATE OF ADMINISTRATION

- IV infusion: 2.5–4 mg/minute, maximum 500 mg/hour

COMMENTS

–

Other information

- Suxamethonium is predominantly excreted in the urine as active and inactive metabolites. Patients on dialysis may require a dose at the lower end of the range due to reduced plasma cholinesterase activity
- Use with caution in hyperkalaemia as potassium is released from depolarised muscle
- Hyperkalaemia may occur when suxamethonium is used in ESRF

Synercid (quinupristin 150 mg/dalfopristin 350 mg)

Clinical use

Antibacterial agent

Dose in normal renal function

7.5 mg/kg every 8 hours

Pharmacokinetics

Molecular weight (daltons)	1183 (quinupristin), 787 (dalfopristin)
% Protein binding	55–78 (quinupristin), 11–26 (dalfopristin)
% Excreted unchanged in urine	15 (quinupristin), 19 (dalfopristin)
Volume of distribution (L/kg)	1
Half-life – normal/ESRF (hrs)	0.9 (quinupristin), 0.75 (dalfopristin)

Dose in renal impairment GFR (mL/min)

20–50	5–7.5 mg/kg 8–12-hourly
10–20	5–7.5 mg/kg 8–12-hourly
<10	5 mg/kg 8–12-hourly

Dose in patients undergoing renal replacement therapies

CAPD	Not dialysed. Dose as in GFR = <10 mL/min
HD	Not dialysed. Dose as in GFR = <10 mL/min
CAV/VVHD	Unlikely dialysability. Dose as in GFR = 10–20 mL/min

Important drug interactions

POTENTIALLY HAZARDOUS INTERACTIONS WITH OTHER DRUGS

• Anti-arrhythmics: increased risk of ventricular arrhythmias with disopyramide, lidocaine and quinidine – avoid concomitant use

• Antihistamines: increased risk of ventricular arrhythmias with terfenadine – avoid concomitant use

• Anxiolytics and hypnotics: increased plasma concentration of midazolam – risk of profound sedation; metabolism of zopiclone inhibited

• Calcium-channel blockers: increased plasma concentration of nifedipine

• Ciclosporin: increased levels of ciclosporin

• Tacrolimus: tacrolimus levels increased by 15%

• Ergotamine and ergometrine: avoid concomitant use

Administration

RECONSTITUTION

• With 5 mL glucose 5% or water for injection

ROUTE

• IV infusion through a central line

RATE OF ADMINISTRATION

• Over 60 minutes

COMMENTS

• Dilute reconstituted solution further in 250 mL glucose 5% for peripheral access for emergency administration or 100 mL for central access

• Central access is recommended

• Stable for 5 hours at room temperature and 24 hours if refrigerated

• Incompatible with saline solutions

Other information

• After the infusion flush the line with glucose 5% to minimise venous irritation

• Has been administered IP at a dose of 25 mg/L in alternate bags in combination with intravenous treatment

• Synercid is an inhibitor of CYP 3A4. Caution is recommended when co-administering any drug also metabolised by this route

Tacrolimus

Clinical use

Immunosuppressive agent: prophylaxis and treatment of acute rejection in liver and kidney transplantation

Dose in normal renal function

Oral:
Liver transplantation: 0.1–0.2 mg/kg/day in two divided doses. Maximum 0.3 mg/kg/day
Kidney transplantation: 0.15–0.3 mg/kg/day in two divided doses
IV:
Liver transplantation: 0.01–0.05 mg/kg as a continuous 24-hour infusion, starting 6 hours post surgery
Kidney transplantation: 0.05–0.10 mg/kg as a continuous 24-hour infusion, starting within 24 hours of surgery

Pharmacokinetics

Molecular weight (daltons)	822
% Protein binding	>98
% Excreted unchanged in urine	<1
Volume of distribution (L/kg)	1300 litres
Half-life – normal/ESRF (hrs)	12–16/probably unchanged

Dose in renal impairment GFR (mL/min)

20–50	Dose as in normal renal function
10–20	Dose as in normal renal function
<10	Dose as in normal renal function

Dose in patients undergoing renal replacement therapies

CAPD	Not dialysed. Dose as in normal renal function
HD	Not dialysed. Dose as in normal renal function
CAV/VVHD	Not dialysed. Dose as in normal renal function

Important drug interactions

POTENTIALLY HAZARDOUS INTERACTIONS WITH OTHER DRUGS

- Tacrolimus may increase the half-life of ciclosporin and exacerbate any toxic effects. The two should not be prescribed concomitantly. Care should be taken when converting from ciclosporin to tacrolimus
- Tacrolimus levels increased by: grapefruit juice, imidazole antifungals, macrolides, danazol, diltiazem, omeprazole, bromocriptine, cortisone, dapsone, ethinyloestradiol, gestodene, lidocaine, nicardipine, nifedipine, quinidine, ritonavir, verapamil
- Tacrolimus levels decreased by: rifampicin, phenytoin, phenobarbital, carbamazepine, isoniazid
- Increased nephrotoxicity with: amphotericin, ibuprofen, aminoglycosides, vancomycin, cotrimoxazole, NSAIDs, ganciclovir, aciclovir
- Increased risk of hyperkalaemia with potassium-sparing diuretics and potassium salts
- Tacrolimus potentiates effects of oral anticoagulants and antidiabetic drugs

Administration

RECONSTITUTION

–

ROUTE

- IV, oral, topical

RATE OF ADMINISTRATION

- Continuous infusion over 24 hours

COMMENTS

- Dilute in glucose 5% to a concentration of 4–100 micrograms/mL, e.g. 5 mg in 50–1000 mL
- Incompatible with PVC. Add to either glucose 5% in polyethylene or glass containers, or sodium chloride 0.9% in polyethylene containers
- Contains polyethoxylated castor oil which has been associated with anaphylaxis

Other information

- When converting from oral to IV give one-fifth of the dose and monitor levels
- Also available as a 0.03% and 0.1% ointment for eczema and anal Crohn's disease

Tadalafil

Clinical use

Treatment of erectile dysfunction

Dose in normal renal function

10–20 mg, 30 minutes to 12 hours before sexual activity

Pharmacokinetics

Molecular weight (daltons)	389.4
% Protein binding	94
% Excreted unchanged in urine	36
Volume of distribution (L/kg)	63 litres
Half-life – normal/ESRF (hrs)	17.5/increased

Dose in renal impairment GFR (mL/min)

20–50	Dose as in normal renal function
10–20	10 mg initially and use with caution
<10	10 mg initially and use with caution

Dose in patients undergoing renal replacement therapies

CAPD	Unlikely dialysability. Dose as in GFR < 10 mL/min
HD	Unlikely dialysability. Dose as in GFR < 10 mL/min
CAV/VVHD	Unlikely dialysability. Dose as in GFR = 10–20 mL/min

Important drug interactions

POTENTIALLY HAZARDOUS INTERACTIONS WITH OTHER DRUGS

- Nitrates: enhanced hypotensive effect
- Antifungals, macrolide antibiotics, protease inhibitors, grapefruit juice, other drugs that inhibit CYP 3A4: may increase tadalafil concentrations
- Rifampicin, phenobarbital, phenytoin, carbamazepine, other CYP 3A4 inducers: may reduce tadalafil concentrations

Administration

RECONSTITUTION

–

ROUTE

- Oral

RATE OF ADMINISTRATION

–

COMMENTS

–

Other information

- Maximum dosing frequency is once daily
- Maximum dose is 10 mg in severe renal impairment due to lack of studies, therefore the higher dose may be used with caution
- Protein binding is not affected by renal impairment

Tamoxifen

Clinical use

Treatment of breast cancer and anovulatory infertility

Dose in normal renal function

Oral: 10–40 mg daily

Pharmacokinetics

Molecular weight (daltons)	372
% Protein binding	>99
% Excreted unchanged in urine	<10
Volume of distribution (L/kg)	20
Half-life – normal/ESRF (hrs)	7 days/probably unchanged

Dose in renal impairment GFR (mL/min)

20–50	Dose as in normal renal function
10–20	Dose as in normal renal function
<10	Dose as in normal renal function

Dose in patients undergoing renal replacement therapies

CAPD	Unknown dialysability. Dose as in normal renal function
HD	Unknown dialysability. Dose as in normal renal function
CAV/VVHD	Unknown dialysability. Dose as in normal renal function

Important drug interactions

POTENTIALLY HAZARDOUS INTERACTIONS WITH OTHER DRUGS

• Warfarin: effects enhanced

Administration

RECONSTITUTION

–

ROUTE

• Oral

RATE OF ADMINISTRATION

–

COMMENTS

–

Other information

–

Tamsulosin

Clinical use

Treatment of benign prostatic hyperplasia

Dose in normal renal function

400 micrograms in the morning after breakfast

Pharmacokinetics

Molecular weight (daltons)	445
% Protein binding	99
% Excreted unchanged in urine	9
Volume of distribution (L/kg)	0.2
Half-life – normal/ESRF (hrs)	4–5.5 (M/R: 14–15)/ increased

Dose in renal impairment GFR (mL/min)

20–50	Dose as in normal renal function
10–20	Dose as in normal renal function
<10	Dose as in normal renal function. Use with caution

Dose in patients undergoing renal replacement therapies

CAPD	Not dialysed. Dose as in GFR = <10 mL/min
HD	Not dialysed. Dose as in GFR = <10 mL/min
CAV/VVHD	Not dialysed. Dose as in GFR = 10–20 mL/min

Important drug interactions

POTENTIALLY HAZARDOUS INTERACTIONS WITH OTHER DRUGS

- Anaesthetics: enhanced hypotensive effect
- Beta-blockers: enhanced hypotensive effect; increased risk of first-dose hypotensive effect
- Calcium-channel blockers: enhanced hypotensive effect; increased risk of first-dose hypotensive effect
- Diuretics: enhanced hypotensive effect; increased risk of first-dose hypotensive effect
- Moxisylyte: possibly severe postural hypotension

Administration

RECONSTITUTION

–

ROUTE

- Oral

RATE OF ADMINISTRATION

–

COMMENTS

–

Other information

- Swallow whole with 150 mL of water while sitting or standing
- Protein binding is increased in renal impairment

Tazocin (piperacillin/tazobactam)

Clinical use

Antibacterial agent

Dose in normal renal function

4.5 g every 8 hours

Pharmacokinetics

Molecular weight (daltons)	861.8
% Protein binding	piperacillin 30; tazobactam 22
% Excreted unchanged in urine	piperacillin 75–90; tazobactam 65
Volume of distribution (L/kg)	piperacillin 0.18–0.3; tazobactam 0.21
Half-life – normal/ESRF (hrs)	piperacillin 0.8–1.5/3.3–5.1; tazobactam 1/7

Dose in renal impairment GFR (mL/min)

20–50	Dose as in normal renal function
10–20	4.5 g every 12 hours
<10	4.5 g every 12 hours

Dose in patients undergoing renal replacement therapies

CAPD	Dialysed. Dose as in GFR = <10 mL/min
HD	Dialysed. Dose as in GFR = <10 mL/min
CAV/VVHD	Dialysed. Dose as in GFR = 10–20 mL/min

Important drug interactions

POTENTIALLY HAZARDOUS INTERACTIONS WITH OTHER DRUGS

- Reduced excretion of methotrexate, monitor methotrexate levels during concomitant treatment
- Prolonged action of vecuronium and similar neuromuscular blocking agents

Administration

RECONSTITUTION

- Reconstitute each 4.5 g with 20 mL sterile water for injection or sodium chloride 0.9%

ROUTE

- IV

RATE OF ADMINISTRATION

- IV: bolus over 3–5 minutes
- Infusion over 20–30 minutes

COMMENTS

- May be given as an infusion in glucose 5% or sodium chloride 0.9%

Other information

- Each 4.5-g vial contains 9.37 mmol sodium
- Has been used IP for treatment of PD peritonitis at a concentration of 250 mg/L
- Patients with renal impairment are at a greater risk of neuromuscular excitability or convulsions which are associated with overdosage

Teicoplanin

Clinical use

Antibacterial agent

Dose in normal renal function

IM/IV: 3–6 mg/kg/day to 12 mg/kg/day (higher in some reports) in life-threatening infections

Pharmacokinetics

Molecular weight (daltons)	1993
% Protein binding	90–95
% Excreted unchanged in urine	>97
Volume of distribution (L/kg)	0.94–1.4
Half-life – normal/ESRF (hrs)	150/270–490

Dose in renal impairment GFR (mL/min)

20–50	Give 50% of normal dose daily or 100% every 48 hours
10–20	Give 30% of normal dose daily or 100% every 72 hours
<10	Give 30% of normal dose daily or 100% every 72 hours

Dose in patients undergoing renal replacement therapies

CAPD	Not dialysed. Dose as in GFR = <10 mL/min
HD	Not dialysed. Dose as in GFR = <10 mL/min
CAV/VVHD	Unknown dialysability. Dose as in GFR = 10–20 mL/min

Important drug interactions

POTENTIALLY HAZARDOUS INTERACTIONS WITH OTHER DRUGS

• None known

Administration

RECONSTITUTION

• Use water for injection provided

ROUTE

• IV, IM

RATE OF ADMINISTRATION

• IV bolus: 2–3 minutes; IV infusion: 30 minutes

COMMENTS

• **USE IN CAPD**
    • Give 400 mg IV stat dose then 20 mg/L/bag IP for 7 days, then 20 mg/L/**alternate** bags for 7 days, then 20 mg/L/**night** bag only for 7 days

Other information

• TDM optimises therapy, but not essential. Troughs not less than 10 mg/L. Peaks 1 hour after 400 mg IV dose 20–50 mg/L

• Relationship between blood level and toxicity not established

• For patients with impaired renal function reduction in dose not required until fourth day of therapy. Measurement of serum levels may help

• Long-term concurrent use of gentamicin with teicoplanin causes additive toxicity

Telmisartan

Clinical use

AT-II antagonist, used for hypertension

Dose in normal renal function

20–80 mg daily

Pharmacokinetics

Molecular weight (daltons)	514.6
% Protein binding	>99.5
% Excreted unchanged in urine	<1
Volume of distribution (L/kg)	500 litres
Half-life – normal/ESRF (hrs)	24/unchanged

Dose in renal impairment GFR (mL/min)

20–50	Dose as in normal renal function
10–20	Dose as in normal renal function
<10	Start with a low dose and adjust according to response

Dose in patients undergoing renal replacement therapies

CAPD	Not dialysed. Dose as in GFR = <10 mL/min
HD	Not dialysed. Dose as in GFR = <10 mL/min
CAV/VVHD	Unlikely dialysability. Dose as in normal renal function

Important drug interactions

POTENTIALLY HAZARDOUS INTERACTIONS WITH OTHER DRUGS

- Ciclosporin: increased risk of hyperkalaemia and nephrotoxicity
- Epoetin: increased risk of hyperkalaemia; antagonism of hypotensive effect
- Lithium levels may be increased
- NSAIDs: antagonism of hypotensive effect; increased risk of hyperkalaemia and renal damage
- Diuretics: enhanced hypotensive effect; increased risk of hyperkalaemia with potassium-sparing diuretics
- Potassium supplements: increased risk of hyperkalaemia
- Anaesthetics: enhanced hypotensive effects
- Cardiac glycosides: plasma concentration of digoxin increased
- Tacrolimus: increased risk of hyperkalaemia and nephrotoxicity

Administration

RECONSTITUTION

–

ROUTE

- Oral

RATE OF ADMINISTRATION

–

COMMENTS

–

Other information

- Hyperkalaemia and other side-effects are more common in patients with impaired renal function
- Close monitoring of renal function during therapy necessary in those patients with renal insufficiency
- Renal failure has been reported in association with AT-II inhibitors in patients with renal artery stenosis, post renal transplant, or those with congestive heart failure

Temazepam

Clinical use

Benzodiazepine: insomnia (short-term use),
pre-med anxiolytic prior to minor procedures

Dose in normal renal function

Insomnia: 5–20 mg at night, up to 40 mg in severe
cases
Premedication: 20–40 mg, 30–60 minutes prior to
procedure

Pharmacokinetics

Molecular weight (daltons)	300.7
% Protein binding	96–98
% Excreted unchanged in urine	1
Volume of distribution (L/kg)	1.3–1.5
Half-life – normal/ESRF (hrs)	2–4/ unchanged

Dose in renal impairment GFR (mL/min)

20–50	Dose as in normal renal function
10–20	Dose as in normal renal function. Start with small doses. Up to 20 mg per day
<10	Dose as in normal renal function. Start with small doses. Up to 10 mg per day (20 mg if single dose)

Dose in patients undergoing renal replacement therapies

CAPD	Unknown dialysability. Dose as in GFR = <10 mL/min
HD	Not dialysed. Dose as in GFR = <10 mL/min
CAV/VVHD	Unknown dialysability. Dose as in GFR = 10–20 mL/min

Important drug interactions

POTENTIALLY HAZARDOUS INTERACTIONS WITH
OTHER DRUGS

• Temazepam toxicity reported with disulfiram

Administration

RECONSTITUTION

–

ROUTE

• Oral

RATE OF ADMINISTRATION

–

COMMENTS

–

Other information

• Liquid available
• Increased CNS sensitivity in renal impairment
• Long-term use may lead to dependence and
  withdrawal symptoms in certain patients
• 80% of metabolites excreted in the urine

Tenecteplase

Clinical use

Thrombolytic, used for acute myocardial infarction

Dose in normal renal function

30–50 mg depending on patient weight
(500–600 micrograms/kg)

Pharmacokinetics

Molecular weight (daltons)	70,000
% Protein binding	No data
% Excreted unchanged in urine	Minimal
Volume of distribution (L/kg)	2.02–14 litres (weight- and dose-related)
Half-life – normal/ESRF (hrs)	90–130 minutes/ unchanged

Dose in renal impairment GFR (mL/min)

20–50	Dose as in normal renal function
10–20	Dose as in normal renal function
<10	Dose as in normal renal function

Dose in patients undergoing renal replacement therapies

CAPD	Unknown dialysability. Dose as in normal renal function
HD	Unknown dialysability. Dose as in normal renal function
CAV/VVHD	Unknown dialysability. Dose as in normal renal function

Important drug interactions

POTENTIALLY HAZARDOUS INTERACTIONS WITH OTHER DRUGS

• Drugs that affect coagulation or platelet function: increased risk of bleeding

Administration

RECONSTITUTION

• Water for injection

ROUTE

• IV

RATE OF ADMINISTRATION

• Over 10 seconds

COMMENTS

• Incompatible with glucose

Other information

• It has an initial half-life of 20–24 minutes
• Cleared mainly by hepatic metabolism
• Re-administration is not recommended due to lack of experience

Tenofovir

Clinical use

Nucleoside reverse transcriptase inhibitor, used for treatment of HIV infection

Dose in normal renal function

300 mg tenofovir disoproxil fumarate equivalent to 245 mg tenofovir disoproxil once daily

Pharmacokinetics

Molecular weight (daltons)	635.5 (as disoproxil fumarate ester)
% Protein binding	0.7–7.2
% Excreted unchanged in urine	(IV) 70–80, (Oral) 32
Volume of distribution (L/kg)	1.3 ± 0.6
Half-life – normal/ESRF (hrs)	10–14/unknown

Dose in renal impairment GFR (mL/min)

30–50	300 mg every 48 hours
10–30	300 mg every 72–96 hours
<10	300 mg every 7 days

Dose in patients undergoing renal replacement therapies

CAPD	Unknown dialysability. Dose as in GFR < 10 mL/min
HD	Dialysed. Dose as in GFR < 10 mL/min
CAV/VVHD	Dialysed. Dose as in GFR = 10–30 mL/min

Important drug interactions

POTENTIALLY HAZARDOUS INTERACTIONS WITH OTHER DRUGS

- Co-administration with other drugs that are actively secreted via the tubular anionic transporter, e.g. cidofovir – increased concentrations of both drugs

Administration

RECONSTITUTION

–

ROUTE

- Oral, IV

RATE OF ADMINISTRATION

- In sodium chloride 0.9% over 1 hour

COMMENTS

–

Other information

- Lactic acidosis, sometimes fatal, and usually associated with severe hepatomegaly and steatosis, has been reported in patients receiving nucleoside reverse transcriptase inhibitors
- Following a single 300 mg dose of tenofovir, subjects with a calculated CL_{CR} <50 mL/min, and those with ESRF requiring dialysis, had substantial reductions in renal elimination of tenofovir, resulting in high systemic exposures necessitating an adjustment in dose
- A 4-hour high-flux haemodialysis session was found to efficiently remove tenofovir from serum with a median extraction coefficient of 54%
- Renal impairment, which may include hypophosphataemia, has been reported with the use of tenofovir. The majority of these cases occurred in patients with underlying systemic or renal disease, or in patients taking nephrotoxic agents
- Proteinuria has occurred infrequently after IV administration
- IV dose = 1–3 mg/kg daily

Terazosin

Clinical use

Alpha-adrenoceptor blocker: hypertension,
benign prostatic hyperplasia

Dose in normal renal function

Oral: 2–10 mg daily (hypertension); 5–10 mg daily
(benign prostatic hyperplasia)

Pharmacokinetics

Molecular weight (daltons)	459.9
% Protein binding	90–94
% Excreted unchanged in urine	10
Volume of distribution (L/kg)	0.5–0.9
Half-life – normal/ESRF (hrs)	9–12/unchanged

Dose in renal impairment GFR (mL/min)

20–50	Dose as in normal renal function
10–20	Dose as in normal renal function
<10	Dose as in normal renal function

Dose in patients undergoing renal replacement therapies

CAPD	Not dialysed. Dose as in normal renal function
HD	Not dialysed. Dose as in normal renal function
CAV/VVHD	Unknown dialysability. Dose as in normal renal function

Important drug interactions

POTENTIALLY HAZARDOUS INTERACTIONS WITH
OTHER DRUGS

- Increased hypotensive effect with beta-blockers,
  calcium-channel blockers, diuretics, general
  anaesthetics, antidepressants, linezolid
- Moxisylyte: possibly severe postural hypotension

Administration

RECONSTITUTION

–

ROUTE

- Oral

RATE OF ADMINISTRATION

–

COMMENTS

–

Other information

- Therapy should be initiated with a single dose of
  1 mg given at bedtime
- In severe renal impairment use doses above 5 mg
  with caution

Terbinafine

Clinical use

Antifungal agent: fungal infections of the skin and nails

Dose in normal renal function

250 mg daily

Pharmacokinetics

Molecular weight (daltons)	327.9
% Protein binding	99
% Excreted unchanged in urine	0
Volume of distribution (L/kg)	1000 litres
Half-life – normal/ESRF (hrs)	17/24

Dose in renal impairment
GFR (mL/min)

20–50	50% of normal dose or 100% on alternate days
10–20	50% of normal dose or 100% on alternate days
<10	50% of normal dose or 100% on alternate days

Dose in patients undergoing renal replacement therapies

CAPD	Unlikely dialysability. Dose as in GFR = <10 mL/min
HD	Unlikely dialysability. Dose as in GFR = <10 mL/min
CAV/VVHD	Unknown dialysability. Dose as in GFR = 10–20 mL/min

Important drug interactions

POTENTIALLY HAZARDOUS INTERACTIONS WITH OTHER DRUGS

• None known

Administration

RECONSTITUTION

–

ROUTE

• Oral, topical

RATE OF ADMINISTRATION

–

COMMENTS

–

Other information

• Terbinafine is hepatically metabolised to two major metabolites, 80% of which are renally excreted
• Little information is available regarding the handling of terbinafine in renal failure
• In ESRF use with caution and monitor for side-effects

Terbutaline

Clinical use

Beta$_2$-adrenoceptor agonist: reversible airways obstruction

Dose in normal renal function

Oral: 2.5–5 mg three times daily

SC/IM: 250–500 micrograms up to four times daily

IV: Slow injection, 250–500 micrograms up to four times daily. Infusion, 1.5–5 micrograms/minute for 8–10 hours

Aerosol: 250–500 micrograms (1–2 puffs) up to 3–4 times daily

Turbohaler: 500 micrograms (1 inhalation) up to four times daily

Nebulisation: 5–10 mg 2–4 times daily or more frequently

Pharmacokinetics

Molecular weight (daltons)	274.3
% Protein binding	15–25
% Excreted unchanged in urine	90
Volume of distribution (L/kg)	1.6
Half-life – normal/ESRF (hrs)	3/–

Dose in renal impairment GFR (mL/min)

20–50   50% of normal parenteral dose. Other routes dose as in normal renal function

10–20   50% of normal parenteral dose. Other routes dose as in normal renal function

<10   Avoid parenteral dose. Other routes dose as in normal renal function

Dose in patients undergoing renal replacement therapies

CAPD	Likely to be dialysed. Dose as in GFR = <10 mL/min
HD	Likely to be dialysed. Dose as in GFR = <10 mL/min
CAV/VVHD	Likely to be dialysed. Dose as in GFR = 10–20 mL/min

Important drug interactions

POTENTIALLY HAZARDOUS INTERACTIONS WITH OTHER DRUGS

• Effect may be diminished by beta-blockers
• Theophylline: increased risk of hypokalaemia

Administration

RECONSTITUTION

–

ROUTE

• IV, SC, IM, oral, inhaled, nebulised

RATE OF ADMINISTRATION

• IV infusion: 1.5–5 micrograms/minute

COMMENTS

• For IV infusion add 3–5 mL to 500 mL glucose 5% or sodium chloride 0.9% (3–5 micrograms/mL)

Other information

–

Terfenadine

Clinical use

Antihistamine: symptomatic relief of allergy and pruritus

Dose in normal renal function

Oral: 60–120 mg daily

Pharmacokinetics

Molecular weight (daltons)	471.7
% Protein binding	97
% Excreted unchanged in urine	0
Volume of distribution (L/kg)	–
Half-life – normal/ESRF (hrs)	16–23/probably unchanged

Dose in renal impairment GFR (mL/min)

20–50	Dose as in normal renal function
10–20	Dose as in normal renal function
<10	Dose as in normal renal function

Dose in patients undergoing renal replacement therapies

CAPD	Not dialysed. Dose as in normal renal function
HD	Not dialysed. Dose as in normal renal function
CAV/VVHD	Not dialysed. Dose as in normal renal function

Important drug interactions

POTENTIALLY HAZARDOUS INTERACTIONS WITH OTHER DRUGS

• Increased risk of ventricular arrhythmias with amiodarone, disopyramide, procainamide, quinidine, erythromycin, clarithromycin, tricyclic antidepressants, SSRIs, imidazole and triazole antifungals, cisapride, antipsychotics, sotalol, quinine, pentamidine, antivirals and diuretics

• Metabolism inhibited by erythromycin and other macrolides, imidazoles (and possibly thiazides)

• Concomitant use with mizolastine not recommended

Administration

RECONSTITUTION
–

ROUTE
• Oral

RATE OF ADMINISTRATION
–

COMMENTS
–

Other information

• Hypokalaemia increases risk of ventricular arrhythmias

• Rare hazardous arrhythmias are associated with terfenadine, particularly with increased blood concentrations. Do not exceed recommended dose. Terfenadine is not recommended in patients in whom electrolyte imbalance or prolonged QT interval are known or suspected

Tetracycline

Clinical use

Antibacterial agent

Dose in normal renal function

250–500 mg four times a day

Acne: 500 mg twice daily

Pharmacokinetics

Molecular weight (daltons)	444.44
% Protein binding	20–90
% Excreted unchanged in urine	30–60
Volume of distribution (L/kg)	1.5
Half-life – normal/ESRF (hrs)	6–12/57–120

Dose in renal impairment GFR (mL/min)

20–50	Normal dose 12–24-hourly
10–20	Normal dose 12–24-hourly
<10	Normal dose 24-hourly

Dose in patients undergoing renal replacement therapies

CAPD	Not dialysed. Dose as in GFR = <10 mL/min
HD	Not dialysed. Dose as in GFR = <10 mL/min
CAV/VVHD	Unlikely dialysability. Dose as in GFR = 10–20 mL/min

Important drug interactions

POTENTIALLY HAZARDOUS INTERACTIONS WITH OTHER DRUGS

• Retinoids: possible increased risk of benign intracranial hypertension with tetracyclines and acitretin, isotretinoin and tretinoin; avoid concomitant use

• Other nephrotoxic drugs: avoid concomitant use

• Methoxyflurane: increased risk of nephrotoxicity

Administration

RECONSTITUTION

–

ROUTE

• Oral

RATE OF ADMINISTRATION

–

COMMENTS

–

Other information

• 10% is removed by haemodialysis and 7% by peritoneal dialysis

• Avoid, if possible, in renal impairment due to its potential nephrotoxicity and increased risk of azotaemia, hyperphosphataemia and acidosis

• May cause an increase in blood urea which is dose related

• Avoid in SLE

Thalidomide (unlicensed product)

Clinical use

Treatment of erythema nodosum leprosum

Also been used for lupus erythematosus, aphthous ulceration, stomatitis, graft-versus-host disease, AIDS-associated waste syndrome, myeloma, rheumatoid arthritis and other acute inflammatory conditions

Dose in normal renal function

100–800 mg daily

Pharmacokinetics

Molecular weight (daltons)	258.2
% Protein binding	Highly protein bound
% Excreted unchanged in urine	0.6 ± 0.2
Volume of distribution (L/kg)	120.69 ± 45.36 litres
Half-life – normal/ESRF (hrs)	8.7 ± 4.11

Dose in renal impairment GFR (mL/min)

20–50	Dose as in normal renal function
10–20	Dose as in normal renal function
<10	Dose as in normal renal function

Dose in patients undergoing renal replacement therapies

CAPD	Unknown dialysability. Dose as in normal renal function
HD	Unknown dialysability. Dose as in normal renal function
CAV/VVHD	Unknown dialysability. Dose as in normal renal function

Important drug interactions

POTENTIALLY HAZARDOUS INTERACTIONS WITH OTHER DRUGS

• Thalidomide enhances the effects of barbiturates, alcohol, chlorpromazine and reserpine

• Sedative action is antagonised by methylphenidate and methylamphetamine

Administration

RECONSTITUTION

–

ROUTE

• Oral

RATE OF ADMINISTRATION

–

COMMENTS

–

Other information

• Major route of elimination is non-renal (i.e. by spontaneous non-enzymatic hydrolytic cleavage) therefore normal doses may be given in renal failure

• Has been used to treat uraemic pruritis in haemodialysis patients unresponsive to other therapy. (Silva SR et al. (1994) Thalidomide for the treatment of uremic pruritis: a crossover randomised double-blind trial. Nephron. 67(3): 270–3)

Thioridazine

Clinical use

Schizophrenia (second-line treatment)

Dose in normal renal function

Schizophrenia: 50–300 mg daily (maximum 600 mg in hospitalised patients)

Pharmacokinetics

Molecular weight (daltons)	407
% Protein binding	97–99
% Excreted unchanged in urine	<1
Volume of distribution (L/kg)	10
Half-life – normal/ESRF (hrs)	16–36/probably unchanged

Dose in renal impairment GFR (mL/min)

20–50	Dose as in normal renal function, use lower initial doses and increase more gradually
10–20	Dose as in normal renal function, use lower initial doses and increase more gradually
<10	Dose as in normal renal function, use lower initial doses and increase more gradually

Dose in patients undergoing renal replacement therapies

CAPD	Unlikely to be dialysed. Dose as in normal renal function
HD	Unlikely to be dialysed. Dose as in normal renal function
CAV/VVHD	Unlikely to be dialysed. Dose as in normal renal function

Important drug interactions

POTENTIALLY HAZARDOUS INTERACTIONS WITH OTHER DRUGS

- Increased risk of ventricular arrhythmias with anti-arrhythmics, sotalol, pentamidine, lithium, diuretics, antivirals, quinine and terfenadine
- Plasma concentrations of tricyclic antidepressants may be increased
- Increased cardiac depressant effects with quinidine
- Antagonises effect of anti-epileptics (reduced convulsive threshold)
- Anaesthetics: enhanced hypotensive effect
- Analgesics: enhanced hypotensive and sedative effect with opioid analgesics
- Sibutramine: increased risk of CNS toxicity – avoid concomitant use

Administration

RECONSTITUTION

–

ROUTE

- Oral

RATE OF ADMINISTRATION

–

COMMENTS

–

Other information

- Elimination of metabolites mainly via the bile with <10% of the dose appearing in the urine

Thyroxine (levothyroxine)

Clinical use

Hypothyroidism

Dose in normal renal function

Oral: 25–200 micrograms daily

Pharmacokinetics

Molecular weight (daltons)	798.9
% Protein binding	99.97
% Excreted unchanged in urine	–
Volume of distribution (L/kg)	8.7–9.7
Half-life – normal/ESRF (hrs)	6–7 days/–

Dose in renal impairment GFR (mL/min)

20–50	Dose as in normal renal function
10–20	Dose as in normal renal function
<10	Dose as in normal renal function

Dose in patients undergoing renal replacement therapies

CAPD	Not dialysed. Dose as in normal renal function
HD	Not dialysed. Dose as in normal renal function
CAV/VVHD	Not dialysed. Dose as in normal renal function

Important drug interactions

POTENTIALLY HAZARDOUS INTERACTIONS WITH OTHER DRUGS

• Effect of warfarin enhanced

Administration

RECONSTITUTION

–

ROUTE

• Oral

RATE OF ADMINISTRATION

–

COMMENTS

–

Other information

• Uraemic toxins may result in inhibition of the enzyme associated with conversion of levothyroxine to liothyronine

Tiagabine

Clinical use

Anti-epileptic agent

Dose in normal renal function

15–45 mg daily in three divided doses if dose >30 mg

Pharmacokinetics

Molecular weight (daltons)	412
% Protein binding	96
% Excreted unchanged in urine	<2
Volume of distribution (L/kg)	1
Half-life – normal/ESRF (hrs)	7–9 (2–3 in patients on enzyme-inducing drugs)

Dose in renal impairment GFR (mL/min)

20–50	Dose as in normal renal function
10–20	Dose as in normal renal function
<10	Dose as in normal renal function

Dose in patients undergoing renal replacement therapies

CAPD	Unknown dialysability. Dose as in normal renal function
HD	Not dialysed. Dose as in normal renal function
CAV/VVHD	Unknown dialysability. Dose as in normal renal function

Important drug interactions

POTENTIALLY HAZARDOUS INTERACTIONS WITH OTHER DRUGS

• Antidepressants: antagonism of anticonvulsant effect (convulsive threshold lowered)
• Anti-epileptic drugs that induce liver enzymes (e.g. phenytoin, carbamazepine, phenobarbital, primidone): enhance metabolism of tiagabine, levels may be reduced by 1.5–3-fold
• Anti-malarials: mefloquine antagonises anticonvulsant effect; chloroquine and hydroxychloroquine occasionally reduce convulsive threshold

Administration

RECONSTITUTION

–

ROUTE

• Oral

RATE OF ADMINISTRATION

–

COMMENTS

–

Other information

• Although there is no evidence of withdrawal seizures, it is recommended to taper off treatment over a period of 2–3 weeks

Ticlopidine

Clinical use

Antiplatelet. Prophylaxis of major ischaemic events in patients with intermittent claudication; in combination with aspirin for prevention of sub-acute stent occlusion after intra-coronary stenting

Dose in normal renal function

250 mg twice daily with meals

Pharmacokinetics

Molecular weight (daltons)	300.2
% Protein binding	98
% Excreted unchanged in urine	<1
Volume of distribution (L/kg)	Probably quite low
Half-life – normal/ESRF (hrs)	30–50/probably unchanged

Dose in renal impairment GFR (mL/min)

20–50	Dose as in normal renal function
10–20	Dose as in normal renal function
<10	Dose as in normal renal function but use with caution. See 'Other information'

Dose in patients undergoing renal replacement therapies

CAPD	Unlikely dialysability. Dose as in GFR = <10 mL/min
HD	Unlikely dialysability. Dose as in GFR = <10 mL/min
CAV/VVHD	Unknown dialysability. Dose as in GFR = 10–20 mL/min

Important drug interactions

POTENTIALLY HAZARDOUS INTERACTIONS WITH OTHER DRUGS

- Anticoagulants and antiplatelets: enhanced effect with warfarin, heparin, aspirin and NSAIDs
- Ciclosporin: rare cases of reduced ciclosporin blood levels have been reported, monitor levels
- Phenytoin: use with caution, phenytoin toxicity has been reported
- Theophylline: increases theophylline levels

Administration

RECONSTITUTION

–

ROUTE

- Oral

RATE OF ADMINISTRATION

–

COMMENTS

–

Other information

- Ticlopidine has been used in a couple of studies in haemodialysis patients to prevent the clotting of fistulae, grafts etc at a dose of 250–500 mg daily
- Duration of inhibition of platelet aggregation does not correlate with plasma drug levels
- Inhibition of platelet aggregation is detected within 2 days of initiating therapy, reaching maximum effect in 5–8 days. In most patients, bleeding time and other platelet function tests returned to normal within 1 week of discontinuing therapy
- Increased risk of haemorrhage in uraemic patients

Tiludronic acid

Clinical use

Paget's disease of bone

Dose in normal renal function

400 mg daily for 12 weeks

Pharmacokinetics

Molecular weight (daltons)	318.6
% Protein binding	91
% Excreted unchanged in urine	40–80
Volume of distribution (L/kg)	No data
Half-life – normal/ESRF (hrs)	>100/increased

Dose in renal impairment GFR (mL/min)

60–90	Use with caution
30–60	Use with caution
<30	Avoid

Dose in patients undergoing renal replacement therapies

CAPD	Unlikely dialysability. Avoid
HD	Unlikely dialysability. Avoid
CAV/VVHD	Unlikely dialysability. Avoid

Important drug interactions

POTENTIALLY HAZARDOUS INTERACTIONS WITH OTHER DRUGS

• Calcium salts: reduced absorption

Administration

RECONSTITUTION

–

ROUTE

• Oral

RATE OF ADMINISTRATION

–

COMMENTS

–

Other information

• Take as a single dose with a glass of water at least 2 hours before or after meals, calcium supplements or aluminium- or magnesium-containing antacids

• Patients should ensure their calcium and vitamin D intake is adequate

• Calcium metabolism disorders should be corrected before starting therapy

• Biphosphonates are mainly eliminated by excretion of unchanged drug in the urine

Timentin (ticarcillin/clavulanic acid)

Clinical use

Antibacterial agent

Dose in normal renal function

3.2 g every 6–8 hours. Maximum every 4 hours

Pharmacokinetics

Molecular weight (daltons)	ticarcillin 428; clavulanic acid 199.2
% Protein binding	ticarcillin 45–60; clavulanic acid 22
% Excreted unchanged in urine	ticarcillin 85–90; clavulanic acid 60
Volume of distribution (L/kg)	ticarcillin 0.14–0.21; clavulanic acid 0.3
Half-life – normal/ESRF (hrs)	ticarcillin 1.2/11–16; clavulanic acid 0.8–1

Dose in renal impairment GFR (mL/min)

>30	3.2 g every 8 hours
10–30	1.6 g every 8 hours
<10	1.6 g every 12 hours

Dose in patients undergoing renal replacement therapies

CAPD	Unknown dialysability. Dose as in GFR = <10 mL/min
HD	Dialysed. Dose as in GFR = <10 mL/min
CAV/VVHD	Unknown dialysability. Dose as in GFR = 10–30 mL/min

Important drug interactions

POTENTIALLY HAZARDOUS INTERACTIONS WITH OTHER DRUGS

• None known

Administration

RECONSTITUTION

• With 10 mL water for injection and add to 100 mL glucose 5%

ROUTE

• IV

RATE OF ADMINISTRATION

• 30–40 minutes

COMMENTS

• Each 3.2 g of ticarcillin/clavulanic acid contains 16 mmol of sodium and 1 mmol of potassium

Other information

–

Timolol

Clinical use

Beta-adrenoceptor blocker: hypertension, angina, glaucoma and migraine prophylaxis

Dose in normal renal function

Oral: 10–60 mg daily

Pharmacokinetics

Molecular weight (daltons)	317
% Protein binding	60
% Excreted unchanged in urine	5–20
Volume of distribution (L/kg)	1–3.5
Half-life – normal/ESRF (hrs)	3–5/unchanged

Dose in renal impairment GFR (mL/min)

20–50	Dose as in normal renal function
10–20	Dose as in normal renal function, start with lowest dose and titrate according to response
<10	Dose as in normal renal function, start with lowest dose and titrate according to response

Dose in patients undergoing renal replacement therapies

CAPD	Not dialysed. Dose as in GFR = <10 mL/min
HD	Not dialysed. Dose as in GFR = <10 mL/min
CAV/VVHD	Unknown dialysability. Dose as in GFR = 10–20 mL/min

Important drug interactions

POTENTIALLY HAZARDOUS INTERACTIONS WITH OTHER DRUGS

- Anti-arrhythmics: increased risk of myocardial depression and bradycardia
- Calcium-channel blockers: increased risk of bradycardia and AV block with diltiazem; severe hypotension, asystole and heart failure with verapamil
- Anaesthetics: enhanced hypotensive effect
- NSAIDs: antagonise hypotensive effect
- Sympathomimetics: severe hypertension
- MAOIs: enhanced hypotensive effect
- Moxisylyte: possibly severe postural hypotension

Administration

RECONSTITUTION

–

ROUTE

- Oral, topical

RATE OF ADMINISTRATION

–

COMMENTS

–

Other information

- Timolol is more hydrophilic than lipophilic

Tinidazole

Clinical use

Antibacterial agent

Dose in normal renal function

Oral: 1–4 g daily

Pharmacokinetics

Molecular weight (daltons)	247
% Protein binding	8–12
% Excreted unchanged in urine	25
Volume of distribution (L/kg)	0.7
Half-life – normal/ESRF (hrs)	12–14/unchanged

Dose in renal impairment GFR (mL/min)

20–50	Dose as in normal renal function
10–20	Dose as in normal renal function
<10	Dose as in normal renal function

Dose in patients undergoing renal replacement therapies

CAPD	Unknown dialysability, but likely to be dialysed. Dose as in normal renal function
HD	Dialysed. Dose as in normal renal function
CAV/VVHD	Unknown dialysability. Dose as in normal renal function

Important drug interactions

POTENTIALLY HAZARDOUS INTERACTIONS WITH OTHER DRUGS

• None known

Administration

RECONSTITUTION

–

ROUTE

• Oral

RATE OF ADMINISTRATION

–

COMMENTS

–

Other information

• Dosage adjustment in renal failure is not necessary as a decrease in renal clearance is compensated for by increased faecal excretion of tinidazole

Tinzaparin sodium (LMWH)

Clinical use

1 Peri- and post-operative surgical thromboprophylaxis

2 Treatment of DVT and PE

3 Prevention of thrombus formation in extra-corporeal circulation during HD

Dose in normal renal function

General surgery: (low-moderate risk): 3500 IU SC 2 hours prior to surgery, thereafter 3500 IU SC daily for 7–10 days

Orthopaedic surgery: (high risk): 50 IU/kg body-weight SC 2 hours prior to surgery, thereafter 50 IU/kg SC daily for 7–10 days (or fixed dose of 4500 IU 12 hours before surgery followed by 4500 IU once daily dose)

DVT and PE: 175 IU/kg body-weight once daily for at least 6 days and until adequate oral anticoagulation is established

Pharmacokinetics

Molecular weight (daltons)	5500–7500 (average 6500)
% Protein binding	14
% Excreted unchanged in urine	80–90
Volume of distribution (L/kg)	3.1–5 litres
Half-life – normal/ESRF (hrs)	1.5/2.5 (detectable antifactor Xa activity persists for 24 hours)

Dose in renal impairment GFR (mL/min)

30–50	Dose as in normal renal function
<30	See 'Other information'

Dose in patients undergoing renal replacement therapies

CAPD	Not dialysed. Dose as in GFR = <30 mL/min
HD	Not dialysed. Dose as in GFR = <30 mL/min
CAV/VVHD	Not dialysed. Dose as in GFR = <30 mL/min

Important drug interactions

POTENTIALLY HAZARDOUS INTERACTIONS WITH OTHER DRUGS

• Anticoagulants/antiplatelet agents, e.g. aspirin, dextran, warfarin and NSAIDs may enhance effects of tinzaparin

• Nitrates: increased excretion of GTN infusion

Administration

RECONSTITUTION

–

ROUTE

• SC injection

• IV bolus/infusion

RATE OF ADMINISTRATION

• See 'Other information'

COMMENTS

–

Other information

• Tinzaparin is also indicated for prevention of clotting in the extra-corporeal circulation during haemodialysis. The dialyser may be primed with 5000 IU tinzaparin in 500–1000 mL sodium chloride 0.9%

• Dose for >4-hour session: IV bolus (into arterial side of the dialyser or intravenously) of 2500 IU followed by 750 IU/hour

• Dose for <4-hour session: IV bolus of 2000–2500 IU

• The bolus dose may be adjusted by 250 IU until a satisfactory response is obtained

• Additional tinzaparin (500–1000 IU) may be given if concentrated RBCs or blood transfusions are given during dialysis or additional treatment beyond the normal dialysis duration is employed

• Heparin can suppress adrenal secretion of aldosterone leading to hypercalcaemia particularly in patients with chronic renal impairment and diabetes mellitus

• Determination of plasma antifactor Xa may be used to monitor the tinzaparin dose during haemodialysis. Plasma antifactor Xa one hour after dosing should be within the range 0.4–0.5 IU/mL

• Low molecular weight heparins are renally excreted and hence accumulate in severe renal impairment. While the doses recommended for prophylaxis against DVT and prevention of thrombus formation in extra-corporeal circuits are well tolerated in patients with ESRF, the doses recommended for treatment of DVT and PE have been associated with severe, sometimes fatal, bleeding episodes in such patients. Hence the use of unfractionated heparin would be preferable in these instances

Tiotropium

Clinical use

Maintenance treatment of chronic obstructive pulmonary disease

Dose in normal renal function

18 micrograms daily – inhaled

Pharmacokinetics

Molecular weight (daltons)	472.4
% Protein binding	72
% Excreted unchanged in urine	14 of inhaled dose
Volume of distribution (L/kg)	32
Half-life – normal/ESRF (hrs)	5–6 days/ increased

Dose in renal impairment GFR (mL/min)

20–50	Dose as in normal renal function
10–20	Dose as in normal renal function. Use with caution
<10	Dose as in normal renal function. Use with caution

Dose in patients undergoing renal replacement therapies

CAPD	Unknown dialysability. Dose as in normal renal function. Use with caution
HD	Unknown dialysability. Dose as in normal renal function. Use with caution
CAV/VVHD	Unknown dialysability. Dose as in normal renal function. Use with caution

Important drug interactions

POTENTIALLY HAZARDOUS INTERACTIONS WITH OTHER DRUGS

• Avoid administration with other anticholinergic drugs

Administration

RECONSTITUTION

–

ROUTE

• Inhalation

RATE OF ADMINISTRATION

–

COMMENTS

–

Other information

• Not to be used for acute episodes of bronchospasm

Tizanidine

Clinical use

Spasticity associated with multiple sclerosis or spinal cord injury/disease

Dose in normal renal function

2–36 mg daily in up to 3–4 divided doses (depending on response)

Pharmacokinetics

Molecular weight (daltons)	290.2
% Protein binding	30
% Excreted unchanged in urine	I
Volume of distribution (L/kg)	2.4
Half-life – normal/ESRF (hrs)	2–5/–

Dose in renal impairment GFR (mL/min)

25–50	Dose as in normal renal function
<25	Initial dose 2 mg once daily and slowly increase by 2 mg increments. Increase once-daily dose before increasing frequency of administration

Dose in patients undergoing renal replacement therapies

CAPD	Unknown dialysability. Dose as in GFR = <25 mL/min
HD	Unknown dialysability. Dose as in GFR = <25 mL/min
CAV/VVHD	Unknown dialysability. Dose as in GFR = 25–50 mL/min

Important drug interactions

POTENTIALLY HAZARDOUS INTERACTIONS WITH OTHER DRUGS

• Oral contraceptives: clearance of tizanidine reduced by 50%
• Anti-arrhythmics: enhance muscle relaxant effect
• Antihypertensives: enhance hypotensive effect

Administration

RECONSTITUTION

–

ROUTE

• Oral

RATE OF ADMINISTRATION

–

COMMENTS

–

Other information

• Pharmacokinetic data suggest that renal clearance in the elderly may be decreased by up to 3-fold
• May induce hypotension, therefore may potentiate the effect of antihypertensive drugs, including diuretics, so exercise caution
• With beta-blockers or digoxin may potentiate hypotension or bradycardia
• LFTs should be monitored monthly for the first 4 months
• Tizanidine undergoes rapid and extensive first-pass metabolism. The metabolites (mainly inactive) constitute 70% of the administered dose and are excreted via the renal route

Tobramycin

Clinical use

Antibacterial agent

Dose in normal renal function

IM/IV: 3 mg/kg/day in three divided doses
Maximum 5 mg/kg/day in 3–4 divided doses

Pharmacokinetics

Molecular weight (daltons)	468
% Protein binding	<10
% Excreted unchanged in urine	90
Volume of distribution (L/kg)	0.25
Half-life – normal/ESRF (hrs)	2–3/≥ 70

Dose in renal impairment GFR (mL/min)

20–50	Give 1 mg/kg then dose according to serum levels
10–20	Give 1 mg/kg then dose according to serum levels
<10	Give 1 mg/kg then dose according to serum levels

Dose in patients undergoing renal replacement therapies

CAPD	Unlikely to be dialysed. Dose as in GFR = <10 mL/min
HD	Dialysed. Dose as in GFR = <10 mL/min
CAV/VVHD	Dialysed. Dose as in GFR = 10–20 mL/min

Important drug interactions

POTENTIALLY HAZARDOUS INTERACTIONS WITH OTHER DRUGS

• Ciclosporin: increased risk of nephrotoxicity
• Loop diuretics: increased risk of ototoxicity
• Botulinum toxin: neuromuscular block enhanced
• Neostigmine and pyridostigmine: antagonism of effects
• Cisplatin: increased risk of nephrotoxicity and possibly ototoxicity
• Non-depolarising muscle relaxants: effects enhanced
• Tacrolimus: increased risk of nephrotoxicity

Administration

RECONSTITUTION

• Add to 50–100 mL sodium chloride 0.9% or glucose 5% for IV infusion

ROUTE

• IV, IM, nebulised

RATE OF ADMINISTRATION

• 20–60 minutes

COMMENTS

• Plasma concentrations should be measured frequently. Trough ≤ 2 mg/L. Peak 60 minutes post dose = 4–6 mg/L. Avoid prolonged peaks above 12 mg/L

Other information

• Dosing nomograms (patient's weight and renal function) are available which detail either reduced dose administered every 8 hours or normal dose (1 mg/kg) given at an increased interval. Doses must be adjusted according to serum levels

• As a rough guide to calculate the reduced dose given every 8 hours, divide the normal dose by serum creatinine (mg/dL). An extended dosage interval in hours can be calculated by multiplying the serum creatinine (mg/dL) by 6. NB: mg/dL x 88.4 = micromol/L

• Used via nebuliser for chronic pulmonary P_s aeruginosa infection in cystic fibrosis: 300 mg every 12 hours for 28 days, repeat after 28 days

Tolbutamide

Clinical use

Hypoglycaemic agent for non-insulin dependent diabetes

Dose in normal renal function

0.5–2 g daily

Pharmacokinetics

Molecular weight (daltons)	270
% Protein binding	95
% Excreted unchanged in urine	<10
Volume of distribution (L/kg)	0.1–0.15
Half-life – normal/ESRF (hrs)	5–11/prolonged

Dose in renal impairment GFR (mL/min)

20–50	Dose as in normal renal function. Use with caution
10–20	Dose as in normal renal function. Use with caution
<10	Dose as in normal renal function. Use with caution

Dose in patients undergoing renal replacement therapies

CAPD	Insignificantly dialysed. Dose as in GFR = <10 mL/min
HD	Insignificantly dialysed. Dose as in GFR = <10 mL/min
CAV/VVHD	Unknown dialysability. Dose as in GFR = 10–20 mL/min

Important drug interactions

POTENTIALLY HAZARDOUS INTERACTIONS WITH OTHER DRUGS

• Enhanced effect with phenylbutazone, azapropazone, chloramphenicol, sulphonamides, sulfinpyrazone, 4-quinolones, trimethoprim, co-trimoxazole

• Decreased effect with rifampicin

Administration

RECONSTITUTION

–

ROUTE

• Oral

RATE OF ADMINISTRATION

–

COMMENTS

–

Other information

• Tolbutamide is contra-indicated in severe renal impairment. It is not removed by dialysis and should be used with great caution in mild to moderate renal impairment because of risk of hypoglycaemia

Tolfenamic acid

Clinical use

NSAID, used for the treatment of migraine

Dose in normal renal function

200 mg when first symptoms appear, repeat once after 1–2 hours if satisfactory response is not obtained

Pharmacokinetics

Molecular weight (daltons)	261.7
% Protein binding	>99
% Excreted unchanged in urine	8 (90% as metabolites)
Volume of distribution (L/kg)	0.16
Half-life – normal/ESRF (hrs)	2.5/–

Dose in renal impairment GFR (mL/min)

20–50	Dose as in normal renal function
10–20	Use with caution and monitor renal function
<10	Avoid

Dose in patients undergoing renal replacement therapies

CAPD	Removal unlikely. Use with caution
HD	Not dialysed. Use with caution
CAV/VVHD	Removal unlikely. Avoid

Important drug interactions

POTENTIALLY HAZARDOUS INTERACTIONS WITH OTHER DRUGS

• Ciclosporin: increased risk of nephrotoxicity
• Excretion of lithium reduced
• Cytotoxic agents: reduced excretion of methotrexate
• Anticoagulants: effects of acenocoumarol and warfarin enhanced
• Antidiabetic agents: effects of sulphonylureas enhanced
• Anti-epileptic agents: effects of phenytoin enhanced

• ACE inhibitors and AT-II antagonists: antagonism of hypotensive effect; increased risk of hyperkalaemia and renal damage
• Uricosurics: probenecid delays excretion of NSAIDs
• Diuretics: increased risk of nephrotoxicity. Hyperkalaemia with potassium-sparing diuretics
• Tacrolimus: increased risk of nephrotoxicity
• Other analgesics: increased risk of side-effects with two or more NSAIDs
• Antibacterials: increased risk of convulsions with quinolones
• Antivirals: increased risk of haematological toxicity with zidovudine; plasma concentration possibly increased by ritonavir
• Tacrolimus: increased risk of nephrotoxicity

Administration

RECONSTITUTION

–

ROUTE

• Oral

RATE OF ADMINISTRATION

–

COMMENTS

–

Other information

• Contra-indicated in significantly impaired kidney or liver function
• The urine may, due to coloured metabolites, become a little more lemon-coloured
• Use only with extreme caution (or not at all) in haemodialysis patients with some preserved diuresis, especially if other risk factors, e.g. nephrotic syndrome, diabetes mellitus or treatment with loop diuretics, are present
• Inhibition of renal prostaglandin synthesis by NSAIDs may interfere with renal function, especially in the presence of existing renal disease. Avoid NSAIDs if possible; if not, check serum creatinine 48–72 hours after starting NSAID. If increased, discontinue therapy
• Use normal doses in patients with ESRD on dialysis
• Use with caution in renal transplant recipients as can reduce intra-renal autocoid synthesis

Tolterodine

Clinical use

Treatment of urinary frequency, urgency and
incontinence

Dose in normal renal function

1–2 mg twice daily
M/R: 4 mg daily

Pharmacokinetics

Molecular weight (daltons)	325
% Protein binding	96
% Excreted unchanged in urine	<1
Volume of distribution (L/kg)	0.9–1.6
Half-life – normal/ESRF (hrs)	2–3 (10 hours in poor metabolisers)

Dose in renal impairment GFR (mL/min)

20–50	Dose as in normal renal failure. Use with caution
10–20	Dose as in normal renal failure. Use with caution
<10	Dose as in normal renal failure. Use with caution

Dose in patients undergoing renal replacement therapies

CAPD	Unlikely to be dialysed. Dose as in GFR = <10 mL/min
HD	Unlikely to be dialysed. Dose as in GFR = 10 mL/min
CAV/VVHD	Unlikely to be dialysed. Dose as in GFR = 10–20 mL/min

Important drug interactions

POTENTIALLY HAZARDOUS INTERACTIONS WITH OTHER DRUGS

• None known

Administration

RECONSTITUTION

–

ROUTE

• Oral

RATE OF ADMINISTRATION

–

COMMENTS

–

Other information

• Active metabolites may accumulate in renal failure
• Modified-release preparation is not suitable for renal patients

Topiramate

Clinical use

Anti-epileptic agent

Dose in normal renal function

200–800 mg daily in two divided doses

Pharmacokinetics

Molecular weight (daltons)	339.4
% Protein binding	9–17
% Excreted unchanged in urine	50–80
Volume of distribution (L/kg)	0.6–0.8
Half-life – normal/ESRF (hrs)	20–30/48–60
	(12–15 hours if used with another enzyme-inducing anti-epileptic drug)

Dose in renal impairment GFR (mL/min)

20–50	Dose as in normal renal function
10–20	50% of normal dose and increase according to response
<10	25–50% of normal dose and increase according to response

Dose in patients undergoing renal replacement therapies

CAPD	Unknown dialysability. Dose as for GFR = <10 mL/min
HD	Dialysed. Dose as for GFR = <10 mL/min
CAV/VVHD	Unknown dialysability. Dose as for GFR = 10–20 mL/min

Important drug interactions

POTENTIALLY HAZARDOUS INTERACTIONS WITH OTHER DRUGS

- Antidepressants: antagonism of anticonvulsant effect
- Anti-malarials: mefloquine antagonises anticonvulsant effect; chloroquine and hydroxychloroquine occasionally reduces convulsive threshold
- Phenytoin and carbamazepine: may reduce topiramate levels; may increase phenytoin concentration
- Oral contraceptives: reduced contraceptive effect

Administration

RECONSTITUTION

–

ROUTE

- Oral

RATE OF ADMINISTRATION

–

COMMENTS

–

Other information

- Patients with moderate to severe renal impairment may take 10–15 days to reach steady state, compared to 4–8 days in patients with normal renal function
- A higher frequency of renal stones has been noted in topiramate-treated patients, although the risk is not related to dose or duration of therapy. Adequate hydration is recommended to reduce this risk

Topotecan

Clinical use

Treatment of metastatic ovarian cancer

Dose in normal renal function

1.5 mg/m² for 5 days, repeated every 3 weeks

Pharmacokinetics

Molecular weight (daltons)	457.9
% Protein binding	35
% Excreted unchanged in urine	20–60
Volume of distribution (L/kg)	132 ± 57 litres
Half-life – normal/ESRF (hrs)	2–3/4.9 (in moderate renal failure)

Dose in renal impairment GFR (mL/min)

40–59	Dose as in normal renal function (see 'Other information')
20–39	0.75 mg/m²/day (see 'Other information')
<20	Use with caution (see 'Other information')

Dose in patients undergoing renal replacement therapies

CAPD	No data. Use with caution (see 'Other information')
HD	No data. Use with caution (see 'Other information')
CAV/VVHD	No data. 0.5–0.75 mg/m²/day and monitor closely

Important drug interactions

POTENTIALLY HAZARDOUS INTERACTIONS WITH OTHER DRUGS

• None known

Administration

RECONSTITUTION

• Add 4 mL of water for injection to each 4 mg vial

ROUTE

• IV infusion

RATE OF ADMINISTRATION

• Over 30 minutes

COMMENTS

• Dilute further in sodium chloride 0.9%, glucose 5% to obtain a concentration of 25–50 micrograms/mL

• Once reconstituted use within 12 hours if stored at room temperature and 24 hours if stored at 2–8°C, if made under aseptic conditions

Other information

• It has also been used to treat small-cell lung cancer, cancers of the breast and uterus and acute and chronic myelogenous leukaemia

• If the patient has received extensive prior therapy it has been suggested that 1 mg/m²/day can be used in mild renal impairment and 0.5 mg/m²/day in moderate renal impairment

• In renal failure there is an increased risk of haematological toxicity (even at low doses, e.g. 0.5 mg/m²/day), therefore if it is to be used in severe renal failure start at doses less than 0.5 mg/m²/day and monitor closely

• An alternative dosing schedule is:
  CL_{CR} 60 mL/min: 80% of dose
  CL_{CR} 45 mL/min: 75% of dose
  CL_{CR} 30 mL/min: 70% of dose
  Kintzel PE, Dorr RT (1995) Cancer Treat Rev. 21: 33–64

• Bennett suggests:
  GFR > 50 mL/min: 75% of dose
  GFR = 10–50 mL/min: 50% of dose
  GFR < 10 mL/min: 25% of dose

Torasemide

Clinical use

Loop diuretic, used for hypertension and oedema due to congestive heart failure, pulmonary or renal oedema

Dose in normal renal function

Oral: 2.5–40 mg (varies according to indication)
Maximum dose: 200 mg

Pharmacokinetics

Molecular weight (daltons)	348.4
% Protein binding	>99
% Excreted unchanged in urine	25
Volume of distribution (L/kg)	0.09–0.33
Half-life – normal/ESRF (hrs)	3–4/unchanged

Dose in renal impairment GFR (mL/min)

20–50	Dose as in normal renal function
10–20	Dose as in normal renal function
<10	Dose as in normal renal function

Dose in patients undergoing renal replacement therapies

CAPD	Unlikely removal. Dose as in normal renal function
HD	Not dialysed. Dose as in normal renal function
CAV/VVHD	Not dialysed. Dose as in normal renal function

Important drug interactions

POTENTIALLY HAZARDOUS INTERACTIONS WITH OTHER DRUGS

- ACE inhibitors and AT-II antagonists: enhanced hypotensive effect
- Analgesics: increased risk of nephrotoxicity with NSAIDs
- Anti-arrhythmics: cardiac toxicity of amiodarone, disopyramide, flecainide and quinidine increased if hypokalaemia occurs; action of mexiletine and lidocaine antagonised by hypokalaemia

- Antibacterials: increased risk of ototoxicity with aminoglycosides, colistin and vancomycin; may increase nephrotoxicity of cephalosporins
- Anti-epileptics: increased risk of hyponatraemia with carbamazepine
- Antihistamines: hypokalaemia increases risk of ventricular arrhythmias with terfenadine
- Antihypertensives: enhanced hypotensive effect; increased risk of first-dose hypotensive effect of post-synaptic alpha-blockers
- Antipsychotics: hypokalaemia increases risk of ventricular arrhythmias with pimozide or thioridazine (avoid concomitant use)
- Cardiac glycosides: increased toxicity if hypokalaemia occurs
- Lithium: reduced excretion of lithium

Administration

RECONSTITUTION

–

ROUTE

- Oral

RATE OF ADMINISTRATION

–

COMMENTS

–

Other information

- Contra-indicated in renal failure with anuria
- Torasemide 10 mg is equivalent to furosemide 20–40 mg
- In patients with renal failure, the renal clearance is reduced but total plasma clearance is not significantly altered
- Approximately 80% of dose is excreted renally as parent drug and metabolites

Toremifene

Clinical use

Hormone-dependent metastatic breast cancer in post-menopausal women

Dose in normal renal function

60 mg daily

Pharmacokinetics

Molecular weight (daltons)	406
% Protein binding	>99.5
% Excreted unchanged in urine	10% as metabolites
Volume of distribution (L/kg)	457–958 litres
Half-life – normal/ESRF (hrs)	5 days/unchanged

Dose in renal impairment GFR (mL/min)

20–50	Dose as in normal renal function
10–20	Dose as in normal renal function
<10	Dose as in normal renal function

Dose in patients undergoing renal replacement therapies

CAPD	Unlikely dialysability. See 'Other information'
HD	Unlikely dialysability. See 'Other information'
CAV/VVHD	Unlikely dialysability. See 'Other information'

Important drug interactions

POTENTIALLY HAZARDOUS INTERACTIONS WITH OTHER DRUGS

• Anticoagulants: enhanced anticoagulant effect

Administration

RECONSTITUTION

–

ROUTE

• Oral

RATE OF ADMINISTRATION

–

COMMENTS

–

Other information

• As it is not renally excreted it may possibly be administered in dialysis patients at a normal dose but it has not been used in this population before

Tramadol

Clinical use

Analgesic

Dose in normal renal function

Oral: 50–100 mg at intervals of not less than
4 hours. Maximum 400 mg daily
IM/IV: 50–100 mg hourly. Total daily dose 600 mg

Pharmacokinetics

Molecular weight (daltons)	300
% Protein binding	4
% Excreted unchanged in urine	30
Volume of distribution (L/kg)	–
Half-life – normal/ESRF (hrs)	6/11

Dose in renal impairment
GFR (mL/min)

20–50	Dose as in normal renal function
10–20	50–100 mg every 12 hours
<10	50 mg every 12 hours

Dose in patients undergoing renal replacement therapies

CAPD	Unknown dialysability. Dose as in GFR = <10 mL/min
HD	Dialysed. Dose as in GFR = <10 mL/min
CAV/VVHD	Dialysed. Dose as in GFR = 10–20 mL/min

Important drug interactions

POTENTIALLY HAZARDOUS INTERACTIONS WITH OTHER DRUGS

• Carbamazepine: tramadol metabolism increased

Administration

RECONSTITUTION
–

ROUTE

• IV, IM, oral

RATE OF ADMINISTRATION

• Slow bolus or continuous IV infusion/PCA

COMMENTS
–

Other information

• Tramadol is a centrally acting opioid agonist which also acts on inhibitory pain pathways
• It should be used with caution in moderate renal impairment and is not recommended in severe impairment

Trandolapril

Clinical use

ACE inhibitor: hypertension

Dose in normal renal function

0.5 mg once daily increased to 1–2 mg once daily (maximum 4 mg daily)

Pharmacokinetics

Molecular weight (daltons)	430
% Protein binding	>80
% Excreted unchanged in urine	10–15
Volume of distribution (L/kg)	–
Half-life – normal/ESRF (hrs)	16–24/–

Dose in renal impairment GFR (mL/min)

20–50	Dose as in normal renal function
10–20	Dose as in normal renal function
<10	Maximum: 2 mg daily

Dose in patients undergoing renal replacement therapies

CAPD	Unknown dialysability. Dose as in GFR = <10 mL/min
HD	Dialysed. Dose as in GFR = <10 mL/min
CAV/VVHD	Unknown dialysability. Dose as in GFR = 10–20 mL/min

Important drug interactions

POTENTIALLY HAZARDOUS INTERACTIONS WITH OTHER DRUGS

• Ciclosporin: increased risk of hyperkalaemia and nephrotoxicity

• Potassium supplements: risk of hyperkalaemia
• Epoetin: risk of hyperkalaemia
• Lithium levels may be increased
• NSAIDs: antagonism of hypotensive effect; increased risk of renal damage and hyperkalaemia
• Diuretics: enhanced hypotensive effect; increased risk of hyperkalaemia with potassium-sparing diuretics
• Anaesthetics: enhanced hypotensive effect
• Tacrolimus: increased risk of hyperkalaemia and nephrotoxicity

Administration

RECONSTITUTION

–

ROUTE

• Oral

RATE OF ADMINISTRATION

–

COMMENTS

–

Other information

• Hyperkalaemia and other side-effects are more common in patients with impaired renal function
• Close monitoring of renal function during therapy necessary in those patients with renal insufficiency
• Renal failure has been reported in association with ACE inhibitors in patients with renal artery stenosis, post renal transplant, or those with congestive heart failure
• A high incidence of anaphylactoid reactions has been reported in patients dialysed with high-flux polyacrylonitrile membranes and treated concomitantly with an ACE inhibitor – this combination should therefore be avoided
• Normal doses can be used in ESRD

Tranexamic acid

Clinical use

Haemostatic agent

Dose in normal renal function

Depends on indication

Oral: 1–1.5 g every 6–12 hours *or* 15–25 mg/kg every 6–12 hours

IV: 0.5–1 g every 8 hours *or* 7.5–15 mg/kg every 8 hours

Pharmacokinetics

Molecular weight (daltons)	157
% Protein binding	3
% Excreted unchanged in urine	90
Volume of distribution (L/kg)	1
Half-life – normal/ESRF (hrs)	1.5/–

Dose in renal impairment GFR (mL/min)

20–50	IV: 10 mg/kg 12-hourly PO: 25 mg/kg 12-hourly
10–20	IV: 10 mg/kg 24-hourly PO: 25 mg/kg 24-hourly
<10	IV: 5 mg/kg 24-hourly PO: 12.5 mg/kg 24-hourly

Dose in patients undergoing renal replacement therapies

CAPD	Unknown dialysability. Dose as in GFR = <10 mL/min
HD	Unknown dialysability. Dose as in GFR = <10 mL/min
CAV/VVHD	Unknown dialysability. Dose as in GFR = 10–20 mL/min

Important drug interactions

POTENTIALLY HAZARDOUS INTERACTIONS WITH OTHER DRUGS

• None known

Administration

RECONSTITUTION

–

ROUTE

• IV, oral

RATE OF ADMINISTRATION

• Slow bolus = 100 mg/minute or continuous IV infusion in glucose 5% or sodium chloride 0.9%

COMMENTS

–

Other information

• A 5% topical solution can be made up using the IV preparation mixed with water for injection. This can be used after dental surgery to stop bleeding as a mouthwash or placed on a swab to reduce bleeding at fistulae or other bleeding sites if conventional measures have not worked

Trazodone

Clinical use

Antidepressant

Dose in normal renal function

Oral: 150–300 mg daily. Maximum 600 mg for hospital patients

Pharmacokinetics

Molecular weight (daltons)	372
% Protein binding	89–95
% Excreted unchanged in urine	<5
Volume of distribution (L/kg)	0.8–1.3
Half-life – normal/ESRF (hrs)	6–14/–

Dose in renal impairment GFR (mL/min)

20–50	Dose as in normal renal function
10–20	Dose as in normal renal function, start with small doses and increase gradually
<10	Avoid or use half dose or half the frequency

Dose in patients undergoing renal replacement therapies

CAPD	Unlikely dialysability. Dose as in GFR = <10 mL/min
HD	Unlikely dialysability. Dose as in GFR = <10 mL/min
CAV/VVHD	Unknown dialysability. Dose as in GFR = 10–20 mL/min

Important drug interactions

POTENTIALLY HAZARDOUS INTERACTIONS WITH OTHER DRUGS

• Anti-epileptics: antagonism of anticonvulsant effect

• Sibutramine: increased risk of CNS toxicity – avoid concomitant use

• Other antidepressants: CNS excitation and hypertension with MAOIs

• Anti-malarials: manufacturer advises avoid concomitant use with artemether with lumefantrine

Administration

RECONSTITUTION

–

ROUTE

• Oral

RATE OF ADMINISTRATION

–

COMMENTS

–

Other information

• Use lower doses in elderly patients

• The majority of a dose (75%) is excreted by the kidney, mainly as metabolites

Triamcinolone

Clinical use

Corticosteroid

Dose in normal renal function

IM: 40 mg of acetonide, maximum single dose 100 mg

Intra-articular: 2.5–40 mg of acetonide

Pharmacokinetics

Molecular weight (daltons)	394 [acetonide (Kenalog) = 435]
% Protein binding	Low
% Excreted unchanged in urine	<1
Volume of distribution (L/kg)	99.5–148 litres
Half-life – normal/ESRF (hrs)	1.5–5/unchanged

Dose in renal impairment GFR (mL/min)

20–50	Dose as in normal renal function
10–20	Dose as in normal renal function
<10	Dose as in normal renal function

Dose in patients undergoing renal replacement therapies

CAPD	Unknown dialysability. Dose as in normal renal function
HD	Unknown dialysability. Dose as in normal renal function
CAV/VVHD	Unknown dialysability. Dose as in normal renal function

Important drug interactions

POTENTIALLY HAZARDOUS INTERACTIONS WITH OTHER DRUGS

• Metabolism increased by rifampicin, carbamazepine, phenytoin, primidone

Administration

RECONSTITUTION

–

ROUTE

• Oral, IM, intra-articular, topical, nasal spray, intradermal

RATE OF ADMINISTRATION

–

COMMENTS

–

Other information

• Use with caution in severe renal impairment as sodium retention may occur

Triamterene

Clinical use

Diuretic

Dose in normal renal function

Oral: 150–250 mg daily in divided doses. Reduce to alternate days after 1 week

Pharmacokinetics

Molecular weight (daltons)	253
% Protein binding	45–70
% Excreted unchanged in urine	5–10
Volume of distribution (L/kg)	2.2–3.7
Half-life – normal/ESRF (hrs)	2/10

Dose in renal impairment GFR (mL/min)

20–50	Dose as in normal renal function
10–20	Avoid
<10	Avoid

Dose in patients undergoing renal replacement therapies

CAPD	Unknown dialysability. Avoid
HD	Unknown dialysability. Avoid
CAV/VVHD	Unknown dialysability. Avoid

Important drug interactions

POTENTIALLY HAZARDOUS INTERACTIONS WITH OTHER DRUGS

- Ciclosporin: increased risk of hyperkalaemia
- Tacrolimus: increased risk of hyperkalaemia
- Risk of hyperkalaemia with: ACE inhibitors and AT-II antagonists, indometacin and possibly other NSAIDs, potassium salts
- Lithium: excretion reduced

Administration

RECONSTITUTION

–

ROUTE

- Oral

RATE OF ADMINISTRATION

–

COMMENTS

–

Other information

- Hyperkalaemia is common when GFR <30 mL/min. May cause ARF
- Potassium-sparing diuretics are weak diuretics and are ineffective in moderate to severe renal failure

Trifluoperazine

Clinical use

Schizophrenia and other psychoses, anxiety, severe
nausea and vomiting

Dose in normal renal function

Oral: Schizophrenia: initially 5 mg twice daily,
increased by 5 mg after 1 week, then at intervals
of 3 days according to response

Anxiolytic and anti-emetic: 2–4 mg daily in divided
doses (maximum 6 mg)

Pharmacokinetics

Molecular weight (daltons)	408
% Protein binding	>99
% Excreted unchanged in urine	<1
Volume of distribution (L/kg)	160
Half-life – normal/ESRF (hrs)	7–18/–

Dose in renal impairment
GFR (mL/min)

20–50	Dose as in normal renal function
10–20	Dose as in normal renal function
<10	Dose as in normal renal function

Dose in patients undergoing renal replacement therapies

CAPD	Not dialysed. Dose as in normal renal function
HD	Not dialysed. Dose as in normal renal function
CAV/VVHD	Unlikely to be dialysed. Dose as in normal renal function

Important drug interactions

POTENTIALLY HAZARDOUS INTERACTIONS WITH
OTHER DRUGS

• Anaesthetics: enhanced hypotensive effect
• Antidepressants: increased plasma concentrations
  and increased antimuscarinic effects with
  tricyclics
• Anti-epileptics: antagonism (convulsive threshold
  lowered)
• Antihistamines: increased risk of ventricular
  arrhythmias with terfenadine and mizolastine
• Beta-blockers: increased risk of ventricular
  arrhythmias with sotalol
• Sibutramine: increased risk of CNS toxicity –
  avoid concomitant use
• Anti-malarials: manufacturer advises avoid
  concomitant use with artemether and
  lumefantrine

Administration

RECONSTITUTION
–

ROUTE
• Oral

RATE OF ADMINISTRATION
–

COMMENTS
–

Other information

• Reduce starting dose in elderly or frail patients
  by at least half

Trimeprazine (alimemazine)

Clinical use

Urticaria and pruritus, pre-med in children

Dose in normal renal function

10 mg every 8–12 hours (maximum 100 mg/day); elderly: 10 mg once or twice daily

Pharmacokinetics

Molecular weight (daltons)	298
% Protein binding	>90
% Excreted unchanged in urine	20
Volume of distribution (L/kg)	–
Half-life – normal/ESRF (hrs)	4.8/–

Dose in renal impairment GFR (mL/min)

20–50	Dose as in normal renal function
10–20	Use with caution
<10	Use with caution

Dose in patients undergoing renal replacement therapies

CAPD	Unlikely to be dialysed. Dose as in GFR = <10 mL/min
HD	Unlikely to be dialysed. Dose as in GFR = <10 mL/min
CAV/VVHD	Unlikely to be dialysed. Dose as in GFR = 10–20 mL/min

Important drug interactions

POTENTIALLY HAZARDOUS INTERACTIONS WITH OTHER DRUGS

• Antidepressants: MAOIs and tricyclics increase antimuscarinic and sedative effects

Administration

RECONSTITUTION

–

ROUTE

• Oral

RATE OF ADMINISTRATION

–

COMMENTS

–

Other information

• Significant amounts of trimeprazine are excreted in urine. It is therefore contra-indicated in renal failure; reduced clearance and elevated serum levels will occur in patients with impaired renal function

• However, it can be used at a dose of 10 mg at night to treat uraemic pruritus

Trimethoprim

Clinical use

Antibacterial agent

Dose in normal renal function

Oral: treatment: 200 mg every 12 hours
Prophylaxis: 100 mg at night
IV: 200 mg every 12 hours

Pharmacokinetics

Molecular weight (daltons)	290
% Protein binding	30–70
% Excreted unchanged in urine	40–70
Volume of distribution (L/kg)	1–2.2
Half-life – normal/ESRF (hrs)	9–13/20–49

Dose in renal impairment GFR (mL/min)

>25	Dose as in normal renal function
15–25	Dose as in normal renal function for 3 days, then 50% of dose every 18 hours
<15	Give 50% of normal dose every 24 hours

Dose in patients undergoing renal replacement therapies

CAPD	Not dialysed. Dose as in GFR = <15 mL/min
HD	Dialysed. Dose as in GFR = <15 mL/min
CAV/VVHD	Probably dialysed. Dose as in GFR = 15–25 mL/min

Important drug interactions

POTENTIALLY HAZARDOUS INTERACTIONS WITH OTHER DRUGS

• Ciclosporin: IV trimethoprim lowers ciclosporin blood levels. Increased risk of nephrotoxicity
• Cytotoxics: increased risk of haematological toxicity with azathioprine and mercaptopurine; antifolate effect of methotrexate increased
• Anti-malarials: increased risk of antifolate effect with pyrimethamine

Administration

RECONSTITUTION

–

ROUTE

• IV, oral

RATE OF ADMINISTRATION

• 3–4 minutes (infusion over 15 minutes)

COMMENTS

–

Other information

• Serum creatinine may rise due to competition for renal secretion
• Monitor trimethoprim serum levels in patients with reduced renal function requiring chronic therapy or high doses of trimethoprim

Trimetrexate

Clinical use

Treatment of moderate to severe PCP in AIDs patients intolerant to other treatments

Dose in normal renal function

45 mg/m^2 daily for 21 days

Pharmacokinetics

Molecular weight (daltons)	563.6
% Protein binding	>97
% Excreted unchanged in urine	10–20
Volume of distribution (L/kg)	0.6
Half-life – normal/ESRF (hrs)	11/increased

Dose in renal impairment
GFR (mL/min)

20–50	Dose as in normal renal function
10–20	Dose as in normal renal function but monitor closely
<10	Avoid

Dose in patients undergoing renal replacement therapies

CAPD	Unlikely dialysability. Dose as in GFR = <10 mL/min
HD	Unlikely dialysability. Dose as in GFR = <10 mL/min
CAV/VVHD	Unknown dialysability. Dose as in normal renal function but monitor closely

Important drug interactions

POTENTIALLY HAZARDOUS INTERACTIONS WITH OTHER DRUGS

- Imidazole antifungals: inhibits metabolism of trimetrexate
- Drugs metabolised by CYP 450: may alter plasma concentration of trimetrexate
- Cimetidine: inhibits metabolism of trimetrexate

Administration

RECONSTITUTION

- Reconstitute with 2 mL glucose 5% or water for injection

ROUTE

- IV infusion

RATE OF ADMINISTRATION

- Over 60–90 minutes

COMMENTS

- Dilute in glucose 5% to obtain a concentration of 0.25–2 mg/mL
- Incompatible with sodium chloride
- Calcium folinate must be administered during treatment with trimetrexate and for 72 hours after last dose to avoid potentially serious or life-threatening complications including bone marrow suppression, oral and GI mucosal ulceration and renal and hepatic dysfunction
- Do not give calcium folinate in the same line as trimetrexate infusion

Other information

- Therapy should be discontinued if creatinine >200 micromol/L
- Adjust dose according to haematological toxicity

Triptorelin

Clinical use

Treatment of advanced prostate cancer,
endometriosis, uterine fibroids prior to surgery

Dose in normal renal function

3–4.2 mg every 4 weeks

Pharmacokinetics

Molecular weight (daltons)	1311.4
% Protein binding	–
% Excreted unchanged in urine	–
Volume of distribution (L/kg)	113.4 ± 21.6 litres
Half-life – normal/ESRF (hrs)	2.8/6–7

Dose in renal impairment GFR (mL/min)

20–50	Dose as in normal renal function
10–20	Dose as in normal renal function, but monitor carefully
<10	Dose as in normal renal function, but monitor carefully

Dose in patients undergoing renal replacement therapies

CAPD	Unlikely dialysability. Dose as in normal renal function, but monitor carefully
HD	Unlikely dialysability. Dose as in normal renal function, but monitor carefully
CAV/VVHD	Unlikely dialysability. Dose as in normal renal function, but monitor carefully

Important drug interactions

POTENTIALLY HAZARDOUS INTERACTIONS WITH OTHER DRUGS

• None known

Administration

RECONSTITUTION

• With 2 mL diluent provided

ROUTE

• IM

RATE OF ADMINISTRATION

–

COMMENTS

–

Other information

–

Urokinase (unlicensed product)

Clinical use

Fibrinolytic agent: thrombosed arteriovenous shunts and intravenous cannulas

Dose in normal renal function

Instillation: 5,000–25,000 IU in 2–3 mL sodium chloride 0.9%

Pharmacokinetics

Molecular weight (daltons)	33,000–54,000
% Protein binding	–
% Excreted unchanged in urine	Low
Volume of distribution (L/kg)	–
Half-life – normal/ESRF (hrs)	11–16 minutes/–

Dose in renal impairment GFR (mL/min)

20–50	Dose as in normal renal function
10–20	Dose as in normal renal function
<10	Dose as in normal renal function

Dose in patients undergoing renal replacement therapies

CAPD	Not dialysed. Dose as in normal renal function
HD	Not dialysed. Dose as in normal renal function
CAV/VVHD	Not dialysed. Dose as in normal renal function

Important drug interactions

POTENTIALLY HAZARDOUS INTERACTIONS WITH OTHER DRUGS

• None known

Administration

RECONSTITUTION

• 2–3 mL of sodium chloride 0.9% to 5000 IU

ROUTE

–

RATE OF ADMINISTRATION

–

COMMENTS

• Use 2500 IU up each side of shunt and leave for 2–4 hours
• Venous side: 5000 IU in 200 mL run in over 30 minutes – less satisfactory than more concentrated solution

Other information

• Care in patients with uraemic coagulopathies or bleeding diatheses
• Some units mix 5000 IU with 1.5 mL heparin 1000 units/mL
• Available from Syner-Med (Pharmaceutical Products) Ltd and IDIS in various strengths

Ursodeoxycholic acid

Clinical use

Dissolution of radiolucent cholesterol gallstones

Dose in normal renal function

8–12 mg/kg/day in 2–3 divided doses

Pharmacokinetics

Molecular weight (daltons)	393
% Protein binding	96–99
% Excreted unchanged in urine	–
Volume of distribution (L/kg)	–
Half-life – normal/ESRF (hrs)	–

Dose in renal impairment GFR (mL/min)

20–50	Dose as in normal renal function
10–20	Dose as in normal renal function
<10	Dose as in normal renal function

Dose in patients undergoing renal replacement therapies

CAPD	Unknown dialysability. Dose as in normal renal function
HD	Unknown dialysability. Dose as in normal renal function
CAV/VVHD	Unknown dialysability. Dose as in normal renal function

Important drug interactions

POTENTIALLY HAZARDOUS INTERACTIONS WITH OTHER DRUGS

• None known

Administration

RECONSTITUTION

–

ROUTE

• Oral

RATE OF ADMINISTRATION

–

COMMENTS

–

Other information

• Completely metabolised in the liver and excreted via the faecal route

Valaciclovir

Clinical use

Antiviral for herpes zoster and herpes simplex

Dose in normal renal function

Herpes simplex: 500 mg twice daily for 5–10 days

Herpes zoster: 1 g three times a day for 7 days

Herpes simplex suppression: 500 mg daily in
1–2 divided doses (500 mg twice daily in the
immunocompromised)

Pharmacokinetics

Molecular weight (daltons)	360.8
% Protein binding	15
% Excreted unchanged in urine	<1
Volume of distribution (L/kg)	0.7
Half-life – normal/ESRF (hrs)	3/14

Dose in renal impairment
GFR (mL/min)

30–50	Dose as in normal renal function
15–30	Herpes simplex: dose as in normal renal function
	Herpes zoster: 1 g every 12–24 hours
<15	Herpes simplex: 500 mg daily
	Herpes zoster: 500 mg – 1 g every 24 hours
	Herpes simplex suppression:
	Immunocompetent – 250 mg daily
	Immunocompromised – 500 mg daily

Dose in patients undergoing renal replacement therapies

CAPD	Probably dialysed. Dose as for GFR = <15 mL/min
HD	Dialysed. Dose as for GFR = <15 mL/min post dialysis
CAV/VVHD	Probably dialysed. Dose as for GFR = 15–30 mL/min

Important drug interactions

POTENTIALLY HAZARDOUS INTERACTIONS WITH OTHER DRUGS

• MMF: higher plasma concentrations of valaciclovir and MMF on concomitant administration

Administration

RECONSTITUTION

–

ROUTE

• Oral

RATE OF ADMINISTRATION

–

COMMENTS

–

Other information

• Almost completely (80%) converted to aciclovir – see aciclovir monograph for further information

• Bioavailability of aciclovir from 1-g oral dose of valaciclovir is 54%

• Mean peak aciclovir concentrations occur 1–2 hours post dose. Peak plasma concentrations of valaciclovir are 4% of aciclovir levels, occur at a median of 30–100 minutes post dose, and are at or below the limit of quantification 3 hours post dose

Valganciclovir

Clinical use

Induction and maintenance treatment of CMV retinitis in AIDS patients

Treatment (unlicensed indication) and prophylaxis of CMV disease in transplant patients, i.e. prophylaxis is now licensed but treatment is still unlicensed

Dose in normal renal function

Induction/treatment: 900 mg twice daily for 21 days
Maintenance/prophylaxis: 900 mg daily

Pharmacokinetics

Molecular weight (daltons)	390.8
% Protein binding	<2 (as ganciclovir)
% Excreted unchanged in urine	90–100 (as ganciclovir)
Volume of distribution (L/kg)	0.680 ± 0.161
Half-life – normal/ESRF (hrs)	4.1 ± 0.9/67.5

Dose in renal impairment GFR (mL/min)

40–59	Induction/treatment: 450 mg twice daily Maintenance/prophylaxis: 450 mg daily
25–39	Induction/treatment: 450 mg daily Maintenance/prophylaxis: 450 mg every 48 hours
10–24	Induction/treatment: 450 mg every 48 hours Maintenance/prophylaxis: 450 mg twice weekly
<10	Transplant patients, treatment: 450 mg twice weekly. See 'Other information'

Dose in patients undergoing renal replacement therapies

CAPD	Dialysed. Avoid
HD	Dialysed. Avoid
CAV/VVHD	Probably dialysed. Dose as in GFR = 10–24 mL/min

Important drug interactions

POTENTIALLY HAZARDOUS INTERACTIONS WITH OTHER DRUGS

- Increased risk of myelosuppression with other myelosuppressive drugs
- Antivirals: profound myelosuppression with zidovudine; possibly increased plasma levels of didanosine
- Generalised seizures reported with imipenem-cilastatin
- MMF: possibly increased plasma concentrations of both drugs

Administration

RECONSTITUTION

–

ROUTE

- Oral

RATE OF ADMINISTRATION

–

COMMENTS

–

Other information

- 900 mg valganciclovir twice daily is therapeutically equivalent to 5 mg/kg intravenous ganciclovir twice daily
- Valganciclovir is a pro-drug of ganciclovir
- Take with food if possible
- There is not a small enough tablet to allow dosing in severe renal impairment
- Avoid in severe renal impairment due to increased risk of bone marrow suppression
- Approximately 50% of ganciclovir is removed by haemodialysis

Valsartan

Clinical use

AT-II antagonist, used for hypertension

Dose in normal renal function

40–160 mg daily

Pharmacokinetics

Molecular weight (daltons)	435.5
% Protein binding	94–97
% Excreted unchanged in urine	13
Volume of distribution (L/kg)	17 litres
Half-life – normal/ESRF (hrs)	5–9/unchanged

Dose in renal impairment GFR (mL/min)

20–50	Dose as in normal renal function
10–20	Initial dose 40 mg, titrate according to response
<10	Initial dose 40 mg, titrate according to response

Dose in patients undergoing renal replacement therapies

CAPD	Removal unlikely. Dose as in GFR = <10 mL/min
HD	Not dialysed. Dose as in GFR = <10 mL/min
CAV/VVHD	Removal unlikely. Dose as in GFR = 10–20 mL/min

Important drug interactions

POTENTIALLY HAZARDOUS INTERACTIONS WITH OTHER DRUGS

• Ciclosporin: increased risk of hyperkalaemia and nephrotoxicity

• Epoetin: increased risk of hyperkalaemia; antagonism of hypotensive effect

• Lithium levels may be increased

• NSAIDs: antagonism of hypotensive effect; increased risk of hyperkalaemia and renal damage

• Diuretics: enhanced hypotensive effect; increased risk of hyperkalaemia with potassium-sparing diuretics

• Potassium supplements: increased risk of hyperkalaemia

• Anaesthetics: enhanced hypotensive effects

• Tacrolimus: increased risk of hyperkalaemia and nephrotoxicity

Administration

RECONSTITUTION

–

ROUTE

• Oral

RATE OF ADMINISTRATION

–

COMMENTS

–

Other information

• Side-effects, e.g. hyperkalaemia, metabolic acidosis, are more common in patients with impaired renal function

• Close monitoring of renal function during therapy is necessary in those with renal insufficiency

• Renal failure has been reported in association with AT-II antagonists in patients with renal artery stenosis, post renal transplant, and in those with severe congestive heart failure

Vancomycin

Clinical use

Antibacterial agent

Dose in normal renal function

IV: 1 g every 12 hours

Oral: 125–250 mg four times daily (not significantly absorbed by this route)

Pharmacokinetics

Molecular weight (daltons)	1486
% Protein binding	10–50 (19 ESRF)
% Excreted unchanged in urine	90–100
Volume of distribution (L/kg)	0.47–1.1 (0.88 ESRF)
Half-life – normal/ESRF (hrs)	6/200–250

Dose in renal impairment GFR (mL/min)

See 'Other information' for alternative method in moderate and severe renal impairment

20–50	500 mg every 12–24 hours
10–20	500 mg every 24–48 hours
<10	500 mg every 48–96 hours

Dose for patients undergoing renal replacement therapies

CAPD	Not dialysed. Dose as in GFR = <10 mL/min
HD	Not dialysed. Dose as in GFR = <10 mL/min
CAV/VVHD	Unknown dialysability. Dose as in GFR = 10–20 mL/min

Important drug interactions

POTENTIALLY HAZARDOUS INTERACTIONS WITH OTHER DRUGS

• Ciclosporin: variable response

Administration

RECONSTITUTION

• 10 mL water for injection then dilute to 100 mL (1 g) with sodium chloride 0.9% (50 mL if giving centrally)

ROUTE

• IV peripherally or centrally. Oral

RATE OF ADMINISTRATION

• Not faster than 10 mg/minute

COMMENTS

• **Use in CAPD peritonitis:**
  • 12.5–25 mg/L per bag (see local protocol)
  • Various other regimens used in CAPD ranging from IV dosing to high dose stat IP use
  • Some units use the following:

    patient's weight >60 kg, stat dose of 2 g IP on days 1 and 7 in one bag 6-hour dwell; patient's weight <60 kg, 1.5 g IP on days 1 and 7

Other information

• **Second line** to metronidazole in treatment of pseudomembranous colitis
• Not absorbed via oral route
• Injection solution may be given orally, however, oral capsules available
• **Alternative dosage adjustment in moderate and severe renal impairment:**

  Give 1-g loading dose and monitor serum levels at 24-hour intervals. When level <10 mg/L give another 1-g dose. Peak levels, 2 hours after dose, should be in range 18–26 mg/L. Some units use a 500-mg loading dose
• Anephric/dialysis patients usually need 1 g once or twice weekly

Vardenafil

Clinical use

Treatment of erectile dysfunction

Dose in normal renal function

5–20 mg approximately 25–60 minutes before sexual activity

Pharmacokinetics

Molecular weight (daltons)	488.6
% Protein binding	95
% Excreted unchanged in urine	2–6
Volume of distribution (L/kg)	208 litres
Half-life – normal/ESRF (hrs)	4–5/–

Dose in renal impairment GFR (mL/min)

30–50	Dose as in normal renal function
10–30	Initial dose 5 mg and adjust accordingly
<10	Initial dose 5 mg and adjust accordingly

Dose in patients undergoing renal replacement therapies

CAPD	Not dialysed. Dose as in GFR < 10 mL/min. Use with caution
HD	Not dialysed. Dose as in GFR < 10 mL/min. Use with caution
CAV/VVHD	Not dialysed. Dose as in GFR = 10–30 mL/min

Important drug interactions

POTENTIALLY HAZARDOUS INTERACTIONS WITH OTHER DRUGS

• Nitrates, alpha-blockers: avoid concomitant administration
• Antifungals, macrolide antibiotics, protease inhibitors, grapefruit juice, other drugs that inhibit CYP 3A4: do not exceed a dose of 5 mg of vardenafil, avoid if the concomitant medication is a potent enzyme inhibitor

Administration

RECONSTITUTION
–

ROUTE
• Oral

RATE OF ADMINISTRATION
–

COMMENTS
–

Other information

• Contra-indicated in dialysis patients due to lack of information, therefore suggest use with caution and monitor patients closely

Vecuronium

Clinical use

Non-depolarising muscle relaxant

Dose in normal renal function

Intubation: 80–100 micrograms/kg, with maintenance of 20–30 micrograms/kg

IV infusion: 40–100 micrograms/kg bolus followed by 50–80 micrograms/kg/hour

Pharmacokinetics

Molecular weight (daltons)	638
% Protein binding	30
% Excreted unchanged in urine	25
Volume of distribution (L/kg)	0.18–0.27
Half-life – normal/ESRF (hrs)	0.5–1.2/ unchanged

Dose in renal impairment GFR (mL/min)

20–50	Dose as in normal renal function
10–20	Dose as in normal renal function
<10	Dose as in normal renal function

Dose in patients undergoing renal replacement therapies

CAPD	Unlikely dialysability. Dose as in normal renal function
HD	Unlikely dialysability. Dose as in normal renal function
CAV/VVHD	Unknown dialysability. Dose as in normal renal function

Important drug interactions

POTENTIALLY HAZARDOUS INTERACTIONS WITH OTHER DRUGS

- Enhances neuromuscular block of botulinum toxin
- Effects increased by aminoglycosides, clindamycin, colistin, quinidine, procainamide and piperacillin

Administration

RECONSTITUTION

- 5 mL water for injection to reconstitute 10-mg vial. Up to 10 mL sodium chloride 0.9% or glucose 5% may be used
- May be added to sodium chloride 0.9%, glucose 5% or Ringer's solution to give a final concentration of 40 mg/L

ROUTE

- IV

RATE OF ADMINISTRATION

- See dose

COMMENTS

–

Other information

- Vecuronium is largely excreted via the liver. Use normal doses with caution in renal failure

Venlafaxine

Clinical use

Antidepressant, used for depressive illness and generalised anxiety disorders

Dose in normal renal function

37.5–75 mg twice daily

XL: 75–225 mg daily

Pharmacokinetics

Molecular weight (daltons)	277 (313.9 as hydrochloride)
% Protein binding	27
% Excreted unchanged in urine	5
Volume of distribution (L/kg)	8
Half-life – normal/ESRF (hrs)	3.8/10.6

Dose in renal impairment GFR (mL/min)

30–50	Dose as in normal renal function
10–30	Reduce total dose by 50% and administer daily
<10	Reduce total dose by 50% and administer daily

Dose in patients undergoing renal replacement therapies

CAPD	Not dialysed. Dose as in GFR = <10 mL/min
HD	Not dialysed. Dose as in GFR = <10 mL/min
CAV/VVHD	Not dialysed. Dose as in GFR = 10–20 mL/min

Important drug interactions

POTENTIALLY HAZARDOUS INTERACTIONS WITH OTHER DRUGS

- MAOIs and linezolid: increased risk of toxicity
- Sibutramine: increased risk of CNS toxicity – avoid concomitant use
- Antimalarials: avoid concomitant use with artemether with lumefantrine
- Antipsychotics: possibly increases plasma concentrations of clozapine
- Anticoagulants: effects of warfarin possibly enhanced

Administration

RECONSTITUTION

–

ROUTE

- Oral

RATE OF ADMINISTRATION

–

COMMENTS

–

Other information

- Withhold dose until after haemodialysis to minimise nausea and any other side-effects
- May be used to treat peripheral diabetic neuropathy in haemodialysis patients. Dose is up to 75 mg daily
- The XL preparation is not suitable for patients with moderate to severe renal impairment

Verapamil

Clinical use

Calcium-channel blocker: supraventricular arrhythmias, angina, hypertension

Dose in normal renal function

Oral: 120–480 mg daily in 2–3 divided doses
IV: 5–10 mg followed by 5 mg 5–10 minutes later if required

Pharmacokinetics

Molecular weight (daltons)	454.6
% Protein binding	83–93
% Excreted unchanged in urine	<10
Volume of distribution (L/kg)	4–7
Half-life – normal/ESRF (hrs)	2–7/2.4–4

Dose in renal impairment GFR (mL/min)

20–50	Dose as in normal renal function. Monitor carefully
10–20	Dose as in normal renal function. Monitor carefully
<10	Dose as in normal renal function. Monitor carefully

Dose in patients undergoing renal replacement therapies

CAPD	Not dialysed. Dose as in GFR = <10 mL/min
HD	Not dialysed. Dose as in GFR = <10 mL/min
CAV/VVHD	Dialysability minimal. Dose as in GFR = 10–20 mL/min

Important drug interactions

POTENTIALLY HAZARDOUS INTERACTIONS WITH OTHER DRUGS

- Ciclosporin: variable reports of decreased nephrotoxicity and potentiated effect. May also increase ciclosporin levels
- Anaesthetics: increased hypotensive effect
- Antiarrhythmics: increased risk of amiodarone-induced bradycardia, AV block and myocardial depression. Increased risk of myocardial depression and asystole with disopyramide and flecainide. Plasma levels of quinidine raised
- Anti-epileptics: enhances effect of carbamazepine. Effect of verapamil reduced by phenobarbital and phenytoin
- Beta-blockers: asystole, severe hypotension and heart failure
- Cardiac glycosides: increased levels of digoxin. Increased AV block and bradycardia
- Theophylline: enhances effect
- Rifampicin: reduces verapamil levels

Administration

RECONSTITUTION

–

ROUTE

- Oral or IV

RATE OF ADMINISTRATION

- 5–10 mg over 2 minutes (3 minutes in elderly)

COMMENTS

–

Other information

- Monitor BP and ECG
- Active metabolites may accumulate in renal impairment

Vigabatrin

Clinical use

Anti-epileptic agent

Dose in normal renal function

2 g daily in one or two doses. Maximum 3 g daily, unless exceptional circumstances

Pharmacokinetics

Molecular weight (daltons)	130
% Protein binding	Negligible
% Excreted unchanged in urine	50–80
Volume of distribution (L/kg)	0.8
Half-life – normal/ESRF (hrs)	7–8/13–15

Dose in renal impairment GFR (mL/min)

20–50	Give 50% of normal dose
10–20	Give 50% of normal dose
<10	Give 25% of normal dose

Dose in patients undergoing renal replacement therapies

CAPD	Unknown dialysability. Dose as for GFR = <10 mL/min
HD	Dialysed. Dose as for GFR = <10 mL/min Give post dialysis on dialysis days
CAV/VVHD	Unknown dialysability. Dose as for GFR = 10–20 mL/min

Important drug interactions

POTENTIALLY HAZARDOUS INTERACTIONS WITH OTHER DRUGS

• Other anti-epileptics: risk of enhanced toxicity and may reduce plasma concentrations of phenytoin, phenobarbital and primidone
• Anti-malarials: mefloquine antagonises anticonvulsant effect; chloroquine and hydroxychloroquine occasionally reduce convulsive threshold

Administration

RECONSTITUTION

–

ROUTE

• Oral

RATE OF ADMINISTRATION

–

COMMENTS

–

Other information

–

Vinblastine

Clinical use

Antineoplastic agent

Dose in normal renal function

6 mg/m^2 (maximum of once a week)

Testicular tumours: up to 0.2 mg/kg on each of 2 consecutive days every 3 weeks

Consult relevant local protocol

Pharmacokinetics

Molecular weight (daltons)	811
% Protein binding	99
% Excreted unchanged in urine	35
Volume of distribution (L/kg)	8–27
Half-life – normal/ESRF (hrs)	20/–

Dose in renal impairment GFR (mL/min)

20–50	Dose as in normal renal function
10–20	Dose as in normal renal function
<10	Dose as in normal renal function

Dose in patients undergoing renal replacement therapies

CAPD	Unlikely to be dialysed. Dose as in normal renal function
HD	Unlikely to be dialysed. Dose as in normal renal function. Give post dialysis on dialysis days
CAV/VVHD	Unlikely to be dialysed. Dose as in normal renal function

Important drug interactions

POTENTIALLY HAZARDOUS INTERACTIONS WITH OTHER DRUGS

• Phenytoin levels may be reduced

Administration

RECONSTITUTION

• Add 10 mL of diluent to 10-mg vial. May be administered into fast-running drip of sodium chloride 0.9%

ROUTE

• IV

RATE OF ADMINISTRATION

• 1 minute

COMMENTS

• Do not dilute with large volumes (e.g. 100–250 mL) or give over long periods (30–60 minutes) as thrombophlebitis and extravasation may occur

Other information

• Vinblastine is metabolised and excreted principally by the liver. No modification of dosage is recommended in patients with impaired renal function

Vincristine

Clinical use

Antineoplastic agent

Dose in normal renal function

IV: 1.4–1.5 mg/m² weekly (maximum 2 mg)
Consult relevant local protocol

Pharmacokinetics

Molecular weight (daltons)	825
% Protein binding	75
% Excreted unchanged in urine	12–15
Volume of distribution (L/kg)	8.4
Half-life – normal/ESRF (hrs)	1–2.5/unchanged

Dose in renal impairment GFR (mL/min)

20–50	Dose as in normal renal function
10–20	Dose as in normal renal function
<10	Dose as in normal renal function

Dose in patients undergoing renal replacement therapies

CAPD	Unlikely to be dialysed. Dose as in normal renal function
HD	Unlikely to be dialysed. Dose as in normal renal function
CAV/VVHD	Unlikely to be dialysed. Dose as in normal renal function

Important drug interactions

POTENTIALLY HAZARDOUS INTERACTIONS WITH OTHER DRUGS

• Phenytoin levels may be reduced

Administration

RECONSTITUTION

–

ROUTE

• IV

RATE OF ADMINISTRATION

• Slow bolus

COMMENTS

• May be administered into fast-running drip of sodium chloride 0.9% or glucose 5%

Other information

• Most of an IV dose is excreted into the bile after rapid tissue binding

Vinorelbine

Clinical use

Treatment of advanced breast cancer (where other anthracyclines have failed) and non-small-cell lung cancer

Dose in normal renal function

25–30 mg/m^2 once a week

Maximum 60 mg per dose

Pharmacokinetics

Molecular weight (daltons)	1079.1
% Protein binding	13.5 (78% bound to platelets)
% Excreted unchanged in urine	18.5
Volume of distribution (L/kg)	>40
Half-life – normal/ESRF (hrs)	>40/–

Dose in renal impairment GFR (mL/min)

20–50	Dose as in normal renal function and monitor closely
10–20	Dose as in normal renal function and monitor closely
<10	Dose as in normal renal function and monitor closely

Dose in patients undergoing renal replacement therapies

CAPD	Removal unlikely. Dose as in normal renal function and monitor closely
HD	Removal unlikely. Dose as in normal renal function and monitor closely
CAV/VVHD	Unknown dialysability. Dose as in normal renal function and monitor closely

Important drug interactions

POTENTIALLY HAZARDOUS INTERACTIONS WITH OTHER DRUGS

• None known

Administration

RECONSTITUTION

–

ROUTE

• IV bolus, infusion

RATE OF ADMINISTRATION

• Bolus: 5–10 minutes
• Infusion: 20–30 minutes

COMMENTS

• Dilute bolus in 20–50 mL of sodium chloride 0.9%
• Dilute infusion in 125 mL of sodium chloride 0.9%
• Stable for 24 hours at 2–8°C

Other information

• Flush line with saline after infusion
• Dose-limiting toxicity is mainly neutropenia
• In patients where >75% of the liver volume has been replaced by metastases, it is empirically suggested that the dose be reduced by one-third, with close haematological follow-up

Vitamin B & C preparations

Clinical use

Vitamin B and C supplementation

Dose in normal renal function

One daily

Pharmacokinetics

Molecular weight (daltons)	N/A
% Protein binding	N/A
% Excreted unchanged in urine	N/A
Volume of distribution (L/kg)	N/A
Half-life – normal/ESRF (hrs)	N/A

Dose in renal impairment GFR (mL/min)

20–50	Dose as in normal renal function
10–20	Dose as in normal renal function
<10	Dose as in normal renal function

Dose in patients undergoing renal replacement therapies

CAPD	Dialysed. Dose as in normal renal function
HD	Dialysed. Dose as in normal renal function
CAV/VVHD	Dialysed. Dose as in normal renal function

Important drug interactions

POTENTIALLY HAZARDOUS INTERACTIONS WITH OTHER DRUGS

• None known

Administration

RECONSTITUTION

–

ROUTE

• Oral

RATE OF ADMINISTRATION

–

COMMENTS

–

Other information

• **Not prescribable on FP10 prescription**

• Supplement in HD patients due to loss on dialysis and poor diet

• Available as Nephrovite (Kimal) and Dialyvit (Vitaline), each tablet contains:

Vitamin B_1 (thiamine)	1.5 mg
Vitamin B_2 (riboflavin)	1.7 mg
Vitamin B_3 (niacinamide)	20 mg
Vitamin B_6 (pyridoxine)	10 mg
Vitamin B_{12} (cyanocobalamin)	6 micrograms
Vitamin C	60 mg
Biotin	300 micrograms
Pantothenic acid	10 mg
Folic acid	800 micrograms

• Ketovite, each tablet contains:

Vitamin B_1 (thiamine)	1 mg
Vitamin B_2 (riboflavin)	1 mg
Acetomenaphthone	500 micrograms
Vitamin B_6 (pyridoxine)	330 micrograms
Nicotinamide	3.3 mg
Vitamin C	16.6 mg
Biotin	170 micrograms
Pantothenic acid	1.16 mg
Alpha tocopheryl acetate	5 mg
Inositol	50 mg
Folic acid	250 micrograms

Voriconazole

Clinical use

Treatment of invasive aspergillosis, fluconazole-resistant serious invasive fungal infections. Treatment for immunocompromised patients with progressive, possibly life-threatening, infections

Dose in normal renal function

IV: 6 mg/kg 12-hourly for 24 hours, then 3–4 mg/kg 12-hourly

Oral:

- <40 kg, 200 mg 12-hourly for 24 hours, then 100–150 mg twice daily
- >40 kg, 400 mg 12-hourly for 24 hours, then 200–300 mg twice daily

Pharmacokinetics

Molecular weight (daltons)	349.3
% Protein binding	58
% Excreted unchanged in urine	<2
Volume of distribution (L/kg)	4.6
Half-life – normal/ESRF (hrs)	6 (depends on dose)/unchanged

Dose in renal impairment GFR (mL/min)

20–50	Dose as in normal renal function
10–20	Dose as in normal renal function
<10	Dose as in normal renal function. See 'Other information'

Dose in patients undergoing renal replacement therapies

CAPD	Probably dialysed. Dose as in normal renal function
HD	Dialysed. Dose as in normal renal function
CAV/VVHD	Probably dialysed. Dose as in normal renal function

Important drug interactions

POTENTIALLY HAZARDOUS INTERACTIONS WITH OTHER DRUGS

- Ciclosporin: AUC increased, reduce ciclosporin dose by 50% and monitor closely
- Tacrolimus: AUC increased, reduce tacrolimus dose by a third and monitor closely
- Anticoagulants: increased prothrombin time
- HIV protease inhibitors: voriconazole may inhibit metabolism
- Non-nucleoside reverse transcriptase inhibitors: may increase the metabolism of voriconazole and voriconazole may reduce metabolism of NNRTIs
- Sulphonylureas: may increase plasma concentration of sulphonylureas leading to hypoglycaemia
- Benzodiazepines: may inhibit metabolism of midazolam and any other benzodiazepines metabolised by CYP 3A4
- Vinca alkaloids: may increase concentration of vinca alkaloids leading to neurotoxicity
- Omeprazole: omeprazole concentration increased, reduce omeprazole dose by 50%
- Terfenadine, astemizole, cisapride, pimozide, quinidine: prolonged QT interval and rare cases of torsades de pointes due to increased drug concentrations. Avoid concomitant use
- Rifampicin, carbamazepine, phenobarbital: reduces plasma concentration of voriconazole. Avoid concomitant use
- Ergotamine, dihydroergotamine: risk of ergotism. Avoid concomitant use
- Sirolimus: increases sirolimus concentration. Avoid concomitant use
- Statins: increased levels of those metabolised by CYP 3A4, increased risk of rhabdomyolysis
- Phenytoin: reduces voriconazole concentration and voriconazole increases phenytoin concentration – double oral voriconazole dose and increase IV to 5 mg/kg dose if using with phenytoin. Avoid concomitant use if possible
- Rifabutin: increase dose of voriconazole from 200 to 350 mg and 100 to 200 mg (depends on patient's weight) and increase IV dose to 5 mg/kg if used in combination. Avoid concomitant use if possible

Administration

RECONSTITUTION

- 19 mL water for injection

ROUTE

- Oral, IV

RATE OF ADMINISTRATION

- 1–2 hours (3 mg/kg/hour)

COMMENTS

- Not compatible with sodium bicarbonate or TPN solutions

- Dilute to a concentration of 2–5 mg/mL with sodium chloride 0.9%, Hartmann's solution or glucose 5%

Other information

- Haemodialysis clearance is 121 mL/min but this is insufficient to warrant a dose adjustment for a 4-hour haemodialysis session

- Oral bioavailability is 96%

- Only use IV in renal patients if patient is unable to tolerate oral as intravenous vehicle (SBECD) accumulates in renal failure. The vehicle is dialysed at a rate of 55 mL/min

- Take oral dose 1 hour before or an hour after meals

- Monitor renal function as can enhance nephrotoxicity of other drugs and concurrent conditions

- Rare reports of ARF and discoid lupus erythematosus occurring

- Also reports of haematuria, nephritis and tubular necrosis

- In clinical trials, 30% of patients had visual problems, usually with higher doses

Warfarin

Clinical use

Anticoagulant

Dose in normal renal function

Oral: daily maintenance 3–9 mg, dependent on prothrombin time

Pharmacokinetics

Molecular weight (daltons)	330.3
% Protein binding	99.4
% Excreted unchanged in urine	0
Volume of distribution (L/kg)	0.11–0.15
Half-life – normal/ESRF (hrs)	36–42/unchanged

Dose in renal impairment GFR (mL/min)

20–50	Dose as in normal renal function
10–20	Dose as in normal renal function
<10	Dose as in normal renal function

Dose for patients undergoing renal replacement therapies

CAPD	Not dialysed. Dose as in normal renal function
HD	Not dialysed. Dose as in normal renal function
CAV/VVHD	Not dialysed. Dose as in normal renal function

Important drug interactions

POTENTIALLY HAZARDOUS INTERACTIONS WITH OTHER DRUGS

- **There are many significant interactions with warfarin. Prescribe with care with regard to the following**:
- Ciclosporin: lowered ciclosporin blood levels, hypercoagulability

- Anticoagulant effect enhanced by: alcohol, amiodarone, anabolic steroids, aspirin, azithromycin, aztreonam, bicalutamide, cephalosporins, chloramphenicol, cimetidine, ciprofloxacin, clarithromycin, clofibrates, clopidogrel, cotrimoxazole, danazol, dextropropoxyphene, dipyridamole, disulfiram, erythromycin, flutamide, fluvoxamine, ifosfamide, imidazoles, metronidazole, NSAIDs, omeprazole, paracetamol, proguanil, propafenone, quinidine, ritonavir, SSRIs, simvastatin, sulfinpyrazone, sulphonamides, tamoxifen, testosterone, ticlopidine, thyroxine, toremifene, trimethoprim
- Anticoagulant effect decreased by: acitretin, aminoglutethimide, azathioprine, barbiturates, carbamazepine, griseofulvin, oral contraceptives, phenytoin, primidone, rifampicin, sucralfate, vitamin K
- Anticoagulant effects enhanced/reduced by: anion exchange resins, broad-spectrum antibiotics, dietary changes

Administration

RECONSTITUTION

–

ROUTE

- Oral

RATE OF ADMINISTRATION

–

COMMENTS

–

Other information

- Active metabolites renally excreted and may accumulate in renal impairment
- Reduced protein binding in renal impairment

Zafirlukast

Clinical use

Prophylaxis of asthma

Dose in normal renal function

20 mg twice daily

Pharmacokinetics

Molecular weight (daltons)	575.7
% Protein binding	99
% Excreted unchanged in urine	0 (10% as metabolites)
Volume of distribution (L/kg)	70
Half-life – normal/ESRF (hrs)	10/possibly unchanged

Dose in renal impairment GFR (mL/min)

20–50	Dose as in normal renal function
10–20	Dose as in normal renal function, but use with care
<10	Dose as in normal renal function, but use with care

Dose in patients undergoing renal replacement therapies

CAPD	Unlikely dialysability. Dose as in normal renal function, but use with care
HD	Unlikely dialysability. Dose as in normal renal function, but use with care
CAV/VVHD	Unknown dialysability. Dose as in normal renal function, but use with care

Important drug interactions

POTENTIALLY HAZARDOUS INTERACTIONS WITH OTHER DRUGS

- Anticoagulants: may enhance the effects of warfarin
- Analgesics: aspirin increases plasma concentration of zafirlukast
- Antibacterials: erythromycin reduces plasma concentration of zafirlukast
- Antihistamines: terfenadine reduces plasma concentration of zafirlukast
- Theophylline: zafirlukast possibly increases plasma theophylline concentration; plasma-zafirlukast concentration reduced

Administration

RECONSTITUTION

–

ROUTE

- Oral

RATE OF ADMINISTRATION

–

COMMENTS

–

Other information

- Do not take with food as reduces bioavailability

Zanamivir

Clinical use

Treatment of influenza A and B within 48 hours after onset of symptoms

Dose in normal renal function

10 mg twice daily for 5 days

Pharmacokinetics

Molecular weight (daltons)	332.3
% Protein binding	Not protein bound
% Excreted unchanged in urine	100
Volume of distribution (L/kg)	No data
Half-life – normal/ESRF (hrs)	2.6–5/–

Dose in renal impairment GFR (mL/min)

20–50	Dose as in normal renal function
10–20	Dose as in normal renal function
<10	Dose as in normal renal function

Dose in patients undergoing renal replacement therapies

CAPD	Unknown dialysability. Dose as in normal renal function
HD	Unknown dialysability. Dose as in normal renal function
CAV/VVHD	Unknown dialysability. Dose as in normal renal function

Important drug interactions

POTENTIALLY HAZARDOUS INTERACTIONS WITH OTHER DRUGS

• None known

Administration

RECONSTITUTION

–

ROUTE

• Inhalation

RATE OF ADMINISTRATION

–

COMMENTS

–

Other information

• 10–20% of dose is systemically absorbed

Zidovudine

Clinical use

Antiretroviral agent

Dose in normal renal function

Oral: 500–600 mg daily in 2–5 divided doses
IV: 1–2 mg/kg every 4 hours

Pharmacokinetics

Molecular weight (daltons)	267
% Protein binding	10–30
% Excreted unchanged in urine	8–25
Volume of distribution (L/kg)	1.6
Half-life – normal/ESRF (hrs)	1.1–1.4/1.4–3

Dose in renal impairment GFR (mL/min)

20–50	Give 100% of normal dose every 8 hours
10–20	Give 100% of normal dose every 8 hours
<10	Give 50% of normal dose every 12 hours

Dose in patients undergoing renal replacement therapies

CAPD	Not dialysed. Dose as in GFR = <10 mL/min
HD	Not dialysed. Dose as in GFR = <10 mL/min
CAV/VVHD	Not dialysed. Dose as in GFR = 10–20 mL/min

Important drug interactions

POTENTIALLY HAZARDOUS INTERACTIONS WITH OTHER DRUGS

- Phenytoin levels may be raised or lowered
- Ribavirin antagonises in vitro activity of zidovudine
- Clarithromycin reduces absorption of zidovudine
- Profound myelosuppression with ganciclovir
- Extreme lethargy on administration of IV aciclovir
- Fluconazole increases zidovudine levels
- Intracellular activation of stavudine inhibited

Administration

RECONSTITUTION

- Dilute with glucose 5% infusion to give a final concentration of 2 mg/mL or 4 mg/mL

ROUTE

- IV, oral

RATE OF ADMINISTRATION

- 1 hour

COMMENTS

–

Other information

- Dialysis has little effect on zidovudine, presumably because of rapid metabolism. The glucuronide metabolite ($t_{1/2}$ = 1 hour) has no antiviral activity and will be removed by dialysis
- Patients with severe renal failure have 50% higher maximum plasma concentrations
- 90% of a dose is excreted renally, 50–80% as the glucuronide. There is substantial accumulation of this metabolite in renal failure

Zoledronic acid

Clinical use

Hypercalcaemia of malignancy

Dose in normal renal function

4 mg as a single dose

Pharmacokinetics

Molecular weight (daltons)	272.1
% Protein binding	56
% Excreted unchanged in urine	39 ± 16
Volume of distribution (L/kg)	6.1–10.8 litres
Half-life – normal/ESRF (hrs)	146/increased

Dose in renal impairment GFR (mL/min)

20–50	Dose as in normal renal function
10–20	Use with caution if benefit outweighs risk
<10	Use with caution if benefit outweighs risk

Dose in patients undergoing renal replacement therapies

CAPD	Unknown dialysability. Dose as in GFR = <10 mL/min
HD	Unknown dialysability. Dose as in GFR = <10 mL/min
CAV/VVHD	Unknown dialysability. Dose as in GFR = 10–20 mL/min

Important drug interactions

POTENTIALLY HAZARDOUS INTERACTIONS WITH OTHER DRUGS

• Other nephrotoxic drugs: use with caution as can enhance nephrotoxicity

Administration

RECONSTITUTION

• Add 5 mL of water for injection to each 4-mg vial

ROUTE

• IV

RATE OF ADMINISTRATION

• 15 minutes

COMMENTS

• Add to 100 mL sodium chloride 0.9% or glucose 5%

• Reconstituted solutions are stable for 24 hours at room temperature

Other information

• Also administer a calcium supplement of 500 mg daily plus 400 IU of vitamin D daily

• Increased risk of renal deterioration if GFR < 10 mL/min; measure creatinine while on zoledronic acid

• Increased risk of renal failure if 8 mg used

Zolmitriptan

Clinical use

Acute treatment of migraine

Dose in normal renal function

2.5–5 mg. Maximum 15 mg in 24 hours. Repeat after 2 hours if required

Pharmacokinetics

Molecular weight (daltons)	287.4
% Protein binding	25
% Excreted unchanged in urine	60 (as metabolites)
Volume of distribution (L/kg)	2.4
Half-life – normal/ESRF (hrs)	2.5–3/3–3.5

Dose in renal impairment GFR (mL/min)

20–50	Dose as in normal renal function
10–20	Dose as in normal renal function
<10	Dose as in normal renal function

Dose in patients undergoing renal replacement therapies

CAPD	Unknown dialysability. Dose as in normal renal function
HD	Unknown dialysability. Dose as in normal renal function
CAV/VVHD	Unknown dialysability. Dose as in normal renal function

Important drug interactions

POTENTIALLY HAZARDOUS INTERACTIONS WITH OTHER DRUGS

• Antibacterials: quinolones possibly inhibit metabolism, reduce dose of zolmitriptan

• Antidepressants: risk of CNS toxicity with MAOIs; increased risk of CNS toxicity with moclobamide, reduce dose of zolmitriptan to max 7.5 mg; SSRIs inhibit metabolism of zolmitriptan; increased serotonergic effects with St John's Wort (avoid concomitant use)

• Cimetidine: inhibits metabolism of zolmitriptan, maximum dose is 5 mg

• Ergotamine and ergometrine: increased risk of vasospasm

• Linezolid: risk of CNS toxicity, reduce dose of zolmitriptan

Administration

RECONSTITUTION

–

ROUTE

• Oral

RATE OF ADMINISTRATION

–

COMMENTS

–

Other information

–

Zolpidem

Clinical use

Insomnia, short-term treatment

Dose in normal renal function

5–10 mg at night

Pharmacokinetics

Molecular weight (daltons)	764.9
% Protein binding	92.5
% Excreted unchanged in urine	Negligible (56% as active metabolites)
Volume of distribution (L/kg)	0.34–0.54 (depends on age)
Half-life – normal/ESRF (hrs)	0.7–3.5 (average: 2.4)/unchanged

Dose in renal impairment GFR (mL/min)

20–50	Dose as in normal renal function
10–20	Dose as in normal renal function
<10	Dose as in normal renal function

Dose in patients undergoing renal replacement therapies

CAPD	Not dialysed. Dose as in normal renal function
HD	Not dialysed. Dose as in normal renal function
CAV/VVHD	Not dialysed. Dose as in normal renal function

Important drug interactions

POTENTIALLY HAZARDOUS INTERACTIONS WITH OTHER DRUGS

• Ritonavir: increases plasma concentration of zolpidem, risk of extreme sedation and respiratory depression – avoid concomitant use
• Alcohol: avoid concomitant use

Administration

RECONSTITUTION

–

ROUTE

• Oral

RATE OF ADMINISTRATION

–

COMMENTS

–

Other information

• First-pass metabolism by liver is 35%
• Clearance is reduced in renal impairment

Zopiclone

Clinical use

Hypnotic

Dose in normal renal function

7.5 mg at night (3.75 mg in elderly)

Pharmacokinetics

Molecular weight (daltons)	389
% Protein binding	45–80
% Excreted unchanged in urine	<7
Volume of distribution (L/kg)	100 litres
Half-life – normal/ESRF (hrs)	3.5–6/>7

Dose in renal impairment GFR (mL/min)

20–50	Dose as in normal renal function
10–20	Dose as in normal renal function
<10	3.75–7.5 mg at night

Dose in patients undergoing renal replacement therapies

CAPD	Unknown dialysability. Dose as in GFR = <10 mL/min
HD	Unknown dialysability. Dose as in GFR = <10 mL/min
CAV/VVHD	Unknown dialysability. Dose as in normal renal function

Important drug interactions

POTENTIALLY HAZARDOUS INTERACTIONS WITH OTHER DRUGS

• None known

Administration

RECONSTITUTION

–

ROUTE

• Oral

RATE OF ADMINISTRATION

–

COMMENTS

–

Other information

• It is recommended that elderly patients and those with severe renal disease should start treatment with 3.75 mg. However, accumulation has not been observed

Zotepine

Clinical use

Treatment of schizophrenia

Dose in normal renal function

25–100 mg three times a day

Pharmacokinetics

Molecular weight (daltons)	331.9
% Protein binding	97
% Excreted unchanged in urine	As metabolites – 40%
Volume of distribution (L/kg)	109 ± 59
Half-life – normal/ESRF (hrs)	14/increased

Dose in renal impairment GFR (mL/min)

20–50	25 mg twice daily increasing to 75 mg twice daily
10–20	25 mg twice daily increasing to 75 mg twice daily
<10	25 mg twice daily increasing to 75 mg twice daily

Dose in patients undergoing renal replacement therapies

CAPD	Unknown dialysability. Dose as in GFR = <10 mL/min
HD	Unknown dialysability. Dose as in GFR = <10 mL/min
CAV/VVHD	Unknown dialysability. Dose as in GFR = 10–20 mL/min

Important drug interactions

POTENTIALLY HAZARDOUS INTERACTIONS WITH OTHER DRUGS

- Anaesthetics: enhanced hypotensive effect
- Analgesics: enhanced sedative and hypotensive effects with opioid analgesics
- Ritonavir: increased plasma levels of zotepine
- Fluoxetine: increased plasma levels of zotepine
- Sibutramine: increased risk of CNS toxicity – avoid concomitant use
- Anti-malarials: manufacturer advises avoid artemether with lumefantrine
- Anti-epileptics: antagonism as convulsive threshold lowered

Administration

RECONSTITUTION

–

ROUTE

- Oral

RATE OF ADMINISTRATION

–

COMMENTS

–

Other information

- Do not use if there is a history of nephrolithiasis
- Occasionally can increase creatinine levels
- Undergoes extensive first-pass metabolism

Malarial prophylaxis

Mefloquine (Lariam)

- 250 mg (one tablet) once a week, starting 1–3 weeks prior to travelling and continuing for 4 weeks after returning
- No dose changes are required for patients with any degree of renal impairment

Doxycycline

- 100 mg (one capsule) once a day starting 1–3 weeks prior to travelling and continuing for 4 weeks after returning
- CAPD or HD patients: no dose adjustment required
- Transplant patients: doxycycline can double ciclosporin or tacrolimus blood levels. Avoid if at all possible

Chloroquine (Avloclor or Nivaquine) and proguanil (Paludrine)

- Chloroquine: 300 mg (two tablets) once a week
- Proguanil: 200 mg (two tablets) once a day starting 1–3 weeks prior to travelling and continuing for 4 weeks after returning

Chloroquine

- No dose adjustment necessary at prophylactic dose
- NB: for full therapeutic dose to treat malaria, take the following into consideration:
  - Transplant patients: chloroquine increases plasma ciclosporin levels; monitor carefully
  - Treatment dose in patients with renal insufficiency

GFR (mL/min)	Dose
20–59	100% dose
10–19	100% dose
<10	50% dose

Proguanil

- Transplant patients: dose according to function of renal transplant
- CAPD and HD patients: half a tablet (50 mg) once a week
- Patients with renal insufficiency

GFR (mL/min)	Dose
≥60	200 mg OD
20–59	100 mg OD
10–19	50 mg alt days
<10	50 mg once a week

NB: Patients with renal insufficiency receiving proguanil should also be prescribed folic acid 5 mg daily to minimise side-effects

Atovaquone 250 mg + proguanil 100 mg (Malarone)

- One tablet daily starting 24–48 hours before travelling, and continuing for 7 days after returning

GFR (mL/min)	Dose
>30	Normal dose
<30	Not recommended: due to need to reduce dose of proguanil, but give full dose of atovaquone. Use alternative therapy

Vaccines

- Immunosuppressed patients should *not* receive live vaccines – this includes both transplant patients and those on dialysis
- Inactivated vaccines can be administered to immunosuppressed patients, although the response may be reduced

Vaccines that are not recommended:
- Polio oral vaccine (OPV, Sabin), including household contacts of immunosuppressed patients as transmission of the live virus through faeces is possible
- MMR vaccine (Measles, Mumps, Rubella)
- Rubella vaccine
- BCG (Bacillus Calmette-Guérin) vaccine
- Yellow fever vaccine
- Typhoid oral vaccine (Vivotif)

Vaccines that can be administered:
- Adsorbed diphtheria vaccine (including adsorbed D/T/P and adsorbed D/T vaccines)
- Adsorbed Tetanus vaccine
- Haemophilus influenzae vaccine (Hiberix, ACT-HIB, ACT-HIB DTP)
- Hepatitis A vaccine (Avaxim, Havrix Monodose, Epaxal)
- Hepatitis B vaccine (Engerix B, HBvaxPRO)
- Hepatitis A & B vaccine (Twinrix)
- Hepatitis A & Typhoid vaccine (Hepatyrix, ViATIM)
- Polio inactivated vaccine (IPV, Salk)
- Influenza vaccine (Split Virion vaccines and Surface Antigen vaccines)
- Meningococcal Group C conjugate vaccine (Meningitec , Menjugate, NeisVac-C)
- Meningococcal polysaccharide A&C vaccine (AC Vax, Mengivac (A+C))
- Pneumococcal vaccine (Pneumovax II, Pnu-Imune, Prevenar)
- Rabies vaccine
- Typhoid Vi capsular polysaccharide vaccine (Typherix, Typhim-Vi)